W9-BFH-076

Ethics in Clinical Practice

Second Edition

Judith C. Ahronheim, MD
Chief, Eileen E. Anderson Section of Geriatric Medicine
Saint Vincents Hospital and Medical Center
New York, New York
Professor of Medicine
New York Medical College
Valhalla, New York

Jonathan D. Moreno, PhD
Kornfeld Professor and Director
Center for Biomedical Ethics
University of Virginia
Charlottesville, Virginia

Connie Zuckerman, JD
Former Associate Director
Center for Ethics in Medicine
Beth Israel Medical Center
New York, New York

AN ASPEN PUBLICATION
Aspen Publishers, Inc.
Gaithersburg, Maryland
2000

Library of Congress Cataloging-in-Publication Data

Ahronheim, Judith C.
Ethics in clinical practice—2nd ed.
p. cm
Includes bibliographical references and index.
ISBN 0-8342-1075-4
1. Medical ethics. 2. Medical ethics—Case studies.
I. Moreno, Jonathan D. II. Zuckerman, Connie.
[DNLM: 1. Ethics, Medical—Legal Cases. W 50 A287e 1999]
R724.A33 1999
174'.2
99-042872

Orders: (800) 638-8437
Customer Service: (800) 234-1660

Editorial Services: Kathy Litzenberg
Library of Congress Catalog Card Number: 99-42872
ISBN: 0-8342-1075-4

Printed in the United States of America

1 2 3 4 5

Table of Contents

Preface

The rapidly changing landscape of clinical medicine, governmental emphasis on cost containment, and the rise of managed care, have brought dramatic changes to our health care system. These changes have taken place against a backdrop of social and economic trends, immigration and multiculturalism, and an aging population. As with the first edition, this second edition of *Ethics in Clinical Practice* helps professionals in all health care disciplines grapple with ethical issues throughout the life span. This edition also gives heightened attention to newer ethical dilemmas spawned by advances in medical genetics, organ transplantation, HIV medicine, and assisted reproductive technologies, and by complementary/ alternative medicine, managed care, physician-assisted suicide, and other timely issues.

In the first edition of *Ethics in Clinical Practice*, we developed a flexible resource for education in the field of clinical ethics. The second edition maintains this approach. The first six chapters provide a solid foundation in the history and theory of clinical ethics. The remainder of the book is devoted to 31 case studies analyzed from a medical, ethical, and legal perspective. Depending on one's purpose, it is not necessary for all readers to study this book from beginning to end. Those who are interested in an overview of clinical theory, for example, will profit from reading our concise summary of the standard theory in Chapters 1–6, or even from sections or subsections that relate to specific subjects or populations. The Cases can then be used as illustrative material. Those who favor a more case-oriented approach might begin by reading several cases of interest to them and then referring to the relevant sections in the first six chapters.

The case analyses contain extensive discussion of medical, ethical, and legal issues; more philosophical concerns are discussed at greater length earlier in the text. Thus, reference to individual cases may be of more immediate value for the clinician seeking information about the care of a particular patient. However, we strongly discourage the use of case analysis to determine the ethics of any actual patient's care, no matter how great its superficial resemblance to the situation at hand. Rather, case analyses in any textbook provide at most orientation to ethical problems likely to be encountered in practice. As it is often said, actual cases are more difficult than those in textbooks.

Finally, though prepared collaboratively by a physician, a philosopher, and an attorney, this text does not purport to be an introduction to medicine, philosophy, or law. Rather, it is an introduction to a multidisciplinary field known as clinical ethics. We believe that the responsible development of educational material for this field must involve these disciplines, for clinical ethics is distinguished by the deep interplay of medical, philosophical, and legal issues that are encountered in clinical practice.

Judith C. Ahronheim
Jonathan D. Moreno
Connie Zuckerman

Acknowledgments

The authors gratefully acknowledge the following colleagues who offered valuable insights as we prepared the second edition of this work: Toni G. Cesta, Geri Pena, and Kathleen Wardach, of the Department of Case Management, and Jayme L. Radding, the Department of Pediatrics, Saint Vincents Hospital and Medical Center, New York; the physicians and faculty of Saint Vincents Hospital and Medical Center and New York Medical College, Drs. Robert Lahita, Jayne D. Rivas, Frederick Siegel, Barbara Johnston, Allen Astrow, David Cordon, and Geoffrey P. Herzig; Drs. Gerson Weiss, of UMDNJ-Newark, and Karen Berkowitz, of the Hospital of the University of Pennsylvania; and Benjamin Kligler, MD, The Center for Health and Healing, Beth Israel Medical Center, New York. Their time and expertise were much appreciated and useful in the preparation of the manuscript. Connie Zuckerman also acknowledges the kind support she received from her colleague Navah Harlow, MA, Director, Center for Ethics in Medicine, Beth Israel Medical Center, New York, during the time she spent at Beth Israel.

The authors also would like to acknowledge colleagues who provided valuable assistance by reviewing portions of the manuscript as we prepared the first edition of *Ethics in Clinical Practice* in 1994: Drs. Kurt Hirschhorn, Steven M. Fruchtman, and Jonathan Winston of Mount Sinai School of Medicine of the City University of New York; Dr. Julius Korein of New York University School of Medicine, and Dr. Alan R. Fleischman of the Albert Einstein College of Medicine of Yeshiva University and Montefiore Medical Center. Their valuable insights were much appreciated and useful at that time as now. Connie Zuckerman would like to express her heartfelt gratitude to Maryjane Doughterty for her tireless research efforts on behalf of this book and would also like to thank her colleague Alice Herb of SUNY-Brooklyn, for her input and support. Jonathan Moreno thanks his colleague Kathleen Powderly of SUNY-Brooklyn for her suggestions concerning the analysis of several cases. Judy Ahronheim would like to thank her smart brother Gerry Ahronheim of Université de Montréal Faculty of Medicine and Hopital Sainte-Justine for sharing ideas and expertise.

We warmly thank Kalen Conerly and the members of the editorial staff of Aspen Publishers for their support and expertise.

We are grateful for the support and presence of Sarah and Jared Zuckerman, and Jillian and Jarrett Moreno, and our spouses Leslye Fenton, Art Zuckerman, and Gerald Blandford for their continued patience.

1

About Clinical Ethics

DEFINING CLINICAL ETHICS

Although there is no single, universally accepted definition of clinical ethics, by presenting several accounts by leading figures in the field, it is possible to identify some essential characteristics. The first definition is that of Fletcher: "Clinical ethics is an interdisciplinary activity to identify, analyze, and resolve ethical problems that arise in the care of particular patients. The major thrust of clinical ethics is to work for outcomes that best serve the interests and welfare of patients and their families."[1]

A second definition is offered by Jonsen, Siegler, and Winslade: "Clinical ethics . . . is a practical discipline that provides a structured approach to decision making that can assist physicians to identify, analyze, and resolve ethical issues in clinical medicine."[2]

A third definition has been proposed by LaPuma: "Clinical ethics is the process of identifying, analyzing and resolving moral problems of a particular patient's care. The primary goal of clinical ethics is to improve patient care with bedside assistance. Clinical ethics seeks to improve the relationship between the patient and the clinician and the relationships among patient, family, and hospital."[3]

These definitions have much in common. They agree that clinical ethics has to do with ethical problems associated with the care of particular patients. All three also note the systematic nature of work in clinical ethics, with an emphasis on the identification, analysis, and resolution of ethical problems. Interestingly, the three definitions differ the most as to precisely whom and in what manner clinical ethics is to serve: the interests and welfare of patients and families (Fletcher), the needs of physicians in dealing with ethical issues (Jonsen, Siegler, and Winslade), and the improvement of patient care and the relationships among the involved parties (LaPuma).

Drawing on these similarities and differences, clinical ethics may be defined as the systematic identification, analysis, and resolution of ethical problems associated with the care of particular patients. Its goals include protecting the rights and interests of patients, assisting clinicians in ethical decision making, and encouraging cooperative relationships among patients and those close to patients, clinicians, and health care institutions.

In this definition, the systematic and practical nature of clinical ethics remains primary. In addition, three distinct goals are emphasized:

1. Decision making should be patient centered, honoring the rights as well as interests of patients.
2. All clinicians (physicians, nurses, social workers, and other health care professionals) can sometimes benefit from assistance in this complex field.
3. Cooperation among all involved parties, including health care organizations themselves, is an important condition for adequately carrying out plans on behalf of the patient.

It should also be made clear that all who have attempted to define clinical ethics agree that it should be seen not as a mere adjunct to health care practices but rather as an integral part of patient care. Therefore, as is increasingly the case, clinical ethics should also be integrated into every stage of medical training, from premedical to continuing education; a similar goal should be set for the allied health professions.

Clinical ethics can thus be distinguished from a more philosophical approach to ethical issues in health care. While medical, nursing, or health care ethics generally may be of a more theoretical nature, clinical ethics is more applied and activist in orientation. Clinical ethics as a field can also be distinguished from research ethics, which is concerned with the morality of the use of human and animal subjects in the investigation of innovative health care techniques. All of these fields can be regarded as areas within biomedical ethics. Although research ethics is commonly regarded as beginning with the reaction to Nazi exploitation of human subjects, some see clinical ethics as dating back to Hippocrates. In the following sections this question is considered in some detail.

THE NEW CLINICAL ETHICS

Medical ethics is a more traditional term than *clinical ethics*, though both terms are ambiguous. Medical ethics may refer to those rules of conduct that are established by the formal bodies of the medical profession in the course of regulating itself, such as the prohibition of sexual exploitation of one's patients, or it may refer to novel ethical dilemmas as they specifically confront doctors, such as determining the appropriate point to cease life-sustaining measures for dying patients. Similarly, the term *clinical ethics,* which is partly an outgrowth of medical ethics, can refer either to uncontroversial codes of conduct that govern all clinicians or to novel ethical dilemmas. This book mainly concerns issues that fall under latter category.

There are at least two ways to date the advent of clinical ethics. The first contends that clinical ethics is merely a contemporary, applied expression of traditional medical ethics recognized since the time of Hippocrates, and that similar traditions of medical ethics are found in other cultures. In this view there is no specific or necessary identification of clinical ethics with the recent intellectual movement known as biomedical ethics, or bioethics for short. Rather, the virtues and moral norms associated with the practice of medicine, primitive as it once was, have evolved to the present day.

There is more than a quantitative difference between traditional and contemporary clinical ethics, and this difference is associated with a number of scientific, clinical, political, and social developments. First, the scientific basis of modern medicine, which might be dated from the development of germ theory in the latter part of the nineteenth century, has brought with it unprecedented abilities to predict and in some cases deliberately to change the course of disease. Second, these new technical abilities have gradually but certainly altered the physician-patient relationship, as these medical interventions have brought with them benefits and risks for both parties. Third, patients in more technologically advanced societies are now insisting on a greater role in making decisions about their treatment. Fourth, the bioethics movement has tended to consolidate the social and moral concerns about the implications of innovations in the basic life sciences, a consolidation that has within the past two decades migrated to the clinical setting itself. Fifth, traditional clinical ethics has been concerned with the practices proper to a certain guild-like group, whereas modern clinical ethics is concerned with moral dilemmas that confront all health care professionals. Put another way, one might say that traditional clinical ethics had to do only with doctor ethics, but modern clinical ethics pertains to the concerns of all health care workers. A vivid example is the doctrine of informed consent, which obligates all clinicians to respect the right of the patient to decide whether or not to accept treatment.

An important implication of the informed consent doctrine for clinical case management is that the goals of care should be developed with the patient. Often the involvement of family and close friends should be involved, as well. The concept of goals of care can serve as a conceptual framework that helps remind clinicians that the patient's wishes are essential elements of the care plan, and that helps organize interventions as part of a cohesive approach to the patient's medical problems.

THE EMERGENCE OF MODERN CLINICAL ETHICS

In dating the advent of modern clinical ethics (or, to use its full name, clinical biomedical ethics), Jonsen highlights three events.[4] The first is the 1962 article by Shana Alexander in *Life* magazine entitled "They Decide Who Lives, Who Dies."[5] In her article Alexander describes the work of a committee in Seattle, Washington, that was charged with the task of allocating access to hemodialysis, then a scarce resource, for patients who would die without this treatment. The committee was composed of ordinary citizens, rather than physicians, out of a recognition that after the medical questions were settled, difficult moral problems remained in the selection process and that physicians did not have a privileged window on what was the morally right allocation of this resource. The committee discovered, however, that its own decidedly middle-class values were being applied in the selection of those who would live, and it disbanded itself.

The second important event in the emergence of clinical ethics is the 1973 publication in the *New England Journal of Medicine* of Raymond Duff and A.G.M. Campbell's article on ethical problems in the intensive care nursery.[6] This paper describes the deliberate decision to withhold treatment from 43 babies with grave medical problems at Yale-New Haven Hospital, following discussions between parents and physicians.

The third event is the 1976 New Jersey Supreme Court decision that recognized the right of Karen Ann Quinlan's family to withdraw medical treatment that they believed she would not have wanted.[7] The court also recommended that alternative means of resolving ethical dilemmas be developed by health care institutions, specifically mentioning an "ethics committee." Ironically, however, this recommendation really referred to a prognosis committee, for what the court termed an *ethics committee* was to focus on verifying the clinical conditions necessary to resolve the dilemmas according to the *Quinlan* formula.

The Seattle hemodialysis experience marked the first time that many Americans became aware of the tragedy of medical decision making in the context of a scarce high technology, combined with the realization that medical science alone could not resolve the distribution dilemma. The Duff and Campbell article signaled the fact that technological innovation had created an environment in which decisions to end life were frequently made, often in a self-conscious manner. The *Quinlan* case, which was far more widely publicized, illustrated the difficulties that can arise when informal processes designed for a less medically sophisticated era falter in the face of technologically complex interventions, that is, turning to next-of-kin to make decisions on behalf of persons who are mentally incapacitated.

Along with changes in the practice of medicine and in the law that were taking place in this period, the civil rights movements also had an enormous effect on the emergence of bioethics in general and of clinical ethics in particular. The patients' rights movement was perhaps first apparent in the psychiatric hospitals, as those who were incarcerated as mental patients insisted that they did not cede all their civil rights on admission, whether or not their admission was voluntary. Later, the academic study of death and dying became closely identified with a growing popular movement in favor of death with dignity, and, in some more politically conscious quarters, with what came to be called the right to die. At this point it became nearly impossible to refer to the changes in medicine without also referring to those in society, as patients were increasingly viewed as among the vulnerable and disadvantaged citizens whose civil rights had not been adequately recognized.

Finally, academic philosophers during the later 1960s and early 1970s were emerging from a period in which the dominant concern was with technical questions in analytic ethics, or metaethics, the study of the meaning of terms used in moral discourse, such as the words *good* and *right*. A new interest in substantive moral problems, called *normative ethics*, reinvigorated academic philosophy. The moral problems of medicine were a major part of these developments, so much so that one distinguished philosopher said that in the 1970s medicine "saved the life of ethics."[8] Finally, as more and more professors of philosophy (including some theologians) became involved in discussions of biomedical ethics, an identifiable sub-discipline of philosophy, called *applied ethics* was recognized by the profession. As the 1970s drew to a close, many philosophers were participating in teaching medical students and other health care professionals.

In the 1980s, a number of academically trained philosophers and philosophically sophisticated physicians moved biomedical ethics out of the seminar room and into the clinic. A common vehicle was the hospital ethics committee, in which a multidisciplinary group was appointed to advise on hospital policies that had ethical implications or on ethically troubling ongoing cases. Others took the role of ethics consultants, who analyzed and clarified the issues at stake, often in association with an ethics committee. Gradually, greater numbers of lawyers and nurses also came to be recognized as experts in clinical ethics. Thus, like bioethics more generally, clinical ethics emerged as a truly multidisciplinary activity.

WHO PRACTICES CLINICAL ETHICS?

The answer to the question, Who practices clinical ethics? depends largely on one's conception of this new field. If clinical ethics is regarded as an emerging profession, then only those who possess certain credentials should be practitioners. Some have argued that only physicians or nurses can validly claim to have the necessary knowledge base to assess clinical ethics cases, which are often steeped in medical detail. Others argue that formal education in moral philosophy is required and perhaps more important than medical training because there is no shortage of informants on medical facts in hospitals. Still others will see an absolutely essential role for legal knowledge and risk management.

A related question is whether clinical ethicists should be independent actors or associated with an ethics committee. Along these lines, perhaps all members of an ethics committee's case consultation service should be regarded as clinical ethicists, in which case, all need to have a level of sophistication about these issues. Finally, in line with medical tradition, perhaps every attending physician should be a qualified clinical ethicist. This view is attractive because the attending physician still bears the primary moral and legal responsibility for a case and because it makes it clear that the practice of medicine cannot be value free—that ethical issues are not so external from medical concerns, as a separate ethics consult might suggest. As admirable as this ideal of the physician-philosopher might appear, however, future regulation of health care may make it impossible to avoid establishing clinical ethics evaluations as distinct moments in the care of some patients, perhaps distinguishing this function from the rest of the patient's treatment.

These will surely continue to be hotly debated matters in clinical ethics. This book takes no particular position on the question of who should practice clinical ethics or on the question of how these individuals should be trained or, as some have urged, credentialed. A task force of the American Society for Bioethics and Humanities (ASBH) has concluded that there are certain core competencies that all ethics consultants should have. These include ethics assessment skills (ethical assessment, process, and interpersonal) and core knowledge (common bioethical issues and concepts, health care systems, clinical context, the local health care institution and its policies, beliefs and perspectives of local patient and staff populations, relevant codes of ethics and professional conduct, guidelines of accrediting organizations, and relevant health law).[9]

The ASBH guidelines can be helpful in determining what specific training might be required to augment the educational background of particular individuals who may be ethics consultants. This skill-oriented approach supports the conviction that clinical ethics is a deeply multidisciplinary field requiring close collaboration in the education of its practitioners and the development of its educational material.

RELIGION IN CLINICAL ETHICS

It may be surprising that no mention has been made of the role played by theologians and members of the clergy in bioethics and particularly in clinical ethics. Although there have been and continue to be a number of prominent clinical ethicists with a background in religious studies, this professional group was somewhat more influential in the earlier period of bioethics in the late 1960s and early 1970s than they have been more recently. Rather, the term *clinical ethics* now refers to secular bioethics in a pluralistic society such as that of the United States. In specific religious communities in the United States and abroad, religious thinkers and leaders do continue to play a leading role in deliberating on moral dilemmas in the clinical setting.

This point raises an interesting and vitally important question in understanding clinical ethics: Precisely what is the appropriate role for religious beliefs in clinical ethics in a pluralistic society?

The theoretical framework described in Chapter 2, which might be called the received view in contemporary clinical ethics, reserves at least the following place for religious considerations: Competent adult patients are entitled to have their own religious beliefs respected, so long as those beliefs do not unduly restrict or compromise the beliefs of anyone else (including those of health care professionals). In other words, a traditional liberal theory of privacy is applied to the question of religious preferences in the ethics of health care. While this seems straightforward enough for the competent adult patient, in practice the health care professional is often unable to accept the patient's religiously based choice, as in the case of the Jehovah's Witness who rejects a medically indicated blood transfusion. Decision making on behalf of young children by those with pronounced religious views is another aspect of the general issue of religious preference. Clearly, according to the received theory of clinical ethics, it is quite important for health care providers to respect the religious beliefs of competent adult patients. However, the issue is less clear when parents are making decisions for children who have not yet developed their own religious preference.

There is another and rather more interesting role for religious beliefs in clinical ethics. As in the field of bioethics, the various religions can be sources of wisdom in territory uncharted by secular society, even if the religion that is the source of this wisdom is not one to which an individual might subscribe. Thus, it was a pope who first offered the distinction between ordinary and extraordinary treatment of the terminally ill, a distinction that, though not so useful anymore, provided a powerful early orientation for clinical ethics. The Roman Catholic Church has also endorsed the doctrine of double effect, which holds that pain medications such as morphine that also suppress respiration may be given to dying patients, so long as the intention is the relief of suffering rather than active euthanasia. To take an example from another religion, Jewish traditions argue from the absolute uniqueness of each individual life to the conclusion that the preservation of life is a prima facie moral obligation that admits few exceptions.

The role of systematic religious beliefs in clinical ethics should be distinguished from that of spirituality. Individuals may have deeply held spiritual values or attitudes that affect their health care decisions without subscribing to a faith tradition. Clearly, health care professionals, who may be quite sensitive to familiar religious identifications but not so much to spirituality in this sense, should not ignore this possibility. It is especially important to attend to an individual's spiritual orientation in the context of serious illness and discussions of end-of-life care.

CULTURAL COMPETENCE AND CLINICAL ETHICS

Formal religious identification and, to a lesser extent, spiritual orientation are often, but not always, associated with cultural background. Over the past several decades there has been a growing appreciation that clinical care—including patient adherence to treatment regimens—can be enhanced by incorporating cultural practices into a care plan. The professional's ability to identify a patient's culture, and knowledge of its elements that are relevant to efficacious health care, is referred to as cultural competence.

Although a detailed discussion of cultural diversity is beyond the scope of this book, it bears emphasizing that cultural differences are factored into the ethical framework presented in the next few chapters. Incorporating cultural patterns into health care can have a fundamental role in helping to satisfy the ethical principle of patient self-determination as well as in promoting patient well-being.

At the same time, assumptions about individual values or preferences based on a patient's cultural background can be erroneous. Differences in philosophies and medical practices based on culture should be kept in mind, but they should not be presumed to apply to every patient who is or appears to be a member of a particular social group.

LAW IN CLINICAL ETHICS

The place of the law in clinical ethics (including constitutional, statutory, regulatory, and case law) raises even more complex theoretical issues. At one extreme, it could be argued that the law should have no place at all in any discussion of ethics as such; at the other, it could be said that ethical questions are so subjective or theoretical, or so confusing and unclear, that the focus should instead be on the perceived clarity of the regulatory apparatus provided by the law. Clinicians should be particularly wary of the latter. Clearly, not all differences between these extreme points of view will be settled here, but they do point out the need to establish some serviceable position on the significance of the law for clinical ethics.

As a beginning, it should be noted that, although the terms *ethics* and *morals* are often used interchangeably in common speech, technically many philosophers hold them to be related in the following way: Ethics is the study of morality. When the requirements of morality are unclear, various traditions can be consulted, including the law. An appeal to the law as a source of information on morality may be justified on the assumption that the law is by and large reasonable in its methods and that it represents an accumulation of human experience with a wide range of cases and problems. These very modest assumptions can, of course, be challenged, but they appear to provide an adequate basis for proceeding, albeit cautiously, with the law as one source of guidance.

An obvious objection to reference to the law as one source on moral issues (besides the fact that much of the law is irrelevant to morality) is that often the law is itself immoral. The civil rights movement of the 1960s rested on this premise, but it also contended that laws permitting discriminatory treatment were ultimately incompatible with the United States Constitution, and in this contention the civil rights movement was vindicated. Yet if the Constitution did not happen to comport with the demands of morality, that would not be a telling point against morality, but rather against the law itself. Therefore, it is important to recall the logical distinction between the law and ethics, even when appealing cautiously to the law for whatever moral insight it might offer.

It is also important to remember that much of the law is a product of political haggling and compromise. The precise philosophical significance of law's political background will depend on one's moral epistemology. For Plato, this appears decisively to undermine law's moral standing, while for the American philosopher John Dewey morality is anyway a creature of human experience, including the political process. From a practical standpoint, the significance of the law for clinical ethics dilemmas is limited because the law is usually reactive. The legal system is not, on the whole, designed to anticipate the particular forms that controversies may take. Thus, it is not always wise to infer the legality of a proposed action from the law as it stands.

Another sort of objection to the use of the law as one guide on difficult moral questions is that laws vary from one society to another; indeed, in the United States they can differ from one state to another. But this does not mean that moral relativism must be accepted. To the contrary, the fact that there is some variation in, for example, the law governing doctor-patient relations from one country to another does not necessarily imply that the ethics of those relations differ. In addition, on certain fundamental matters the law may not differ as much as might be expected. That under ordinary circumstances a person accused of a crime is entitled to a fair trial seems to be a universal (albeit not always honored) feature of the criminal law. Similarly, the right to decide about participation in clinical research is universally supposed to be honored in the most rigorous fashion. Finally, to the extent that there are important differences between legal systems, these could be revealing about each society's attempt to reckon with difficult issues and provide some insight into the values that are operative or the way various values are weighted in that society.

There is an entirely different line of explanation for the prominent role that the law often plays in discussions about clinical ethics. Professional conduct is heavily regulated; it is often appropriate and even necessary to look no further than to the standards of practice in assessing the ethical obligations of health care providers. Actually, much of regulatory law and tort law is based on the standards of practice that the professions set for themselves. These standards include not only the relevant law, but also policy statements and codes of ethics developed by professional and governmental organizations as well as the implicit standards that may not be articulated as such. Thus, looking beyond standards of practice to more general moral considerations is necessary only when those standards are morally suspect or when they fail to address a particular problem. By contrast, in discussions of philosophical medical ethics the law plays a less prominent role than it does in discussions of clinical ethics.

Because it provides some more or less informative orientation to controversial social questions, the law is often the starting point for discussion in clinical ethics. It is rarely where the ethical discussion concludes, however, and often the results of moral discourse initiated by a reconsideration of the law effect a change in the law itself, or at least in the interpretation of the law. As will be shown, these are familiar patterns in discussions of clinical ethics.

Finally, exaggerated concern for personal legal liability is another impetus for looking to the law. Here, at least, let us call a spade a spade: Defensive medicine has nothing to do with ethics, even though it might happen to be consistent with the morally right outcome. This is not to suggest that a professional should be so naive and imprudent as to ignore the law that bears on his or her activities. Rather, the authority that society grants to professionals rests partly on the assumption that they will in turn be informed about and strive to act in accordance with social regulations that affect their field. At the same time, it is clear that society does not want professionals to be robots, and it affords them the privilege to set their own standards of conduct. The credentialed professional has the right to cite moral limits imposed by his or her individual integrity, but this must be balanced against the normal presumption that he or she will comply with the law. The professional who practices according to the standards of his or her field, who makes a good-faith effort to understand the law, and, as conscience permits, to comply with it, should have little fear of liability.

PUBLIC POLICY AND CLINICAL ETHICS

Traditionally, it has been left to clinicians to arrive at solutions to ethical problems. Occasionally, professional associations would articulate a position, but the ultimate conclusion was still left largely to the individual professional, especially the physician. In recent years, professional independence concerning ethical practices has been reduced for various reasons. Among these is that modern medical technologies have created familiar uncertainties about the application of traditional ethical canons. Public investment in the financing of health care, in both governmental and nongovernmental arrangements, has generated a more sharply defined public interest in the disposition of these funds. These and other factors have helped create pressure to arrive at solutions to ethical problems by more formal strategies than has often been the case in the past.

Two of the more formal approaches to managing ethical controversies are commissions or task forces appointed by executive branches of the federal or state governments and new statutory requirements promulgated by legislative branches, mainly at the state level. Each of these public approaches to problems in clinical ethics possesses advantages and disadvantages. Commissions can be useful in focusing public attention on an issue, gathering diverse expertise, and helping to move toward a consensus. Unfortunately, a conscientious public commission is an expensive and time-consuming process that may not respond efficiently to a perceived crisis.

Legislative approaches are efficient and justifiable on some theories of representative democracy, but the law can be a blunt instrument, especially when sensitive and deeply held values are at stake. Consider the example of physician-assisted suicide. Legislation prohibiting this practice may express an admirable policy goal, to ensure that physicians respect human life and avoid a slippery slope that some fear could follow any legal uncertainty in this regard. But suppose that there are individual circumstances, however rare they may be, in which an intervention intended to reduce suffering by shortening human life is justifiable. Statutory law is in a poor position to recognize exceptional circumstances.

In principle, the most desirable public ethics process would seem to be a combination of a thoughtful commission that builds or reinforces a societal moral consensus with clearly expressed and procedurally fair legislation that issues from the commission's recommendations. An example may be the model statute on determination of death that was developed by the President's Commission for the Study of Ethical Problems in Medicine in the early 1980s and adopted by virtually all the states. A less successful effort was the attempt by the National Bioethics Advisory Commission to generate a consensus on human cloning. The latter effort was hampered by a very short deadline in the face of a startling technical development.

ORGANIZATION ETHICS AND CLINICAL ETHICS

Ethical dilemmas arise not only because of inherent substantive ethical issues in clinical practice, they also come about due to shifts in the manner and locale for the delivery of health care, how it is financed, and how care systems are organizationally structured. These changes have obvious policy implications, but they also influence the ethical tensions and conflicts that surface in the clinical care setting.

The introduction of managed care practices has brought with it problems of medical ethics that are in some ways new, or at least more visible than they were before. Though fee-for-service practice contained the moral hazard of a temptation to overtreat (and hence overcharge), newer financial incentives tend toward undertreatment. When health care professionals enter into contractual arrangements, those contacts may serve the interests of the organization or of the professionals to the detriment of the patient.

Governmental agencies charged with the regulation of business practices, such as the United States Department of Justice, have taken a growing interest in corporate compliance with the criminal law and have encouraged the development of compliance or ethics programs. Among the corporate entities subject to this scrutiny are health care organizations, partly due to the advent and rapid market penetration of managed care. For example, an organization's policies and practices in the presentation and implementation of benefits must not be fraudulent. Health care organizations have thus become more aware of the ethical issues that relate to their business practices.

In order to address the ethical and legal factors that characterize the business environment of the health care organization, the field of organization ethics has emerged. Organization ethics has been defined as "the articulation, application, and evaluation of the consistent values and moral values of an organization by which it is defined, both internally and externally."[10] The Joint Commission for Accreditation of Healthcare Organizations (JCAHO) has defined organization ethics as those elements of the organization that have to do with the "ethical responsibility" of the entity "to conduct its business and patient care practices in an honest, decent and proper manner."[11]

A critical aspect of an organization's ethical orientation is its ethical climate, the "general and pervasive characteristics of [an] organization affecting a broad range of decisions."[12] A positive ethical climate is, among other things, one in which the organization's mission is consistent with its expectations for the professionals it employs. In health care organizations these expectations should include the professionals' commitment to the well-being of those who are enrolled in the plan.

Although there are certain ethical requirements for organizations that must be reflected in their culture and practices, these cannot substitute for the professional obligations of health care professionals themselves. These, too, should be supported by the organization. Nonetheless, there is often tension between the primacy of the individual patient, which is a value frequently upheld by professional ethics, and the contractual obligations to a group of subscribers. Organizations must develop processes for resolving this tension that are well articulated and understood by all who have a stake in its mission.

The next chapter describes the currently predominant theoretical framework of clinical ethics. That framework is the conceptual background for the treatment of the cases presented in the second part of this book.

REFERENCES

1. J. Fletcher, "The Bioethics Movement and Hospital Ethics Committees," *Maryland Law Review* 50 (1991): 859n, note 1.
2. A.R. Jonsen, M. Siegler, and W. Winslade, *Clinical Ethics,* 3rd ed. (New York: McGraw-Hill, 1992), 1.
3. J. LaPuma, "Clinical Ethics, Mission and Vision: Practical Wisdom in Health Care," *Hospital and Health Services Administration* 35 (Fall 1990): 321–326.
4. A.R. Jonsen, *The Birth of Bioethics* (New York: Oxford University Press, 1998).
5. S. Alexander, "They Decide Who Lives, Who Dies," *Life* LI 11, November 9, 1962, 102.
6. R. Duff and A.G.M. Campbell, "Ethical Dilemmas in the Special Care Nursery," *New England Journal of Medicine* 289 (1973): 890.
7. In re Quinlan, 355 A.2d 647 (N.J. 1976); *cert. denied,* 429 U.S. (1992).
8. S. Toulmin, "How Medicine Saved the Life of Philosophy," in *New Directions in Ethics,* eds. J. DeMarco and R. Fox (Boston: Routledge and Kegan Paul, 1986).
9. American Society for Bioethics and Humanities, *Core Competencies for Health Care Ethics Consultation* (Glenview, IL: 1998), 11–21.
10. E.M. Spencer, A. Mills, M.V. Rorty, and P.H. Werhane, *Organization Ethics for HealthCare Organizations* (New York: Oxford University Press, 1999).
11. Joint Commission for Accreditation of Healthcare Organizations, "Patients Rights and Organizational Ethics: Standards for Organizational Ethics," in *1996 Comprehensive Manual for Hospitals* (Chicago: 1996), 95–97.
12. B. Victor and J. Cullen, "The Organizational Bases of Ethical Work Climates," *Administrative Science Quarterly* 33 (1988): 101–125.

2

A Theory of Clinical Ethics

THE DOMINANT MORAL PHILOSOPHIES IN CLINICAL ETHICS: DEONTOLOGY AND UTILITARIANISM

This chapter is an account of what might be called the standard theory of clinical ethics, beginning with a review of the philosophies and ethical principles that have dominated the literature of biomedical ethics. Chapter 5 features a critique and alternatives to the standard theory.

Although it is important for the student of clinical ethics to be aware of the concepts presented in this section, a theory of clinical ethics cannot end simply with a recitation of philosophies and principles and an admonition to apply the philosophies and balance the principles in particular cases. Rather, experience with clinical ethics in the past few years suggests that a more practice-oriented method must be developed.

Two philosophic approaches dominate the literature. One is the deontologic approach, identified most closely with the German philosopher Immanuel Kant (1724–1804). Deontology is, literally, the study of duties that persons have toward one another. Thus, deontologic ethics is often called *duty-based* ethics. The second dominant philosophic approach to ethics is utilitarianism, identified most closely with the English philosophers John Locke (1632–1704) and John Stuart Mill (1806–1873). Utilitarianism is the view that actions or policies are to be morally evaluated according to the extent to which they promote happiness or well-being. To be sure, other important intellectual traditions have been applied to ethical questions in clinical practice, such as natural law, but deontology and utilitarianism have been the most cited. Both are appealing in the medical context, though for different reasons. Deontology is reminiscent of the familiar notion that doctors have certain special duties of care toward their patients, duties that do not usually apply in other relationships. A physician has a duty to treat a patient with whom he or she has established a therapeutic relationship or to help the patient secure suitable treatment; ordinarily, people are not obligated to be solicitous of one another's welfare to this extent. Utilitarianism is consistent with the preoccupation that most health care providers have with the outcomes or consequences of an intervention. Thus, physicians tend to recommend one treatment or another based on the likelihood that one would be more medically beneficial to a patient than the alternatives.

THE PRINCIPLES: SELF-DETERMINATION, BENEFICENCE, AND JUSTICE

Before examining the philosophic bases for the principles that are most often associated with the received view in clinical ethics, it should be noted how this account of the standard theory makes use of the principles. One way to develop a principled theory of clinical ethics would be to perform strict deductions from the ideas implicit in the principles, giving them much the same role that axioms have in a geometric proof. Although this approach has the virtue of intellectual rigor, it is rather formalistic and unappealing for the purpose of introducing clinical ethics, particularly to the practicing clinician. Instead, the principles should be taken in a more informal vein as guidelines. While the logic of the relation between ethical principles and actions or policies may not always be explicit in this informal approach, the assumption is that these relationships could be rendered explicit if needed.

Interestingly, neither deontology nor utilitarianism on its face calls immediate attention to the idea of patient self-determination, the most prominent value in the field of clinical ethics, though both are thought to be compatible with it. The philosophic grounds for self-determination issue rather from another aspect of Kant's philosophy, that of autonomy or self-government. Moral agents are those who can both formulate and appreciate their duties; it might be said that they are equipped both to generate and respect the rational necessity of their moral obligations. Moral agents, in turn, also recognize the respect to which all moral agents are entitled as capable of governing themselves, as autonomous. Another source of this principle of self-determination is the social theory of liberal philosophers such as Adam Smith and the utilitarian John Stuart Mill. In this tradition the legitimacy of the state as sovereign is founded on the sovereignty of the individual. The principle of self-determination is commonly regarded as the first principle of contemporary biomedical ethics. In the discussions that follow, the value of patient self-determination is based on the philosophic concept of autonomy.

The principle of self-determination is usually seen as conceptually balanced by the principle of beneficence, or the obligation to do good for the patient. Beneficence is closely associated with the traditional Hippocratic obligation at least not to harm the patient, or the principle of nonmaleficence. For purposes of this book, beneficence (doing good) includes nonmaleficence (doing no harm). Arguments that establish the moral basis of beneficence and nonmaleficence are also thought to be available in both deontologic and utilitarian moral philosophies. In the discussions that follow, the value of the best interests of the patient rests on the complementary philosophic principles of beneficence and nonmaleficence.

The principle of justice is frequently the point of reference for discussions of access to health care as a matter of social policy. The ancient Greek philosopher Aristotle (384–322 BC) is the classical source of theorizing about justice. An Aristotelian conception of justice as equity, or the principle that similar cases should be treated in a similar fashion, is one basis for the argument that the United States should adopt a universal health care system. Opponents argue that, by the same token, justice would be defeated by any universal system, and that high-quality health care for all should be the goal (defined in terms of a minimum level of basic services), not identical health care (defined as the same services for all, regardless of the need or ability to pay for more). The contemporary American philosopher John Rawls[1] has used a concept of justice as fairness as part of an argument on behalf of the rationality of distributing certain goods so as to maximize benefits to the worst off. Some of his followers have applied his approach to health policy, arguing that health care is such a good.[2]

The particular form of justice that is usually taken to be relevant to biomedical ethics is distributive justice. Distributive justice applies to *macroallocation* decisions (public health policy) and *microallocation* decisions (classically, triage in wartime). The clinician's role includes the second but not the first sort of judgment, and there is even controversy about how involved clinicians should be in microallocation.

Patient Self-Determination: Implementing Autonomy

In the history of biomedical ethics, no doctrine, principle, or proposition has been more influential than the idea that the competent, adult patient has the right to determine the course of his or her own medical treatment. This is the touchstone in the standard account of clinical ethical theory. This thesis has numerous implications and thus numerous problems in applying it.

Philosophic Basis

The philosophic roots of patient self-determination are perhaps even deeper, from a historical standpoint, than the legal background. It may be somewhat surprising that these roots are not derived from the Hippocratic tradition, which has nothing to say on the matter, but rather from medieval and Renaissance ideas about the sovereignty of the state. As has already been noted, autonomy or self-government is a notion that began in political theory and came to be seen, through the work of liberal philosophers such as Adam Smith and John Stuart Mill, as founded on the individual. Similarly, in Kant's philosophy, individuals are seen as moral agents entitled to respect.

Strictly speaking, autonomy refers to the potential for the individual to be self-determining. Self-determination is regarded as a good thing in itself and also as a means to an end. Self-determination is thought to be good in itself because it is the expression of a unique personality. In our society's liberal political philosophy individuality is of inherent value and entitled to respect. Self-determination is thought to be good as a means to the end of identifying that individual's best interests, a determination that involves incorporating the values of that person into the decision, values that the individual is in the best position to assess. In the clinical setting, self-determination is supported and expressed through an informed consent process, through which the patient chooses that option for care that is most individually appropriate, according to the patient's own values. (For a complete discussion of the elements of informed consent, see the following section.)

Clearly, many circumstances could prevent this potential for self-determination from being realized. Since self-determination is regarded as a good thing, certain individuals may be thought to be obligated to foster another's self-determination if they are in certain sorts of relationships with that individual; it can be argued that the relationship between patient and clinician is one of these. Perhaps the best example of such a relationship is that of the parent, who has a unique opportunity to help the developing child realize his or her individuality by helping to prepare the child to make his or her own choices. (It is important to point out that this is not an endorsement of paternalism or "parentalism," which is a distortion of the features of sound parenting.) At first the child tends to make choices that are rather haphazard and poorly considered. These choices are not thought to be truly the results of self-determination until they are considered judgments that reflect the person's reflective deliberation. It is implicit that these judgments would then also be authentic and reliable representations of that person's character and values.

This is a rather tall order; it is not hard to see how many conditions in the health care setting could prevent its realization. One of these is the sense of vulnerability that can accompany illness. Physicians and other health care providers are in very advantageous positions to reduce this sense of vulnerability and promote in the patient a feeling that he or she has some measure of control over the situation. They should also be aware of the potential to exploit this vulnerability, which may arise from the illness or from the imbalance of power between patient and clinician. The professional's support for the patient's efforts to retain or reclaim a sense of control appears to be the first important step in promoting the patient's self-determination. In light of such reassurance, the second important step is helping the patient to identify his or her own authentic preferences among the options available.

Legal Basis and Manifestations of Patient Self-Determination

History and Scope

The Anglo-American common-law notion of the right to determine what shall be done with one's own body emerged in the health care context in a series of surgical cases that resulted in litigation in the United States.[3] These cases often involved the excision of tissue without the consent of the patient, that is, without obtaining the patient's permission for the procedure. When the consent requirement was first articulated, it did not include the need to inform the patient about the risks and benefits of the procedure and alternative therapies, unlike today's legal standards.

As the concept evolved, failure to obtain informed consent has been understood by the courts in two ways. Originally, a legal theory of battery was applied to this line of cases, a gross view of the nature of the contract as merely involving the physical concerns and interaction of the doctor-patient relationship. Later, the concept of consent took on informational aspects as well. Failure to obtain a patient's informed consent came to be regarded as a breach under a negligence theory rather than battery; that is, it came to be viewed as a failure to provide an acceptable standard of care. This approach is today the standard.

Courts have entertained a few exceptions to fully informed consent, varying somewhat in different states. The least controversial exception is that of an emergency, understood as an immediate threat to life or limb; however, it is important to understand that in emergencies, consent is presumed rather than suspended. In particular, it is presumed that the reasonable person would agree to be treated under these emergency conditions. Since the right of self-determination is inalienable, one is never without that right. Thus, once the emergency passes, so, too, does this exception to the need to obtain consent. One may waive the right to consent and assign decision-making authority to someone else, while retaining the right to revoke the waiver at any time. This theoretical possibility of waiver is not, however, frequently encountered in the clinical setting and should never be presumed. Further, these considerations of exceptions to informed consent are based on the model of the competent adult patient. The age of majority, or the attainment of legal competency, is a matter both of the individual's actual decisional capacity and of statutory law, though we will shortly address exceptions. *Competence* in this context is a legal term of art and finally depends on a judicial determination.

Therapeutic Exception

Considerably more doubt surrounds the legitimacy of the doctrine of the therapeutic exception to informed consent, or therapeutic privilege. Once this was a popular rationale for not obtaining informed consent. Under the therapeutic exception, the activity of seeking the patient's consent is suspended because the physician believes that the harm that may befall the patient from the information conveyed would outweigh any benefit the patient would find from being given a comprehensive view of his or her clinical condition (see Case 5, "Don't Tell Mother"). There has recently been a philosophic and legal tendency to constrain the therapeutic exception, which is often regarded as paternalistic and disrespectful of a patient's right to know and ability to handle bad news. The anti-paternalistic trend has been based both philosophically on the view that self-determination is a more powerful consideration in principle and empirically on data that indicate that the vast majority of patients wish to know their medical status and suffer no harm as a result of this knowledge. Where statutory law addresses this question, as in the State of New York do-not-resuscitate (DNR) law, it has required the physician to document the reasons for believing that providing the patient with information about his or her condition would be likely to cause immediate and serious harm to the patient. Moreover, the conditions that would create adequate grounds for this exception are considered rare and time limited.

Advance Directives

Most jurisdictions have also crafted legislation that recognizes the legality of certain advance directives. Advance directives are instructions given by a patient while he or she has decisional capacity concerning medical treatment he or she would or would not like to receive in the event that decisional capacity is lost. In general, there are two types of advance directives: those dealing with substantive concerns that will determine a person's care when he or she can no longer express a preference and those dealing with procedural issues, such as who should make health care decisions if the preferences of the patient are unknown and cannot be ascertained. The living will is the most common form of substantive advance directive, usually used to specify those interventions that are not desired by the patient under certain conditions (see Case 3, "Urgent Surgery in a Stuporous Patient"). Most jurisdictions also allow for a procedural advance directive, usually the assignment of a durable power of attorney for health care, sometimes also called a *surrogate decision maker* or *health care agent,* who has authority to make all or virtually all medical decisions that the patient would have made were he or she able to express a preference. This legislation also typically protects the physician from any potential liability arising from good-faith compliance with the advance directive, whether substantive or procedural.

The authority of advance directives is based on the proposition that the legal right to self-determination, as a reflection of individual self-determination, is not voided by the formerly competent adult's loss of decision-making ability, whether temporary or not. This applies to neurologic conditions such as coma and Alzheimer's disease, as well as psychiatric disorders (not including developmental disabilities and mental retardation, for these individuals have never been able to exercise their self-determination). Clearly, problems will sometimes arise in determining exactly what counts as the faithful execution of an advance directive, particularly of the substantive variety. These will be addressed later, as will the problems the clinician faces in determining the patient's wishes in the absence of an explicit document and the authority to be granted surrogate decision makers, such as close relatives, in the absence of relevant legislation.

Advance directives, it should be noted, are not identical with advance care planning. The former is a mechanism for making treatment decisions; the latter is a form of treatment management for individuals whose loss of decision-making capacity is foreseeable. Advance directives may—and in general should—be an element of advance care planning for such individuals. Advance directives are also not necessarily written documents. They are expressions of a person's wishes, and should be documented for the sake of accuracy, but they may not necessarily involve the execution of a legal instrument by the individual.

This book has emphasized the fundamental legal and moral right of the patient to have his or her preferences respected. The law does not always make honoring these preferences contingent on an explicit document having been rendered. Since the 1976 New Jersey Supreme Court's *Quinlan* case, it has been recognized in some jurisdictions that family members and other close friends are often able to provide information about the patient's likely wishes under his or her current circumstances. This proposition was affirmed by several state courts, and for the first time by the United States Supreme Court in its 1991 decision in the case of Nancy Cruzan, a young woman who, like Karen Ann Quinlan, was in a persistent vegetative state.[4] When a decision is made based on the patient's previously expressed wishes, whether it is made by family or friends or by a court, it is called a substituted judgment, sometimes also known as the *subjective test* for determining the course of a patient's care.

Evidence of a patient's prior wishes may be based either on actual statements the patient made or through an interpretation based on having known the person before incapacity. A few state legal systems, including those of New York and Missouri, currently require that a patient's prior wishes regarding treatment be substantiated by a very high standard of evidence, called "clear and convincing," in order to legally validate, for example, the removal of life-sustaining therapy. The philosophic basis for this requirement is the view that the state's interest in the continued life of its citizens and the vulnerability of people who are profoundly impaired justify extreme caution in interpreting the individual's wishes about forgoing life-sustaining measures. An example of evidence that would meet this standard would be a written statement by a patient that she would not wish to be fed artificially if she should become irreversibly unconscious. In principle, there is nothing to prevent verbal statements from achieving this level of evidence about a person's wishes. In practice, however, verbal statements that people make in conversation about these matters are often not specific concerning types of therapies that should be withheld under particular circumstances. Thus, in these states, attorneys or courts of law understandably regard written or oral advance directives that are not specific enough so as to meet the "clear and convincing" standard with some skepticism.

Sometimes no record or knowledge exists of the patient's preferences or previously held values. In these instances it is generally thought that the decision maker should proceed based on an assessment of the patient's best interests, sometimes also called the *objective test*. Among a number of alternatives, the one that satisfies a person's best interests is usually considered the optimal balance of benefits over burdens for that person. This benefits-burdens analysis is mandatory when a person is deciding on behalf of another. In the absence of guidance about that person's actual wishes or values, as a matter of policy, the appeal to best interests appears to be the most satisfactory alternative available. Another standard of decision making that has been suggested under these circumstances is what a reasonable person would decide under the circumstances. The reasonable person test is, however, less prominent than it once was. In any case, from a pragmatic standpoint it appears that the results of a reasonable person analysis would track very closely those of a best-interests analysis.

Respect for self-determination is normally taken to imply the patient's right to *refuse* unwanted treatment; it has not traditionally encompassed a patient's right to *insist* on access to any particular treatment, especially when physicians believe that it is highly unlikely that such care will benefit the patient. Patient or family insistence on medically useless treatment also has obvious financial implications, considering the continuing increase in the costs of health care in the United States. Thus, the question of whether and under what circumstances requested care may be denied the patient is tied to the question of justice in the distribution of health care and is addressed in Chapter 4 (Clinical Ethics throughout the Life Span).

Respect for patient self-determination does not obligate the physician to intervene in a way that would be harmful to a patient, even if the patient insists. A notable example is the question of whether this general proposition applies to the provision of barbiturates to a terminally ill patient intent on suicide or more direct means of physician-assisted suicide. Some would consider meeting these demands to be expressions of care rather than harmful acts. However, even if one departs from the standard moral and legal view and endorses some cases of physician-assisted suicide, this is not equivalent to rendering physician involvement in such activities obligatory. If there were ever a basis for limits to patient self-determination with respect to demands placed on physicians, surely one exists here.

Finally, some of the limits to patient self-determination have to do with the public interest rather than physician integrity, understood as the right and duty of clinicians to obey the demands of their own conscience. For example, keeping a patient's confidences is normally required as one form of respect for self-determination; to possess intimate information about someone is, after all, to have power over that person. The exception of information about sexually transmissible disease, however, is of such importance that authorities are routinely informed in order to track and prevent the spread of the disease. Here, societal obligations to preserve the public health are considered to outweigh the concern of the individual patient for privacy and self-determination. Of course, the concept of confidentiality also includes the obligation for those who have a legitimate need to know to keep such information private.

Hierarchy of Surrogates

It is necessary to distinguish different senses in which a surrogate may be validly identified, for this is relevant to all situations in which patients cannot speak for themselves (Table 2–1). First, a surrogate may be appointed by a court of law as a guardian for an incompetent patient. Second, a surrogate may have been previously appointed by the patient in an advance directive document such as a durable power of attorney for health care. Third, a surrogate may be identified on the basis of common practice, whether with or without actual legal empowerment. The standard ordering

Table 2–1 Decision-Making Authority for Adults in Order of Priority

Competent adult patient
Competent adult patient's advance directives* (e.g., living will, durable power-of-attorney for health care)
Court-appointed guardian*
Surrogate as empowered according to state statutory or common law*
Court as decision maker

* Check state law for specific requirements.

of such customary surrogates begins first with the spouse, then moves to an adult child, then perhaps to another close relative. Fourth, the correct priority of potential surrogates may be established by statute, as in the New York do-not-resuscitate law.

Parents are the presumptive decision makers for children. When one parent is not reasonably available, a single parent may consent to treatment. On evidence of reasonable suspicion of abuse or neglect, or if neither biologic parent is available, a court may appoint a guardian empowered to make decisions in the best interests of the child. Often this guardian will be the social services commissioner of that jurisdiction. Unlike adoptive parents, foster parents do not automatically have decisional authority for children in their care.

Philosophically, both the identification of the most qualified surrogate and the surrogate's precise decisional role are closely tied to the standard of decision making. If the standard is the previously expressed wishes of the patient who is no longer competent, which is the standard that modern clinical ethics has adopted, then the individual who is most knowledgeable of those wishes is the most desirable surrogate. Further, according to this standard the surrogate's role is to acquaint clinicians with the patient's wishes, so far as they are known, rather than to express his or her own views about what would be best for the patient. Obviously, this would differ from a medical indicators standard, for example, in which case the most qualified surrogate would be the one who could make the most reliable judgment about what treatment was medically indicated, presumably based on the current standard of care for that condition.

For patients whose previous wishes are unknown, or for those who have never had the opportunity to develop the intellectual skills associated with such wishes, the received standard for surrogate decision making is either an objective substituted judgment, based on the likely wishes of a person in this situation, or the patient's best interests. The proper decision-making standard for this population remains a highly controversial area.

Elements of Informed Consent

Philosophically, autonomy and its promotion both undergird and exert greater demands than the legal doctrine of informed consent (Table 2–2). Indeed, the standard philosophic account of informed consent exhibits a much more extensive conceptual scheme than is found in the law, which focuses mainly on the concepts of provision of information and free consent. Another important difference between legal and philosophic accounts of informed consent is that for the law, informed consent as a one-time event is generally sufficient. From a philosophic standpoint, however, a *process* model rather than an *event* model of informed consent is far preferable and often morally required. A process model emphasizes the need for interaction between the clinician and patient, sometimes demands repeated exchanges, and de-emphasizes a written document.

Table 2–2 The Elements of Informed Consent*

Threshold requirement
Competence

Information requirements
Information
Understanding

Consent requirements
Consent
Authorization

* Our interpretation of these elements for our theory of clinical ethics may not in all instances be identical with Beauchamp and Childress.

Source: Data from T. Beauchamp and J.F. Childress, *Principles of Biomedical Ethics 3rd Ed.,* © 1989, Oxford University Press.

Competence

Competence is a legal term, and the theoretical as well as ultimate determination of a patient's competence is in principle made by a court of law. In practice, however, the routine assessment of competence, that is, the determination of whether or not the patient has the capacity to either consent to or refuse a proposed intervention, is usually made by the attending physician, sometimes after having consulted a psychiatrist. There is a strong legal presumption of competence for the patient who has reached the age of majority. Philosophically, self-determination is generally so significant that specific evidence of incapacity is required to call into question an adult's empowerment to make his or her own decisions. However, precisely what the appropriate criteria are for assessing competence is still unclear.

Although competence is often thought to be an intractably ambiguous concept, a clinically useful account of competence is available. The valuable account of Buchanan and Brock emphasizes that much of the apparent obscurity of competence vanishes when it is taken not as an abstraction but as competence for some particular task.[5] Competence is therefore best understood as decision-specific capacity. Thus, rather than use the term *competence*, the terms *decisional capacity* and simply *capacity* will be used here. The capacity to perform a particular decision-making task is further delimited according to the time at which the decision is to be made, and the specific conditions under which it is to be made.

Understood in this way, decisional capacity may call on various abilities, depending on the demands of the task at hand (see Case 2, "Determining If a Patient Has Decisional Capacity"). Yet there appear to be some general abilities required in the process of becoming involved in and in determining treatment decisions. These include the ability to understand or appreciate the nature of various alternatives, as well as the ability to communicate a preference. In reaching a personal preference, one must also be capable of reasoning and deliberation, the latter signaling that this is a process in which the decision maker's own values are gradually brought to bear on the question. Accordingly, too, the competent decision maker's values will be more or less stable and consistent over a period of time; they will be values that the decision maker recognizes as his or her own.[6]

These general attributes that pertain to the decision maker with capacity are consistent with the earlier and overriding observation that decisional capacity involves task-relative abilities. Not only is it important to view competence in functional rather than global terms (and thus as decisional capacity), it is also important to see it as a threshold concept (with clear cases in which it applies and in which it does not), rather than as an incremental one (a concept that increasingly applies to an ordered series of cases). Thus, while it is certainly true that patients will have differing degrees of capacity at different times or with respect to different decisions, nonetheless a basic determination must be made of whether or not a particular patient is capable of deciding on a particular treatment option. Of course, the threshold may shift depending on the circumstances of the decision-making task. On this point, Culver and Gert[7] offer an account of competence that competes with that of Buchanan and Brock. They note that, according to Buchanan and Brock, a patient may be competent to accept treatment but not to reject it, because the decision to reject a low-risk treatment requires a higher threshold of capacity than the decision to accept it. Culver and Gert avoid this result by emphasizing the rationality of the decision rather than the competence of the decision maker. The trouble with this approach is that the competent decision maker's preference could then be overruled in a paternalistic fashion because it is considered irrational. Although this debate is of considerable theoretical significance, these two views of competence will reach the same conclusion about the vast majority of actual cases in which patient competence is an issue.

The arguments in this book rely on the Buchanan and Brock formulation, which brings us squarely up against the following problem. Every clinician will at one time or another experience the frustration of a noncompliant but decisionally capable patient who could benefit from straightforward therapy. According to the approach adopted here, the patient cannot be declared incompetent and thus overruled simply because his or her decision appears to the clinician to be an irrational one. An unavoidable byproduct of a concept of competence founded on the patient's capacity to decide, rather than the rationality of the decision, is that the patient has a right to be "wrong," and that a wrong decision is nonetheless deserving of respect. In this vein, requests for psychiatric consultation concerning decision-making capacity generally should be framed in terms of assessments of decision-specific capacity: not, Can this patient make decisions? but rather, Does this patient have the capacity to make this particular decision?

The clinician is not barred from attempting to persuade the patient to accept the recommended treatment, so long as these efforts do not become coercive. For example, suggestions that other elements of the patient's treatment might be withdrawn or withheld in the light of his or her uncooperative position are clearly coercive. Manipulative strategies to obtain the patient's apparent consent, such as ambiguously worded descriptions of risks associated with a therapy or misleading accounts of benefits, are still more insidious than overt coercion and just as objectionable. Just as the patient nearly always has the right to know the truth about his or her condition, even if the news is bad, so he or she also has the right to know what can be reasonably expected of treatment options even if that information might well lead to a decision his or her caregivers find disagreeable.

Though earlier accounts of decision-making capacity have tended to focus on the patient alone, capacity can vary depending on the way the message is conveyed and the communications skills of the clinician. These skills can be critical in successfully imparting what a patient needs to know, which requires more than simply reciting information. Similarly, patient refusals (or uninformed consents) can often be reexamined through a process of active listening, which requires the clinician to actively engage in dialogue with a patient in order to ensure that the clinician accurately hears and understands the concerns and perspective of the patient.

Matters are still more complicated with respect to patients who have not achieved the legal age of majority, or who would be regarded by the law as never having been capable of making their own decisions in spite of chronological age, such as the developmentally disabled and profoundly retarded. Even if the patient has a biologic parent or a legal guardian, his or her wishes should still be solicited, and in many cases respected, to the extent that he or she is capable of understanding the decision and expressing a preference. The basis for this respectfully solicitous attitude is philosophic rather than legal: A deontologic view (concerned with the role-specific duties of clinicians to patients), holds that there is a prima facie obligation to promote the self-determination of others; a consequentialist view (concerned with optimizing patient outcome) is that, regardless of his or her intellectual condition, the patient will be most directly affected by whatever action is taken or not taken. It might be argued that the patient who is irreversibly unconscious is an exception to this latter consequentialist point, but this refers to patients with some intellectual ability, rather than those with none.

In the case of children, some measure of capacity may be recognized as early as 8 years of age (though not in the law), and certainly by age 15. If the child is an emancipated minor, meaning that he or she is self-supporting and leading a life independent of his or her parents, then the rights that normally accord to adults usually apply. There is also a mature minor exception, recognized in most jurisdictions, which grants decision-making authority at around age 15, depending on the decisional circumstances. Again, these are minimal legal conditions and should not be taken as exhausting the moral obligations of clinicians toward those who are not technically competent adults.

Very young children and others who have never been able to express a preference, such as some developmentally disabled individuals, constitute a somewhat ambiguous area in the law, both in terms of who should make decisions for them and on what basis the decisions should be made. In general, the parents of infants and other very young children are presumed to be in the best position to represent their child's best interests and to make decisions for the child. The best-interests framework is discussed in detail later in this chapter.

Information

The patient with decisional authority, or the properly identified surrogate decision maker, is entitled to all the information available about his or her condition that could be pertinent to a decision about treatment. This formulation of the right to be informed includes the right to know the diagnosis and prognosis of the disease and the known or estimated risks and benefits of proposed therapies and alternatives, as well as the implications for the patient of having no treatment at all. The free flow of information to the patient, however sensitively it may need to be conveyed, is obviously vital for a valid consent process. Special training in holding conversations that deal with sensitive information may be appropriate, including techniques for giving patients a sense of continued control over their lives. The patient's likely quality of life following the intervention, including the nature of any rehabilitation period, is also a proper part of this conversation. Patients are also entitled to information concerning the costs of proposed interventions and of alternatives and of the availability of insurance coverage. Often the question is raised as to whether the financial costs of the care that is proposed should be a part of the information provided. While there is no doubt that the patient should have access to this information, whether or not he or she is insured, it is not at all clear that the physician or any other clinician should be the one to provide it. First, clinicians are rarely well informed themselves about the costs of care, and, second, overt attention to financial matters may well create the appearance of conflict of interest. This area appears to be one in which the health care institution has the primary obligation to provide information on request.

Full information is one of the legal pillars of informed consent, the other being free and uncoerced consent itself. Yet concern is often expressed, particularly by physicians in fields in which terminal illness is common, about the inhumanity of giving the unvarnished truth. It is important, however, to distinguish between the inherently unwelcome nature of bad medical news and the feelings of the vast majority of patients who, surveys demonstrate, desire to have that information. Again, the information should be imparted in a manner that is sensitive to the patient's particular circumstances but fully imparted nonetheless.

At such times it may be tempting to speak first with, for example, the patient's adult child, to enlist his or her support before the encounter with an older patient. For several reasons, this temptation should be avoided. First, certain classes of patients, such as the elderly, are too easily stereotyped as decisionally incapable or unable to manage emotionally powerful information, even though they may be quite functional in other areas of their lives and lack any psychiatric history relevant to this issue. Second, the information is, after all, more the concern of the patient than of anyone else, and he or she should hear it first and has the right to determine who else is privy to this information. Third, the misguided attempt to enlist the adult child's help could backfire in several ways. The grown child may not be prepared for the loss of a parent, may not enjoy the patient's confidence, or may even have a personal agenda that is in conflict with the best interests of the patient. However, there is no barrier to asking the patient whether it would be desirable for the physician to have a conversation with a particular relative or close friend, whether privately or with the patient, so that all three can cooperate in planning for the patient's future. In that case, family or friends should be part of discussions about care as soon as is practicable. In the final analysis, though, the confidentiality of the patient must be respected so far as is possible.

Understanding

A somewhat different objection to the idea of the fully informed patient is the argument that some medical decisions are so complex that the lay patient cannot be expected to integrate them, thus calling into question the foundations of the informed consent notion. Clearly, a medical school education could not be a prerequisite for a workable consent process, but that is not required. Perhaps the best way to think about articulating information for the patient is this: What does the patient need to know about how the available options will affect his or her life? This approach recommends that explanations be given in functional rather than scientific terms, for example, that following a certain procedure a patient may no longer be able to perform a certain physical activity. Some patients will benefit from a more technical presentation, but it is surely not required for the consent process to be valid.

Clinically, the greatest difficulty is often encountered when the clinician is unsure whether the patient fully understands information that has been imparted. Clearly, the timing of the conversation, language barriers, and other extraneous factors will influence patient understanding. The patient in intensive care who is sedated and is drifting in and out of consciousness is the classic (if somewhat extreme) example. To a great extent this problem brings up the issue of competence, for it has been observed that the ability to understand information is one of the general requirements of competence. Often, however, the clinician believes that the patient has until very recently been cogent, and only now, when there is a crucial decision about continuing therapy to be made, is there some doubt.

This uncomfortable situation speaks to the importance of advance planning or preventive ethics. Unfortunately, it is not uncommon for the physician now responsible for a patient's care never to have seen the patient before admission, so that both the patient and physician suffer from the shortcomings of the previous management. In spite of these disadvantages, it should be determined whether or not the patient understands enough to retain decisional authority. The physician should be satisfied that there is no physical basis for ruling out the patient's competence. Consistency of response is another measure.

Especially in the case of gravely ill patients who may be highly medicated, the clinician's communications skills may be critical, as patients who appear to lack understanding may simply be responding as well as they can to the specific query. Questions must be put clearly and unambiguously, as the following anecdote illustrates: When a heavily medicated patient in intensive care was asked, "Do you want to die?" she shook her head from side to side. When the same patient was then asked, "Do you want to live?" she also shook her head. The air of paradox about these exchanges was resolved by a senior psychiatrist who deduced that the patient interpreted the first query as, "Do you want to be killed?" This analysis immediately altered the style of communication with the patient.

Consent

Consent refers to the voluntary and uncoerced choice of the patient. Consent is a more active process than mere assent or dissent. Ideally, it implies deliberation and perhaps also reflection based on one's own values. Obstacles to truly reflective consent in the hospital include the very physical conditions commonly associated with treatment for severe illness. For example, mechanical restraints may be utilized for legitimate or illegitimate purposes, but it is certain that they compromise the sense of control that enables a person to make well-considered choices. Medications may inadvertently exert a more insidious influence over the patient.

Certain sorts of constraints on the patient may not be obvious to the physician. Examples range from pressures associated with familial dynamics to concern with the financial consequences of one alternative or another. In extreme circumstances the physician may be justified in assuming an active role as patient advocate in attempting to determine if a stated choice is truly what the patient would want. Additionally, some patients who are unable to give consent, such as certain elderly with dementia, should nevertheless be interviewed for their assent, meaning a simple "yes" or nod of the head in response to a concise and clearly stated question. When the clinician has the slightest doubt about a patient's remaining capacity, this process does more than express respect for the patient. It may also be important in deciding whether or not to go ahead with a procedure that has only a moderately favorable risk-benefit ratio.

Refusal may be thought of as the obverse of consent, with the same moral implications and authority. Just as the concept of consent entails a higher level of understanding and involvement than simple assent, so the concept of refusal entails a higher level of understanding and involvement than simple dissent. In order for a refusal of treatment to count as truly informed, it should be as competent and informed as a consent to treatment.

Authorization

An action is authorized when the individual with the appropriate authority gives approval. In accordance with the previous discussion, this will either be the patient or some representative of the patient. Normally, the authorization is assumed to be granted via a signed consent form. Unfortunately, in a system preoccupied with documentation and recordkeeping, the signed consent form has tended to substitute for the consent process itself. Of course, a form that purports to represent an actual event but does not is neither ethically nor legally valid. Similarly, verbal consent without a form signed by the patient or surrogate may be valid, though obviously documentation of one kind or another is always advisable.

Besides the tendency in some busy centers to obtain patients' signatures that do not represent a valid consent process, documents that require one or two witnesses often involve another misunderstanding. From a legal standpoint, the act of witnessing a document pertains only to the fact that the individual truly signed on the dotted line. From an ethical standpoint it might be argued that an individual who is not comfortable that a patient truly understands the content expressed in the form should not agree to witness the signing of the document. However, this additional condition on the act of witnessing a consent form has not become part of the ethical consensus on authorization in the informed consent process.

Beneficence: The Place of Patient Interests

The standard theory of clinical ethics takes the position that the competent patient, or the appropriately identified surrogate, is the best judge of patient interests. Implicit in this position is the possibility that the clinician will occasionally disagree with the conclusion reached by a patient or surrogate. Because these situations present a conflict between the clinician's traditional obligation to do good for the patient (to act in a beneficent manner) and the more recently recognized obligation to respect the patient's expressed wishes, these are among the most difficult situations faced by clinicians.

Competent Patient, Wrong Decision

At times clinicians encounter patients who are clearly competent but who make decisions that seem to fly in the face of their medical best interests. An example may be that of the 60-year-old oncology patient who elects not to endure chemotherapy treatment expected to produce a significant remission. As disconcerting as such decisions are, if they are undertaken freely and with full information, they are to be respected. This does not suggest, however, that an initial "no" should be taken as a final answer. Rather, a reasonable effort should be made short of coercion to persuade the patient at least to attempt therapy, along with an offer to help him or her reassess the decision.

A patient's refusal of the most promising course of therapy should be the beginning, not the end, of conversations. These conversations may provide an opportunity to learn ways in which the patient is confused about some information or that the patient's values are not in line with the clinician's assumptions. They can even be the springboard to treatment strategies or negotiations, such as an agreement to undertake a time-limited trial of therapy subject to the patient's choice to continue or not after a certain period has elapsed.

An even more confusing situation may be one in which a patient of identified but marginal competence declines recommended treatment that is known to be efficacious, such as the hospitalized drug addict who refuses dialysis. Such a patient is a likely candidate for being labeled noncompliant; not only does he resist medical advice, he may happen also to be personally unpleasant, so the clinician may be tempted neither to press a recommendation too strongly nor to attempt to override the patient's wishes. The professional's duty is to overcome these tendencies and treat the patient as any other.

Less obvious is the special utility of the psychiatric consultant in these cases, whose assistance should be sought not only with the competency assessment. When special skills are required to impress upon the patient the urgency of recommended treatment, the psychiatrist who is trained to recognize and manage behaviors associated with personality disorders should be enlisted. In this vein, clinicians should carefully distinguish between the goals of an ethics consultation and those of a psychiatric consultation; problems in applying personal values can mask underlying psychiatric issues.[8]

The Uncertain Patient

At least as common as the patient whose views about medical treatment are incompatible with those of the clinician is the patient who is unsure of or who vacillates about his or her wishes. Sometimes this is expressed as a desire for the physician to make the decision, while in other instances the patient is racked with doubt about the best approach. Perhaps the most important tactic, from the patient's standpoint, is for the physician and other professionals to repeatedly assure the patient of their support whatever the decision is, as well as to participate in the decision-making process with the patient.

The familiar scenario of the patient who wants the doctor to make the decision is not tantamount to a transfer of decision-making authority to the physician, who would in any case be an inappropriate surrogate. Rather, the physician is commonly thought to have an obligation not only to respect the patient's self-determination, but also to promote it where possible. Therefore, the first step in such a situation would be to engage the patient in a conversation about what he or she understands and hopes the outcome of alternative interventions, or nonintervention, would be; to help the patient assess his possible futures from his own point of view; and then to suggest the likelihood of the various possibilities. In most cases a therapeutic alternative is not an "all or none" situation, such as a major organ transplant, but resembles cancer chemotherapy in the sense that the intervention ceases whenever the patient wishes. It may be important for the patient to be reassured that an initial decision to proceed with one alternative does not mean that she will lose control over her life. Further, without reducing the opportunity for the patient's own wishes to emerge during the conversation, it is entirely appropriate for the physician to give an opinion as to what is medically the best course.

The doctrine of informed consent does not require a physician to browbeat patients into making their own treatment decisions. Rather, a waiver of the right to be informed about and to consent to treatment is a legitimate option. If the patient genuinely desires a transfer of authority so that he or she does not have to undergo the stress of the decision process, that should be formally executed and documented, an arrangement that the competent patient may terminate at any time. Preferably, the surrogate should be someone familiar with the patient's preferences or at least his or her values. Once again, however, these waivers are rare and their existence must not be presumed.

Expressions of doubt about treatment options are wholly reasonable, especially in instances of major illness. Indeed, one may doubt that a patient who appears to reach a decision too easily has authentically engaged with the facts of his or her situation. Again, reassurance that one can be expected to have reservations about the right step to take and offers of assistance in making a decision may be among the most healing acts in the clinician's repertoire of therapeutic interventions.

How Are Surrogates to Decide?

A consensus has emerged regarding the basis of surrogate decision making, or substituted judgment, in the absence of explicit advance directives, whether written or oral. The preferred standard or, as the *Quinlan* court called it, the "subjective test," is whatever the particular patient would have wanted had he or she been able to decide. Here any evidence about the patient's values, religious beliefs, and lifestyle is considered relevant. In the absence of information about what the patient would have wanted, the surrogate should base the medical decision on the optimal balance of benefits and burdens (the best interests) that pertain to that patient, also known as the objective test. In general, relief of pain and suffering are important goals of the best-interest standard, whichever test of best interest is used.

The philosophical standard that should guide surrogate decision making is an especially important matter in light of data indicating that many surrogates are unfamiliar with patient wishes. Under these conditions advance directives may indeed not be serving the goal of patient self-determination.[9,10] A surrogate who is not proceeding according first to the subjective test and then the objective test is presumably not performing the job properly.

Appropriate Surrogate, Wrong Decision

Consider now a situation in which the appropriate surrogate decision maker makes a decision that the physician believes to be incompatible with the patient's medical best interests, including a situation in which the surrogate insists that the clinicians "do everything" when aggressive treatment is not believed to be medically appropriate. To what extent must the surrogate's decision be respected, in both legal and ethical senses? What avenues are available for the clinician who is convinced that an error is being made?

It may be helpful to distinguish between two different sorts of errors in this type of situation. The first kind of error is that pertaining to a surrogate's failure to act on the patient's previously expressed wishes. The second kind occurs when the patient's wishes are unknown and the surrogate has reached what the physician believes to be an erroneous conclusion about what would be best for the patient.

If a physician or other clinician suspects that a surrogate is failing to respect what are believed to be the previously expressed wishes of the patient, the first kind of error, then the clinician may have a moral obligation to treat the patient according to that understanding. However, the clinician who attempts to override a decision made by a valid surrogate, particularly a patient-appointed agent, carries an extraordinary burden of proof. The legal implications of such a course will depend on the type of surrogate in each case. In the instance of a court-appointed guardian, the professional must be prepared to provide evidence that the guardian's recommendation does not respect the patient's wishes. In the case of a surrogate with a statutory advance directive such as a durable power of attorney for health care, one can only appeal to a court. Protests against customary surrogates may be lodged with other members of the family or friends, but unambiguous identification of a legally empowered surrogate may require judicial intervention.

Statutes establishing the appropriate order of surrogacy may include a dispute mediation system. Even if state law does not specify mediation, there are constructive approaches before a matter such as this is taken to the legal system. One of them is alternative dispute resolution (ADR), which involves a well-described mediation process and techniques for improving communication. Another alternative prior to judicial review is consultation with an ethics committee. Hospital ethics committees should include individuals who are familiar with managing disputes, such as chaplains.[11]

When clinicians attempt to overcome an alleged error of the first type, the burden is on their knowledge of the patient's actual previous wishes. In errors of the second kind, the clinician's burden is to show that, in his or her professional judgment, the surrogate's decision would not be in the patient's best interests. Even surrogates with very strong claims to authority, such as parents of minor children, have in fact sometimes been subject to loss of decision-making authority on such grounds, as in the case of Jehovah's Witnesses who refuse to consent to blood transfusions for their children (see Case 29, "A Religious Objection to a Child's Medical Treatment"). When the alternative is certain death, judges are apt to be impressed by the appeals of physicians. By contrast, when clinicians attempt to wrest control from a traditionally authorized surrogate in order to stop what they regard as inappropriately extending life, as in the case of the parents of a dying child who elect to continue aggressive treatment, they are much less likely to prevail. Court-appointed surrogates may be challenged on the basis of poor judgment, as may statutory surrogates, though the likelihood of success will vary with the nature of the disagreement.

Determining Best Interests without a Surrogate

Frequently, neither advance directives nor surrogate decision makers are available to represent the wishes of a patient who lacks the functional ability to make a treatment decision. In life-threatening emergency situations, of course, there is a valid presumption that the patient will be resuscitated or treated. In some cases, however, when there is opportunity for deliberation and alternative routes of treatment present themselves, the responsible health care professionals may discover that they have no one to whom they can turn for guidance about this particular person's previous preferences. The absence of an informed surrogate may be due to numerous factors: a lack of advance directives from a formerly competent patient; a patient who, though chronologically an adult, has never been competent due to severe cognitive impairments; a patient who is estranged from other people or has no living relatives; or simply one who has never even casually addressed such issues.

There is widespread agreement that judgments on behalf of the noncompetent patient with no advance directives (understood also as the absence of an informed surrogate) should be made by a surrogate with the patient's best interests in mind (see Case 4, "Management of Life-Threatening Illness"). This is also thought to be true if the appropriate surrogate happens also not to have information about the patient's likely wishes. Among the potential treatment alternatives, the alternative that is in the patient's best interest is determined by assessing each option for its net benefit (the result of subtracting burdens from benefits in each option) and then selecting the one with the greatest net benefit for the patient.[5] The concept of net benefit suggests that each option will have both advantages and disadvantages, and will promote some of the patient's interests while reducing or blocking others. The patient's best interests are thus embodied in that option with the greatest net benefit.

Although the best-interests standard may seem the obvious ethical reference point for making decisions on behalf of patients who lack capacity, in fact this standard has many competitors. Instead of the best interests of the patient, for example, our society could have opted for the principle that the best interests of the aggregate community of patients or potential patients, those of the state, those of students of the health care professions, or those of health care professionals themselves should prevail when the patient's wishes are unknown. Very different arrangements would follow from these alternative values. Thus, the best interest of the patient is an orienting principle of some substance in these discussions.

Occasionally, a distinction is drawn between the best interests of the patient generally and the patient's specifically medical best interests, with the implication that the latter comprises only the "objective" factors that argue for one form of treatment, factors that physicians are in a better position to know than are surrogates. This notion is specious. While surely many factors about a patient's medical condition are more fully understood by the clinical specialist than by the layperson, to speak of interests of any sort is to inherently enter subjective territory. Hence, values are necessary features of any assessment of best interests, and in the standard theory of clinical ethics the relevant values are those of the patient.

Among the ideas implicated by those of best interests is the patient's quality of life, which is one kind of subjective consideration. Once the best-interests standard is adopted as the basis for decision making in the absence of patient directives or a surrogate, it does not seem possible to avoid quality-of-life judgments. For example, one could decide that every effort should be made to extend the life of a dying patient come what may, on the grounds that every moment of life is precious. By adopting this strategy, one may hope to avoid making quality-of-life judgments. Even that strategy, however, implies a certain view of quality of life, namely a sanctity-of-life perspective to the effect that any life is qualitatively superior to no life at all. In its extreme form this view is known as *vitalism*.

On the other hand, choosing to base decisions on the patient's best interests would necessarily mean looking not only to the length of time that the life would be extended, but also to the kind of life it would be. Often this more flexible idea of quality of life will not lead to very different practical outcomes from the sanctity-of-life view. For example, in the case of a person with severe cognitive impairments, a life that is not a continuous torment, but rather mostly comfortable albeit terribly limited, may be an entirely acceptable quality of life for that individual and preferable to death (see Case 12, "Resuscitation Decision in a Patient with Lung Cancer").

The notion that one may base end-of-life determinations on assessments of the kind of life to which a patient may look forward has been a source of concern to many. Some fear a slippery slope leading to active euthanasia for those deemed by the individual clinician to be unworthy of continued life or effort to extend that life. Critical here is a distinction between comparative and noncomparative quality-of-life judgments.[12] Comparative quality-of-life judgments rate the subjective character of one person's life against that of another, his or her social worth, whereas noncomparative judgments rate the value of that person's life to that person only. Thus, the former sort of judgment opens the possibility that one person's quality of life will be found less worthwhile than that of another, the kind of conclusion reached by Nazi authorities concerning Jews, Gypsies, and other groups. Noncomparative quality-of-life judgments reflect the humanistic, person-centered principle that each individual is unique and that the value of one life cannot be measured against that of another.

Without realizing that they have slipped into a comparative mode, clinicians sometimes think through treatment alternatives for very ill patients in terms of the sort of life that they, the clinicians, would want for themselves or their loved ones. While this approach almost always stems from compassion rather than venal or "eugenic" impulses, it nevertheless is usually the result of an intellectual confusion on the part of the clinician. The ethically relevant consideration is not how much better it would be if this patient were in a condition that was more like that of someone else, or what condition someone else would want for themselves; rather, the ethically relevant consideration is the value of this life for this patient, given the alternatives available for this individual. With this understanding, the clinician may also feel somewhat relieved that he or she does not have to weigh the patient's quality of life against any factor other than its value for that patient.

Finally, one may raise the question as to whether the difference between formerly competent patients and incompetent patients is morally relevant in the sense that, in some cases, it will entail a different quality-of-life judgment. The classic case in which such an argument was employed was that of Joseph Saikewicz, who in 1976 was diagnosed with leukemia. At the time Saikewicz was 67 years old with an IQ of 10 and a mental age of about 2 years and 8 months. He had resided in state institutions for virtually his entire life. On appeal, the Massachusetts Supreme Court agreed that a probate court had the authority to decide about withholding treatment, and agreed with the probate judge that chemotherapy, which had a 30 to 50 percent chance of producing remission for 2 to 13 months, would have also entailed incomprehensible burdens for Saikewicz while extending his life only briefly. Treatment was not initiated, and Saikewicz died 5 months after he was diagnosed.

Critics of the decision in *Superintendent of Belchertown State School v. Saikewicz* argued that the decision-making process in this case puts an unfair burden on the patient to defend an interest in chemotherapy. Further, the inflexibility of a legal proceeding, while viewed by supporters as the best way to ensure that the incompetent's best interests can be promoted, seems poorly matched with the subtleties of medical decision making. For example, the possibility of prognostic change and the treatment alternative of beginning a trial of therapy subject to regular reassessment are among the variables that can best be considered by a process closer to the clinical setting.[13] Institutional arrangements, including perhaps ethics committees, could provide more timely and flexible review than judicial intervention, while also subjecting the decision process to the sort of public scrutiny that protects the patient's interests. One may wonder why a probate judge, or even a state high court justice, is in a particularly qualified position to perform a benefits-burdens analysis for a person who was never competent. Of course, legal intervention remains the socially sanctioned last resort; the question is whether, in such cases, it should be the first resort.

Apart from the procedural questions in *Saikewicz*, the substantive problem remains of interpolating the significance of cognitive impairment into the best-interests assessment. In that case, the patient's disorientation when even minor changes were introduced into his routine suggests that his emotional suffering during chemotherapy might indeed be so great as to nullify the potential benefits of remission. This possibility is part and parcel of the difficulties that arise in attempting to ascribe or define interests for this kind of individual. The effort to render this assessment in a noncomparative fashion, in terms of the value to Saikewicz of a somewhat extended life along with the discomforts associated with chemotherapy, must remain somewhat speculative in the absence of a trial of therapy. Thus, although the decision in *Saikewicz* surely continues to have its defenders, in retrospect it has evoked a great deal of skepticism in the clinical ethics community (see Case 7, "Painful Treatment for a Severely Retarded Man").

When Best Interests Do Not Apply

The best-interests standard presupposes some capacity to experience pleasure and pain; however, there are patients who are irreversibly unconscious. On the assumption that such patients are incapable of any awareness of their surroundings or their situation, it would seem that the concept of best interests does not easily apply to them whether or not there is a surrogate. Under these circumstances, when best interests cannot be ascertained, the usual approach is to focus on these patients' basic interests as biologic creatures. This might entail the provision of routine nursing care for hygiene and to prevent breakdown of the skin; to treat acute and potentially reversible conditions, such as infections; and to continue routinely to draw blood and to perform other standard procedures to monitor the patient's condition. More invasive and costly interventions, such as dialysis and blood transfusions, might not be provided. This strategy appears to be plausible because it respects the continuing value of a human life even in a profoundly reduced state, though it does not go as far as an extreme sanctity-of-life view would require.

Still, some questions should be asked about care under these circumstances. In general, the goals for the patient should be clear, as should the purpose of specific interventions. For example, if it is virtually certain that the patient will not regain consciousness, is it necessary to continue to monitor blood gases, or are blood samples being taken merely because they are part of the routine? By the same token, nursing care, such as the maintenance of hygiene and the prevention of skin breakdown, may be taken as an expression of respect for the patient, even though he or she will not be aware of these services. Whatever is determined to be appropriate care under these circumstances should be undertaken in light of clarity about both the patient's prognosis and the values that the staff recognizes as important to preserve for patients who are forever lost to consciousness.

Justice: Allocating Resources

Because resource allocation has more to do with macroscopic considerations of justice (having to do with the distribution of goods in the society as a whole) than microscopic considerations about patient self-determination or best interests (having to do with particular clinical encounters), it is not closely related to many of the problems addressed so far. Yet resource allocation decisions have always been part of the practice of medicine, if the term *resources* is construed broadly enough. For example, the time and energy of a busy clinician must often be allocated among his or her many patients in need of attention. Discussions of resource allocation usually focus on more dramatic dilemmas such as a shortage of organs for transplant, but what these examples have in common is that they are genuinely scarce resources. Some items are scarce because they are expensive, like cosmetic surgical procedures, while others are in short supply for reasons that are inherent to the item. Genuinely scarce items may also be expensive, but, unlike cosmetic surgery, their scarcity is a cause of their high cost, and not the other way around.[13] Some resources in the history of medicine have at one time been truly scarce and at another only expensive, such as kidney dialysis machines. In the United States, the End-Stage Renal Disease Program under Medicare ensures that everyone in need has access to dialysis, so that although dialysis machines are expensive, they are not scarce.

The distinction between genuinely scarce resources and expensive resources is important because in one sense it is entirely appropriate for clinicians to make decisions about what categories of patients should have access to resources under their control. So long as the decision is based on patients grouped together due to their common medical need, this is the ethically uncontroversial concept of allocation of scarce resources. Thus, for example, standards have been devised for the admission of patients to intensive care units. So long as these standards are applied fairly to all candidates based on medical need and benefit, the allocation of this scarce resource is a proper part of medical practice. If, however, groups of patients are excluded from the ICU due to the expense of the resource, then it is obvious that medical need is not the criterion. Since physicians are not public policymakers, it is inappropriate for them to decide about ICU admissions on any but a medical basis.

At some point the genuine scarcity of a resource will even impinge on the ability to serve all those who are members of a group that has been defined as medically needy. When this occurs, the situation has been transformed from one of allocation to one of rationing. Rationing is necessary when not all members of an otherwise qualified group can be served. The classic example of rationing is battlefield triage. The injured are first separated into three groups: those beyond help, those who will die without immediate treatment, and those who will survive without immediate treatment.

So far we have described a straightforward allocation scenario, with the groupings for access to the scarce resources of medical attention based on medical need. The second group may also be too large for the available resources to provide immediate attention, and at this point true rationing takes hold; a nonmedical criterion is used to identify those who will be treated immediately. In the military context the criterion is rank, so that officers will be treated first. If further distinctions are needed, they can be made based on the rank of the officers. In civilian life the criterion might be age, number of dependents, contribution to the community, or some other standard based on social worth. Thus, rationing entails discrimination among potential recipients of genuinely scarce resources based on some nonmedical criterion.

Rationing of scarce resources does take place in the health care setting. Again, consider the example of the ICU bed. Even though a new patient is medically qualified for a bed, often none is available. Indeed, sometimes a new patient will stand to gain more medically than one already in the unit. In such cases, the medical profession has in general avoided basing rationing decisions on estimates of relative social worth; the few examples in which that was done, as in the early days of kidney dialysis, produced disconcerting results. Instead, a "first come, first served" rule has prevailed, combined partly with a medical need standard. Admittedly, the first come, first served standard is not itself a purely medical judgment. It might even be considered to be a sort of lottery, with those lucky enough to get to the unit first being the ones who "win." While this might turn out to be a more appealing approach than social worth, it seems usually to be combined with the condition that the patient already in the unit is receiving some medical benefit. Thus, so long as the patient already in the ICU is receiving some medical benefit for intensive care, he or she will continue to be treated there. The inclusion of medical benefit in the calculus of admission to the busy ICU helps remind us that the decision to discontinue treatment for one patient is to be carefully separated from the decision to admit one who is waiting.

By contrast, a decision to deny an expensive but available resource to one who could benefit is an ethically perilous form of rationing. First, physicians are rarely sufficiently sophisticated about the economics and financing of health care to make fiscally sensible decisions. For example, some resources are expensive only in the sense that they are billed at a high rate, such as maternity unit beds, but their dollar cost may be a result of their availability as a profit center to support other hospital services, such as the emergency room. Second, even if a primary care or intensive care unit physician were intellectually equipped to be an informed fiscal gatekeeper, he or she would be moving well beyond his or her socially sanctioned role and into that of a public policy maker. Third, and closely related to the second problem, comparative judgments about worthiness of access to an expensive resource put physicians in a moral position that is at best dubious.

Nonetheless, by all indications clinicians will increasingly be called upon to participate in decisions to limit access to expensive resources. Advances in fields such as assisted reproduction and the development of whole new families of drugs such as protease inhibitors all but guarantee that difficult allocation decisions await the health care system as a whole. It is unlikely that patient interest in these expensive interventions will lessen or that insurers will be able to satisfy demand. Thus the problem of expensive resources, and not merely their scarcity, has surely entered the arena of clinical decision making and seems here to stay.

Depending on the financing arrangements, clinicians may find themselves in a position of divided loyalties that resembles the company doctor of a previous era: physicians whose first obligation was thought to be to the company rather than to the employee-patient. While clinicians in the managed care setting are obliged to use the organization's resources wisely, they are also required to meet the standard of care. Normally, both of these goals can be achieved by avoiding unnecessary tests and treatment. Clinicians also make de facto allocation decisions in the inpatient setting, when deciding about appropriate lengths of stay.

Clinicians are also obligated to resist any effort to compromise a patient's care, even if the alternative is to forfeit reimbursement. Unfortunately, a practical effect of the ethical responsibility to forgo reimbursement for the sake of patient care (an extreme situation to be sure), is that some clinicians will avoid taking patients who could present a bad risk. Nonetheless, failure to treat the patient appropriately is the physician's ethical and legal responsibility, not that of the third-party payer.

Efforts to promote outcomes research and the development of clinical pathways are still in their infancy but hold out the promise of rendering clinical decision making more rational and reliable and care plans more efficient. Moreover, modern health care requires continuity of care across delivery settings, and managed care arrangements do provide an opportunity for integrated services, although that promise has not yet been realized.

A related issue is the extent to which health care organizations avoid financially risky populations owing to the obligations that ensue once an insurance relationship is established. Unlike life and disability insurance, health insurers do not normally underwrite their policies, so individuals are not excluded from coverage due to their history or prospects for illness, although organizations can find ways to avoid risky populations if they choose to do so. Some may urge that the medical profession has an obligation to ensure that society as a whole is served—and that physicians even have an obligation to function in the political arena as advocates for health care access—it is harder to mount that argument for private sector organizations.

There is an undeniable tension between the way that the concept of managed care has often been implemented and the clinician's ethical responsibilities. Yet, whatever one's views about the American experience with managed care, the sorts of limits that have been introduced into our system of health care and delivery are unlikely to recede in the future. Some of these market-driven limits have been modified by legislation, as in the case of required length-of-stay coverage for maternity services, but these measures are too ad hoc and specific to alter the economy of the health care market on a large scale. Large-scale change will probably require another effort at public control of the health care system on a national and universal basis, which does not appear likely under prevailing political conditions.

Resource allocation is thus one of the great unsettled areas of clinical ethics, one in which the standard theory offers rather little guidance beyond discouraging physicians who might be tempted to perform explicit bedside rationing. More than most clinical ethics issues, health care resource allocation will be determined by political processes that require continuous assessment on ethical grounds and the continuous adjustment of clinicians to new institutional realities.

Still more generally, the societal allocation of health care resources, whether controlled by governmental or nongovernmental organizations, is perhaps the greatest practical failure to realize the principle of justice in clinical ethics. The widely recognized and growing class of individuals who do not have access to adequate health care due to a lack of health insurance represents a failure to put our society's philosophic commitment to justice into practice.

REFERENCES

1. J.A. Rawls, *Theory of Justice* (Cambridge, MA: Harvard University Press, 1971).
2. N. Daniels, *Just Health Care* (Cambridge, England: Cambridge University Press, 1985).
3. Cf. *Canterbury v. Spence*, 464 F.2d 772 (D.C. Cir.), *cert. denied,* 409 U.S. 1064 (1972).
4. *Cruzan v. Director, Missouri Department of Health*, 100 S. Ct. 2841 (1990).
5. A.E. Buchanan and D.W. Brock, *Deciding for Others* (New York: Cambridge University Press, 1989).
6. President's Commission, *Making Health Care Decisions* (Washington, DC: US Government Printing Office, 1982).
7. C.M. Culver and B. Gert, "The Inadequacy of Incompetence," *Milbank Quarterly* 68(4) (1990): 619–643.
8. C.P. Leeman, "Ethics Consultation Masking Psychiatric Issues in Medicine," *Archives of Internal Medicine* 155 (1995): 1715–1717.
9. N.R. Zweibel and C.K. Cassel, "Treatment Choices at the End of Life: A Comparison of Decisions by Older Patients and Their Physician-Selected Proxies," *Gerontologist* 29 (1989): 615–621.
10. A.B. Seckler et al., "Substituted Judgment: How Accurate Are Proxy Predictions?" *Annals of Internal Medicine* 112 (1991): 92–98.
11. J. Moreno, *Deciding Together: Bioethics and Moral Consensus* (New York: Oxford University Press, 1995), chapter 8.
12. J. Arras, "Toward an Ethic of Ambiguity," *Hastings Center Report* 14 (1984): 2533.
13. Personal communication.

3

Evaluating Common Distinctions

In this chapter four sets of distinctions that are commonly used in discussions of clinical ethics will be evaluated. In each case two different questions must be asked: Is the distinction logically valid and, if so, is the distinction morally relevant? A distinction is logically valid if it is capable of sorting actions into two different groups without ambiguity. A distinction is morally relevant if one of the sorts of actions it identifies is morally justifiable while the other is not. It should be noted that, of the following distinctions, only that between killing and letting die has any legal standing. The primary concern here is with the logical and ethical status of the distinctions.

ACTIVE AND PASSIVE

The distinction between active and passive means to bring about certain ends is often associated with forms of euthanasia and is sometimes identified as the distinction between commission and omission. The active-passive distinction is different from the distinction between killing and letting die or between withholding and withdrawing treatment, the subjects of later discussions.

Those who use the active-passive distinction intend to differentiate lively participation in bringing about an end from more or less deliberate failure to execute certain behaviors in order to bring about a certain end. It is not clear, however, that the active-passive distinction is valid, for the decision to omit certain medical interventions may entail measures that could be construed as active, such as calling a meeting of those caring for a patient in order to inform them that life-extending measures are to be forgone. Or perhaps the active-passive distinction refers only to certain kinds of physical activity, such as refraining from a resuscitation attempt.

Even if limiting its reference to a narrow range of physical activities can save the active-passive distinction, it is of dubious logical validity. If the distinction can indeed be saved, it is nonetheless subject to similar objections that will be seen to pertain to the killing–letting die distinction on grounds of moral relevance: It can be argued that it is sometimes more justifiable to actively bring about a patient's death than it is to stand by passively while that patient languishes and suffers. Thus, since the logic of the active-passive distinction is at least questionable, and since, even if logically valid, it involves serious questions of moral relevance, it is not recommended for use in a clinical ethics assessment and is not referred to in subsequent discussions.

ORDINARY AND EXTRAORDINARY MEANS

Sometimes expressed as the difference between nonoptional and optional, obligatory and nonobligatory, or nonheroic and heroic therapy, this distinction attempts to identify those interventions that are considered standard of practice and those that are not. The underlying notion is that dying patients and their physicians have no moral obligation to go beyond ordinary means in attempting to extend life, an important tenet of modern Roman Catholic medical ethics.

It is not always easy to determine which therapies are indeed standard of care and which are not. The very concept of standard of care is subject to rapid shifts of meaning in modern medical care, including in particular the arena of end-of-life care. Another problem is that some interventions, though they fall within the standard, are nevertheless not indicated. Practice standards are, after all, merely aggregates of what is in fact done for patients, and they do not necessarily reflect what ought or ought not to be done based on sound scientific principles. Moreover, even if medical and surgical practices were properly grounded in science, it is difficult to find a basis in secular clinical ethics for requiring a patient to accept any and all standard means of extending life. Thus, unless a patient subscribes to the tradition of a particular faith, we do not recommend that this distinction be part of a clinical ethics assessment.

KILLING AND LETTING DIE

In the clinical setting, the term *letting a patient* die refers to permitting a disease process to take its course, while *killing* refers to some deliberate and physically active means, such as giving a lethal injection. It is not generally thought that standing by under these circumstances is equivalent to killing, unless the individual standing by was responsible for setting the process in motion. This leaves open the difficult question of whether an individual (physician or not) who provides barbiturates to a dying patient knowing that he or she intends to overdose is indeed responsible for setting the process in motion, or, if so, whether or not this is morally justifiable. With the exception of the truly difficult question of assisted suicide, which will be taken up shortly, killing and letting die appears to be a serviceable distinction in the clinical setting. Thus, complex scenarios in which person A, knowingly or not, sets in motion processes that have been designed by person B to take person A's life can be set aside. They are too far-fetched to have much force in clinical ethics discussions of killing and letting die.

The moral relevance of the distinction can be expressed in the following way: As a matter of policy, taking the life of another is morally wrong, but one has no moral obligation to rescue another if that attempt would not substantially prolong the other's life, or if in attempting to do so one subjects oneself to substantial risk. Various reasons can be given for the statement that it is generally wrong to take another's life, stemming from various philosophic systems, but perhaps the justification that is most salient for clinical ethics appeals to the so-called slippery slope. According to this argument, even if there were instances in which it would be better for a dying patient to be killed voluntarily rather than to undergo prolonged suffering, as a matter of policy it would be a mistake to allow doctors or others to do this, because it would lessen the respect for life in general and increase the likelihood that such allegedly beneficent killing could be abused. In other words, in this view, even in those instances in which the distinction appears not to be morally relevant, the likely consequences of allowing these exceptions are unacceptable as a matter of policy. Therefore, the moral relevance of the distinction as a matter of policy is affirmed. In its most recent decision examining physician-assisted suicide, the Supreme Court also found important distinctions between allowing patients to die, such as permitting the withholding or withdrawal of life-sustaining treatment, versus actions intended to bring about the death of the patient, such as providing lethal doses of medication or even more directly causing the death of the patient.[1] In subsequent case discussions, the distinction between killing and letting die is taken as logically valid and morally relevant.

This conclusion presupposes that one can distinguish between the moral justification for a policy and the moral justification for a particular action. On this view, for example, one can consistently oppose the institution of a policy that permits clinicians to engage in assisted suicide while admitting that it may be justifiable in particular cases. It does not follow that any cases in fact meet the standards of justifiability, only that as a matter of logic those judgments are independent of judgments about the morally preferable policy.

WITHHOLDING AND WITHDRAWING

That this distinction is of uncertain logical validity can be demonstrated by reference to a scenario developed by the President's Commission.[2] In this scenario, a patient is on a mechanical ventilator when a power failure occurs. One of the clinicians remembers that there is an old manual bellows in a closet down the hall. If the bellows is not used, has treatment been withheld (never started) or withdrawn (stopped)? The fact that there is no right answer to this conundrum shows the distinction to be of dubious logical validity, because it does not clearly sort out the instances of withdrawing treatment from those of withholding treatment. Nevertheless, this distinction is commonly appealed to in the clinical setting, and there are obviously some clear cases of withholding and withdrawing therapy, such as not intubating a patient on the one hand and extubating a patient on the other. Less clear is a decision to interrupt a trial of chemotherapy in midcourse: Has the therapy been withheld or withdrawn? In fact, the distinction holds up only within a very limited range of situations.

Many clinicians believe that, while it is permissible to withhold treatment that is not indicated, treatment that has already been started may not be withdrawn, either for moral or legal reasons, or both. As has been stated, there is no legal basis for the distinction. Further, the moral relevance of the distinction is also unclear. To see this, consider patient A, whose condition is such that a decision is made not to begin treatment. Now consider patient B in the same condition, except that treatment has already begun. In both cases the treatment is not efficacious. From a moral point of view, there does not appear to be any more basis for continuing the treatment for patient B than for initiating it for patient A. Therefore, the distinction does not seem to have moral relevance.

The President's Commission also noted that the policy consequences of following this morally baseless distinction could be worse than confusing—they could even be lethal. Were there a widespread notion among physicians that they are legally or morally committed to an intervention once it has begun, they would sometimes be reluctant to undertake a trial of therapy if its benefits are unclear, for fear of creating a dismal situation from which they could not withdraw. Thus, intellectual confusion could actually deprive some patients of an opportunity to benefit from a trial of therapy (see Case 8, "Withdrawing Mechanical Ventilation at the Request of a Patient with Decisional Capacity").

All this having been said, it must be admitted that in current clinical reality there is not widespread acceptance of this view. In fact, this is perhaps the best example of the difference between medical ethics (as theory) and the current accepted standards of clinical ethics (as application). Clinicians are reluctant to withdraw a technology, however inefficacious with regard to the underlying disease, particularly in the case of treatment that preserves biologic life. If the above analysis is correct, however, then the only basis for this reluctance is psychological, and not rational. However we might respect the strength of this psychological attitude, a goal of clinical ethics should be to educate providers about the moral irrelevance of the withholding-withdrawing distinction.

One final qualification must be added. Orthodox Jewish authorities draw a distinction between withholding and withdrawing treatment on the basis of the following argument: While it is acceptable to remove impediments to the death of a person who is irreversibly dying, it is not permissible to hasten that person's dying.[3] Since in practice it is impossible to tell the difference between removing impediments to the death and hastening the death, no action that could be construed as the latter is permissible. Secular medical ethics has not generally found this metaphysical uncertainty about causation as important as the fact that there would be no difference in the consequences of the act of withdrawing therapy. Thus, unlike the Orthodox Jewish commentators, secular ethicists have not viewed the withholding-withdrawing distinction as morally relevant.

REFERENCES

1. *Vacco v. Quill,* 117 S.Ct. 2293 (1997).
2. President's Commission for the Study of Ethical Problems in Medicine and Biomedical and Behavioral Research, *Deciding To Forgo Life-Sustaining Treatment* (Washington, DC: US Government Printing Office, 1983), 7376.
3. F. Rosner, "Jewish Medical Ethics," *The Journal of Clinical Ethics* 6 (1995): 202–217.

4

Clinical Ethics throughout the Life Span

Patients are usually encountered, from the clinician's perspective, as members of age groups with certain characteristic problems. Characteristic ethical issues are also associated with age groups, and therefore it is useful to summarize these issues in terms of these populations. Once again, the ethical principles will not be applied to these topics in an explicit manner. Patient self-determination, the best interests of the patient, and just distribution of resources guide the themes and emphases of the discussion and could be rendered explicit.

The context of care is another background condition of this discussion. Modern health care is increasingly delivered in a variety of settings besides the hospital: outpatient clinics, day care institutions, rehabilitation centers, nursing homes, and the home itself. Throughout the life span, patients are cared for in several of these settings. Each lends particular nuance and color to the ethical problems that may be encountered by the clinician.

BEFORE PREGNANCY

The advent of carrier screening for genetic disorders, of in vitro fertilization (IVF) and related technologies such as embryo transfer, and perhaps even of human cloning has raised new moral questions for society to ponder. No effort is made here to canvas the myriad related issues, only to give an account of the considerations that seem to be most central, an account that will proceed from the standard theory of biomedical ethics according to patient self-determination. As the remainder of this section unfolds, it will be clear that the legitimate interests of the public in clinical decisions relating to pregnancy, childbirth, and child rearing introduce a new and complicating element to the standard view. [1]

In general, the salient ethical issue concerning preconception planning is whether and to what extent prospective parents should be constrained in their choices. In American society, with its strong libertarian tradition of respect for reproductive freedom, virtually no legal limitations are placed on individuals who choose to produce children themselves, even if they are at high risk of producing a genetically impaired infant, or an infant with another serious disorder, such as human immunodeficiency virus (HIV). Accordingly, the standard philosophy of counseling those who may face such an outcome is a nondirective one: Prospective parents are educated concerning their risks of having an affected child, but the final decision about pregnancy is scrupulously to be left up to them (see Case 24, "Assisted Reproduction in a Woman with Strong Religious Beliefs"). Even some public health screening programs, such as that undertaken for sickle cell anemia in the 1970s, may be viewed as unacceptable if they are regarded as implicitly discouraging certain vulnerable groups from reproducing.

In the AIDS era, it has been suggested, however, that all pregnant women be tested for HIV infection. The risk of maternal transmission of HIV without treatment is between 30 and 50 percent. It is now known that antiretroviral treatment with zidovudine (AZT) can safely and effectively reduce the risk of perinatal transmission by about two-thirds, provided that administration is initiated during pregnancy and continued through the first weeks of life. Elective cesarean section may reduce the risk still further, to perhaps as low as 2 percent in selected cases. The precise risk of transmission overall is uncertain, however, and the possibility that HIV will be transmitted in any particular pregnancy is not an inconsequential risk. AIDS morbidity and mortality for adults and children remain considerable, despite the advent of highly active antiretroviral therapy.

In addition to questions about genetic or infectious disease that could be transmitted to offspring, there has been considerable public curiosity and discussion about various forms of third-party or assisted reproduction. These range from "low-tech" methods such as so-called surrogate motherhood to in vitro fertilization and the extraordinary possibilities for genetic diagnosis and even therapeutic intervention to alter an individual's genetic endowment. Once again, there has been a strong presumption in favor of reproductive freedom, so that only very powerful public interest considerations have been thought to warrant the imposition of constraints.

In the case of surrogate motherhood, most Western societies that have considered the matter have adopted a policy that permits altruistic or noncommercial surrogacy, while some jurisdictions have gone so far as to criminalize surrogacy for hire. Opponents of commercial surrogacy argue that it is de facto baby selling, which is contrary to public policy, while the defenders of commercialism argue that this amounts to banning the practice, and they contend that what is being sold is not a baby but rather gestational services. In any case, the trend has been to view surrogacy arrangements as permissible private matters so long as there are no contractual or commercial elements. Like the surrogate motherhood debate, the early reception to the news in 1978 that a "test tube" baby had been born was sensational. Yet IVF is now widely perceived as ethically acceptable, and today its products are far less likely to be considered "freaks."

The technologies associated with IVF also create the opportunity for performing therapeutic interventions on gametes that carry a gene for a disease or condition, or the elimination of specific traits by engineering the removal of marked strings of DNA. The prospect of widespread gene therapy and genetic engineering has met with all sorts of objections, including worries that respect for variations among humans will be eroded. Once again, in our secular and pluralistic society the crucial question is at what point societal interests will decisively undermine individual prerogatives in the area of reproduction.

There have been some well-publicized instances of postmenopausal motherhood, achieved with a combination of donor eggs, IVF, and embryo transfer technology. Apart from health risks to the older mother, the predominant reservations concern the psychological effects upon the child. Supporters of reproductive freedom note that many societies do not find reproduction problematic in the case of older men, and they further note that women tend to live longer than men so are more likely to live until a child reaches maturity. Granting these facts, questions may still arise about the effects upon the child of having an older parent of either sex and about the wisdom of this use of expensive resources.

The theoretical possibility of human cloning raises still further concerns about the best interests of children produced in this manner. The depth of moral ambiguity about human cloning begins at the earliest stages, with the questions whether the products of "somatic cell nuclear transfer" could even be called embryos and whether the process is one of reproduction or replication. Then there are concerns about the psychological impact upon the products of human cloning, who might well be decades younger than the individual from whom the genetic material was obtained. Yet for individuals who, for example, are unable to have a genetically related offspring in any other way or who have their only child and are no longer able to reproduce, cloning may be a very desirable option. For the time being, however, many commentators agree that the risks entailed by this unfamiliar procedure to the potential human clone render any such efforts unethical.

Even the more familiar assisted reproduction techniques are expensive, time consuming, and of dubious reliability and entail considerable discomfort for the woman. These issues raise questions of the validity of informed consent for people desperate for a genetically related child. Serious justice issues are also raised by these technologies, for as the success rates improve, the cost will continue to be quite high. The social resources applied to efforts to produce more infants when there are so many already born and living in dire circumstances should at least give us pause about the aggregate consequences of many individual choices founded on reproductive freedom.[2]

DURING PREGNANCY

The manipulation of embryos involves the prospective interests of another party, namely the potential child, and therefore is widely regarded as even more ethically complex than preconception arrangements. Some view the entire field of embryo manipulation as unacceptable because of the currently unforeseeable harm that might be done to the future child. The transfer of an embryo from the uterus of a woman capable of conception to one able only to provide a gestational environment arouses this concern. Embryo transfer also usually entails the production of more embryos by the donor than can be transferred and brought to term; thus, the unused embryos are either discarded or stored for possible future use. Even those who endorse abortion under other circumstances might question the morality of producing excess embryos in such a deliberate manner for the sake of one lucky "survivor."

More conventional therapies have also been seen as raising questions of conflicts of interest between a mother and her fetus. Confining ourselves for the moment to pregnancies that the woman intends to bring to term, it would seem that both the prospective mother and her health care providers have an obligation to promote the well-being of the fetus, within reason. Thus, moral objections and legal challenges have been raised concerning women who are substance abusers and continue to abuse drugs during pregnancy. Some jurisdictions have attempted to prosecute women on the basis of laws against the delivery of controlled substances to minors, or based on child protection laws. While the behavior of these women may not be praiseworthy, there are good reasons not to use so blunt an instrument as the criminal law to deal with this social problem. First, many of these women are unable to gain access to drug treatment programs precisely because they are pregnant. Second, knowing the risk of prosecution they may avoid prenatal care and thus aggravate the problem. Third, prosecution is far more likely to focus on poor women than on those who are materially advantaged and whose behaviors are not so subject to scrutiny, thus raising serious questions of equity.

Other circumstances of apparent maternal-fetal conflict do not present themselves as stemming from such obviously questionable maternal behavior. For example, the woman with a horrific fear of surgery may decline a cesarean delivery even though her anatomy puts both her and her fetus at increased risk in a vaginal delivery. A pregnant AIDS patient receiving treatment for opportunistic infections may be putting her fetus at some risk even while accepting medication that could significantly extend her life. Another example is the case of Angela Carder, a woman dying of cancer whose wishes were that her possibly viable fetus not be "rescued" by a surgical delivery.[3] In all of these cases, the bodily integrity of the woman is a profound concern that must be weighed against the interests of the fetus, but it is important that these are cases of wanted pregnancies and that the mother is available to weigh these considerations.

By contrast, the abortion issue identifies the outer limits of the decision-making framework of clinical ethics, for that framework assumes that there is an identifiable patient whose preferences may not be known but whose interests should be determined and in some way respected. In the context of abortion, the issue is whether or not the fetus should be regarded as an individual possessed of interests due respect. The pregnant woman is a clearly identifiable patient, whereas it is at least doubtful that this is true of the previable fetus, and therefore the woman's preferences should be respected as a matter of self-determination, regardless of the consequences for the fetus. However useful, this approach may be increasingly at risk, as the ability to image, diagnose, and even treat the fetus makes it increasingly difficult to decide whether the obstetrician has one patient or two.

Even prenatal diagnosis in the earlier stages of pregnancy does not entirely escape the controversy about abortion. Prenatal diagnosis is intended to inform couples about the possibility of giving birth to a child with Down syndrome or other chromosomal abnormalities, so that they understand their options. Unlike amniocentesis, which usually does not yield results until about the twenty-first week of pregnancy, the more recently developed chorionic villus sampling (CVS) may provide a report of the presence or absence of genetic disease in the fetus as early as the tenth week. The early stage of fetal development, along with the general agreement that couples are entitled to try to avoid having children with genetic diseases, should make prenatal diagnosis by CVS relatively uncontroversial. However, the question has been raised as to whether prospective parents who are known to prefer one sex over another should be told the sex of the fetus following CVS, even if it is determined that the fetus is not affected by any sex-linked disorder. As a matter of the geneticist's clinical ethics, should the parents' right to information about their fetus trump the geneticist's wish to avoid what he or she may regard as the moral repugnance of abortion solely for the purpose of fetal sex selection? It would not be inconsistent for one to support the freedom of choice while at the same time opposing abortion for what may be regarded as frivolous reasons. Because this question potentially engages the interests of a third party whose status is subject to profound disagreement, it cannot readily be managed by the standard clinical decision-making framework. This problem is qualitatively different from other criticisms of fetal sexing, such as consequentialist "slippery slope" concerns about a lack of respect for one sex or the other, which are largely empiric questions rather than conceptual problems.

This having been said, it must still be recognized that, in a very narrow sense, abortion on demand remains legal in the United States, though many jurisdictions require minors contemplating abortion to notify their parents or to undergo a judicial hearing. Yet, again, even those who support a legal and moral right to elective abortion in general may find certain practices that lead to abortion under certain circumstances repugnant. The difficulty this creates for clinical ethics is whether, as a matter of policy, clinicians should refuse to engage in practices that they believe lead to a certain class of unjustifiable abortions in spite of a still prevalent social consensus permitting abortion on demand.

Markers associated with an embryo's risk of developing a certain disease if brought to term may someday be identifiable in prenatal genetic diagnosis. Abortion has been proposed in order to prevent the birth of a fetus that is at risk for a disease in adulthood. If abortions can be performed in order to prevent the birth of a fetus with a lethal genetic anomaly that will be expressed in early childhood, then why would abortion be unethical for later onset diseases, such as Alzheimer's or prostate cancer? Suppose that the confidence level for such tests is high. Is abortion preferable in such cases because it would save the prospective person the suffering associated with serious illness decades later, or is there a critical difference in the fact that this individual will at least have the opportunity to reach maturity and live a life, unlike the individual with a lethal childhood affliction?

A state of affairs that combines the ethics of reproductive technologies with that of abortion is the increasing incidence of multiple gestation. Many of these cases are due to the increased use of drugs that hyperstimulate ovaries. When such pregnancies occur, the implications of multiple births for healthy survival create a dilemma concerning fetal reduction. In this instance, preventive ethics should perhaps be practiced and care taken to transfer fewer rather than more embryos to the uterus. The somewhat lessened chances for a successful pregnancy seem worth the risk and the more responsible course in this instance.

INFANTS

With the exception of individuals in persistent vegetative states (PVS), probably no class of patients has been the subject of more public debate than infants born with severe impairments. As a result of the famous "Baby Doe" controversy of the mid-1980s,[4] the United States Congress adopted amendments to the 1984 Child Abuse Prevention and Treatment Act that require states receiving certain federal funds to ensure that intensive care nurseries provide treatment to infants regardless of the likelihood of cognitive handicap.[5] Failure to provide treatment, except in cases of infants who are "irreversibly comatose" or born dying, or for whom treatment would be futile and inhumane, is considered abuse under the amendments, and federal sanctions may follow as a consequence (see Case 27, "Tracheo-esophageal Fistula in a Newborn with Down Syndrome").

For the vast majority of states that continue to accept federal funds for their child welfare programs, the child abuse amendments have set a very stringent standard of aggressive treatment. Many of the conditions represented in the well-publicized cases since the acceptance of neonatal intensive care, including Down syndrome and meningomyelocele (spina bifida), must clearly be treated under these rules. Yet the moral obligation to treat these infants is a conclusion that had probably been reached by neonatologists independent of the federal legislation. On the other hand, the amendments do not require life-sustaining treatment for babies born with conditions that are expected to be lethal within weeks of birth, such as anencephaly, and they do call for physicians to use their "reasonable medical judgment." Similarly, they do not require aggressive treatment of babies afflicted with other conditions that are both incompatible with life and for which treatment might entail considerable suffering, such as trisomy 13 and 18.

Even within the framework of infants who should presumably be included within the amendments' scope, serious ambiguities are found. For example, it is not clear that the term "irreversibly comatose" applies to infants in the persistent vegetative state, even though "irreversibility" can be more confidently applied to PVS than coma. More significantly, the Baby Doe framework applies most clearly to infants for whom there is some one-time, all-or-none decision to be made, such as surgical correction of esophageal atresia in Down syndrome. It applies far less well, for example, to infants who have been asphyxiated at birth, a leading cause of neonatal impairment. Many of these infants face a difficult course of invasive, complex, and harrowing interventions without a definitive prognosis as to their cognitive or physical potential. In cases such as these, the problem is determining if and when the burden of continued treatment outweighs the foreseeable benefits to the infant of living a certain sort of life. Again, we are reminded how difficult it is to make noncomparative judgments in these sorts of cases, judgments that assess an individual's quality of life in terms of its value to that person and not compared to anyone else.

Thus, in many cases of decision making for newborns it is almost impossible at some point to avoid the quality-of-life judgments that the original Baby Doe rule sought to prohibit. A decision to continue to treat an infant regardless of the suffering entailed and in spite of a grim prognosis is itself a de facto quality-of-life judgment. At this point, and for the vast majority of ambiguous cases that are not covered by the Baby Doe framework or textbook neonatal practice, the question becomes who should have the authority to make that judgment. As in pediatrics generally, the preferred decision makers are the parents, in consultation with physicians (see Case 26, "A Pregnant Woman Using Cocaine," and Case 27, "Tracheoesophageal Fistula in a Newborn with Down Syndrome").

The standard theory described here, modeled on the self-determining, competent adult, obviously cannot be applied to neonatal decision making without substantial modification. Further, unlike those who are no longer competent, the infant has never even had the opportunity to formulate a set of values that can guide a surrogate. Instead, the infant is in much the same position as the mentally disabled adult, for whom decisions can apparently be made only on the basis of a substituted judgment that uses the patient's best interests as the standard. The choice of a patient-centered standard is a significant one, for some will argue that parents should have the latitude to decide about an infant's continued treatment based instead on a family-centered standard that focuses on the best interests of the entire family, not just a single member. In response, it is noted that the infant is not the property of his or her parents, any more than are older children. Instead, parents are regarded in our society as those in the best position to act as trustees of their child's well-being. Only if the parents' actions violate the terms of their implicit trusteeship, as in instances of abuse or neglect, will society, acting through the courts, suspend or revoke that trust. Professionals charged with the care of infants are also social agents who are expected to advocate on behalf of children whose best interests are jeopardized. Rarely will parental decisions in the health care setting warrant this sort of challenge.

In passing, it should be noted that some might advocate a societally centered standard of neonatal decision making that takes into account the considerable costs of caring for infants with a doubtful future. Of course, similar claims can and have been made for other costly patient groups as well. The role of fiscal decision making according to the received view in clinical ethics is considered below.

Parental discretion thus applies to a very broad range of situations in which there is ambiguity about the best alternative for an infant. In some cases, even parents who unquestionably have the best interests of their infant at heart may be regarded as having exceeded the bounds of the authority granted them by society, as may occur when parents decline a lifesaving or other medically indicated intervention on religious grounds. However, within the range of situations in which life-sustaining treatment is not clearly in the child's best interests (i.e., cases that are not clearly covered by the Baby Doe requirements), parental wishes to continue treatment are normally honored, even if only one of the parents wants treatment to continue.

CHILDREN AND ADOLESCENTS

The previous discussion outlined the essential nature of the parental role in decision making for children: that parents, as society's trustees for their children, are the presumptive decision makers, and that their decisions are to be based on the best interests of the child.[6] Only in extreme cases involving neglect or abuse may society exercise its authority to intercede to protect a child's well-being, and even then this authority should be imposed as gingerly and as briefly as possible, so that the bond between parent and child might be retained or, if necessary, repaired.

Because the received view of clinical ethics is founded on patient self-determination, ethical issues involving older children and adolescents pose special problems. Part of the maturation process is the increasing ability both to recognize disease processes and to evaluate alternatives in a more or less independent manner. Thus, the capacity to be self-determining does not suddenly appear, but rather emerges. Further, its emergence is characterized by fits and starts, by periods of self-realization punctuated with episodes of regression to more childish behaviors, as well as times typified by sullenness and rebellion. These normal and finally constructive elements of the maturation process constitute a challenge for an ethic that demands deferral to self-determination if at all possible.

The law has recognized some classes of adolescents as competent by virtue of their "emancipation," including those who are married or who are mothers, and those who are financially and physically independent of their parents (see Case 30, "A Teenager Who Wants Cosmetic Surgery"). In many jurisdictions there are exceptions for "mature minors," usually 15 or older, who may be granted decisional authority by courts of law. Still other exceptions have been made with respect to sex and reproduction. Adolescents are entitled to confidential counseling and treatment of venereal disease, and in most states they may have confidential access to birth control treatment and counseling. Attesting to the authority our society grants parenthood, young teenage mothers are the presumptive decision makers for their infants, even if they are not, in reality, emotionally or intellectually prepared to decide about their own medical care, let alone that of their infant.

It is interesting that each of these exceptions to the general dependence of those who have not reached the age of majority has a somewhat different rationale. These include sheer practicality, the moral importance attributed to the capacity to make one's own decisions, the demands of public health, and the authority of the parental role. There is no single, pervasive basis for these exceptions, which therefore constitute genuinely different categories. As exceptions, they stand against the overriding presumption that until a person reaches a certain age he or she is not fully in command of the faculties necessary for self-determination. The vulnerability associated with immaturity creates an obligation for certain societal agents to assess the best interests of the minor. Normally, again, these agents are the parents.

While adolescents may be old enough to qualify as legal exceptions to the general rule under certain circumstances, no legal exceptions exist for preadolescents and younger children. This being said, clinical practice has recognized circumstances in which even these children may be permitted a voice in their treatment. The most obvious case is one in which a terminally ill child expresses resistance to a surgical procedure or trial of therapy of uncertain benefit. In such a case, appreciating the importance of the patient's attitude in recovering from highly invasive procedures and the delicate emotional condition of a dying child, clinicians are normally loath to proceed (see Case 31, "An Adolescent with Cancer Who Wants To Discontinue Medical Treatment"). One may say that, as the foreseeable benefits of a procedure decrease and the risks increase, even a child as young as 8 or 9 may be given the opportunity to voice a dissent. If a delay with further counseling fails to produce a change in attitude, that dissent is commonly respected. Of course, in some children this age or younger, the expression of dissent is often a generalized protest about his or her situation, a childish albeit understandable cry of anger, fear, and sadness, and not one that will truly complicate recovery from the intervention. It is obviously an important and difficult task for the clinician to evaluate the significance of a child's dissent, which suggests that postponement to permit complete evaluation, with the aid of a pediatric psychiatrist, is frequently a wise decision.

Work that has been done on moral development may provide some rough guidance in assessing the ability of a particular child to participate in decision making concerning his or her medical care.[7] Until about age 9, most children are unable to conceptualize disease entities as processes that take place within their bodies, rather than as discrete "germs" from without. Further, many early adolescents, up to around age 15, are unable to identify a preference that is not unduly influenced by some authority figure. Thus, while the cognitive ability to apprehend the information elements necessary for informed consent may be present, the emotional capacity for voluntary choice is ordinarily not developed until later. These are important considerations for the clinician, part of whose role is to act as an advocate for the child patient.

One reason that the decisional rights of minors receiving medical treatment have not been a subject of much public discussion is that, as a practical matter, they lack the power of the purse. With the telling exception of the emancipated minor, parents or other legal guardians are responsible for paying the bill. From a strictly consumerist standpoint, therefore, most minors lack the authority to authorize the performance of services. Nevertheless, health care is not regarded as just another market item, even in a country such as the United States that lacks a universal care system, and minors in particular are, as has been noted, generally regarded as a social trust. Hence, there is a powerful obligation for the clinician to evaluate the needs and capacities of the minor child independently of his or her standing in the marketplace.

THE ELDERLY

Even more than infants, older people have been enormously affected by the advances of modern health care. Like newborns, the elderly are, for the most part, far better off for these developments. Yet, technical advances have not been an unalloyed blessing for either group, and special ethical concerns are engaged in the care of older patients, the vast majority of whom are capable of participating as full partners in their treatment programs, in many instances even up to the very end of their lives.

There is nevertheless no denying that the aging process is generally accompanied by increasing infirmity, in spite of the compensations of maturity and perspective, and the older person is usually well aware of this process. Moreover, for the most part, members of this population have lived half a century or more as competent adults. Thus, respect for the self-determination of the older patient with capacity has a unique importance for that individual, particularly in a society that does not always recognize this capacity in the elderly. In fact, prejudice against the elderly is as much a problem among health care professionals as among others.

Many of the most important shifts in perspective in modern medical ethics have taken place with regard to geriatric patients, with profound consequences for other populations. An appreciation of the significance of truth telling and confidentiality has altered the approach to health care for the elderly, at least in theory. In practice, unfortunately, there is still a tendency in some quarters to regard advanced age as automatically disqualifying a patient from being told the truth about his or her medical condition, or as reason in itself to violate confidentiality by informing a relative of the patient's condition without the patient's consent. It should be clear that advanced age in itself should at most trigger an assessment of the patient's capacity to participate in decision making, but it is not in itself decisive. Apart from such an assessment, the older person should be treated as any other competent adult, according to the tenets outlined elsewhere in this volume (see Case 5, "Don't Tell Mother").

Respect for the geriatric patient with capacity suggests a further ethical obligation on the part of the health care worker. As with any competent patient facing a period of significant health risks, the clinician has an obligation to practice preventive ethics and engage in planning with the patient for lapses in decision-making capacity. As has been discussed previously, federal law now requires that all adults admitted to hospitals, nursing homes, and health plans be informed of their rights in that state to create advance treatment directives. While many older patients do not fall into this category, they do have regular contact with a physician, practical nurse, or social worker and should be afforded an opportunity, well in advance of hospitalization or nursing home admission, to exercise their legal and moral rights in this regard. Although such conversations should be entered with the greatest sensitivity, "therapeutic privilege" is no longer a valid excuse not to engage in such planning, especially in light of empiric studies that show the elderly to prefer openness in their caregivers.

In the nursing home setting, attitudes toward the use of physical restraints for frail residents have undergone a shift. Many of these individuals have physical and cognitive impairments. The traditional rationale for physical restraints has been that the frail elderly are at risk of falling and sustaining serious injuries. During the past 20 years, however, evidence and experience indicate that the most commonly used restraints, particularly in beds, are themselves the cause of injury and other significant morbidities. Moreover, restraints often seem to be used to benefit the staff rather than the residents themselves, who may otherwise be mobile and thus require more supervision. Thus, even setting aside the fact that many of these individuals are capable of making a decision about their ability to function and accepting attendant risks, there are reasons to find creative alternatives to physical restraints, based on considerations of beneficence as well as self-determination (see Case 9, "Withholding Tube Feeding in a Woman with Advanced Dementia").

Further, because the elderly are at or near the end of life, their care often involves capacity determinations and decisions about life-sustaining treatment. All that has already been said about these matters applies to geriatric patients, with the additional emphasis on advance care planning, or preventive ethics. For older people more than most others, it is often possible to engage in planning for incapacity or terminal illness well in advance of the fact. Institutions and individual practitioners are well advised to make such conversations part of their routine in the care of elderly patients.

TREATING THE FAMILY

One of the most salient features of family practice is the contact with persons of various ages in the family system. Much of what has been discussed will therefore apply in obvious ways to patients encountered by clinicians in family medicine. However, the unique ethical problems in family practice often occur when more than one member of the family is affected, and that dynamic situation is the focus of this section.

Although certain issues are commonly embodied in the classic family medicine practice, they are often applicable to other sorts of practice environments as well. The family as unit of care is a familiar concept in the hospice, for example. All clinicians should be aware of family dynamics as they affect patient care, especially in the context of permanent disability, chronic care, or terminal illness. An analysis of family caregiving roles and responsibilities, and their rights in the caregiving process, therefore has general applicability.[8]

As previously described, the standard theory of clinical ethics tends to proceed from the standpoint of the individual, self-determining patient, and limits to individual self-determination require justification. However, family clinicians normally do not have a concept of the discrete patient, but tend rather to think of patients in terms of their role in a family system. This presents an interesting philosophic difference with an approach based on the autonomous patient, but so long as the rights or interests of the patient are justifiably valued more highly than those of the group (however legitimate they might be), there is no ethical conflict.

That the rights or interests of the individual patient are still presumed to outweigh those of the larger group is true of the ethics of family medicine, according to the standard theory, but it is not necessarily true of all situations in which individual and group interests conflict. For example, there is a well-established principle of public health ethics that patients with highly contagious diseases, such as tuberculosis, must either accept therapy voluntarily or have it imposed on them. In that case the threat to the public is believed to outweigh by far the restriction of liberty of the individual. In the case of family groups, however, the standard approach to clinical ethics holds to a patient-centered view.

This patient-centered ethic is not always easy to sustain for the clinician who treats both the patient and the family unit. Ethical difficulties concerning the family's role often arise in two different types of situations: when the self-determination of the patient is tied to the patient's relationships with close family members, and when the best interests of the patient and those of the family are closely bound up with each other. These two situations may be further complicated by factors that are often more evident in ambulatory care than in the acute care setting. Among these additional factors are specific cultural values, beliefs, and practices that may be unfamiliar to the clinician, extending to a literal inability to communicate in the language of the patient and family. [9]

Some patients are obviously reluctant to make decisions or even to acquire medical information without a family member present or close at hand. In certain traditional societies an elder, religious figure, or other respected member of the clan could be the source of authority on important decisions, including medical decisions. Since the clinician's first obligation is to the patient, it is generally thought that every effort should be made to encourage the patient to assert his or her own wishes and to defend that decision on the patient's behalf. With some traditional cultures, however, not only is it difficult for patients to exercise their self-determination, but the very idea of personal autonomy may be closely tied to values of interdependence. In extreme cases the clinician may have to ascertain that the patient wants freely to submit to the group's influence or authority, much as any competent patient may identify another decision maker.

In a quite different sort of situation, the clinician finds that the family's interests are clear-cut and the patient's interests are not. An example would be a recommendation of one or another therapy when the two are not significantly different from the standpoint of medical benefit but one places more of a burden on family members than the other. In that case the less burdensome therapy may be chosen, since it will indirectly also be of more benefit to the patient for those engaged in at-home care to be able to follow a less stressful regimen. Another example would be that of an elderly family member who may either remain at home under the care of his or her family or be admitted to a nursing home. If it is not clear that the patient's interests would be better served at home, and if his or her continuing care at home present extraordinary burdens to his or her family, then nursing home placement would be justifiable. Far more difficult are those instances in which a patient's best interests clearly entail a certain medical approach that is burdensome to the family for social or financial reasons, such as life-sustaining measures for a severely disabled child. Here the clinician has a duty to make reasonable efforts to identify the problem and secure whatever societal assistance is available (see Case 12, "Resuscitation Decision in a Patient with Lung Cancer," and Case 26, "A Pregnant Woman Using Cocaine").

FUTILITY

In the next two sections, two topics are discussed that, in different ways, occupy the outer limits of the standard theory: futility and brain death. Futility is a seemingly straightforward concept that has recently undergone a great deal of scrutiny. Brain death has been an area of broad but not necessarily deep consensus in clinical ethics. In the clinical setting, both these terms are often used far too loosely. An unresponsive patient may be labeled "brain dead" in a casual manner even though the clinical criteria have not been met, and a very sick patient may be regarded as one for whom treatment is "futile," in spite of the various meanings that can be attributed to the word.

Just as some issues relating to abortion do not seem to fit readily under the rubric of decision making for patients, another class of issues that seems to challenge the conceptual reach of the standard framework is that of medical futility. For while there is agreement that competent patients may decline unwanted interventions, it is not clear what the clinician's obligations are with respect to demands for therapies that are not regarded as medically indicated.

One problem is that determining the futility of an intervention is not necessarily accomplished by finding that it is not medically indicated (see Case 12, "Resuscitation Decision in a Patient with Lung Cancer"). It might be argued, for example, that judgments about futility include reference to values as well as to medical facts, and that the latter are therefore objective scientific matters that fall short of establishing futility. That is, while chronic mechanical ventilation of a patient with end-stage emphysema would be futile in the sense that his or her underlying disease will not be reversed by this means, it will not be futile if the patient wishes to live at least long enough to see a new grandchild. In adopting this view, there is no difficulty in referring to the patient or the appropriate surrogate as the source of information about what counts as futile intervention in a particular case, and the standard decision-making framework is thus preserved. Such appears to have been the result in the case of Helga Wanglie, an 87-year-old woman in a persistent vegetative state whose husband contended that she would have wanted to be maintained in her vegetative state indefinitely. Though the hospital argued that it should not be required by the family to provide care that would not affect Mrs. Wanglie's underlying condition, a probate court judge found no reason to appoint a guardian to take the place of her husband as spokesperson for his wife.

The decision in this case did not settle the question of under what circumstances physicians must comply with the requests of their patients for specific forms of treatment, but it did open the debate about what types of care can be considered futile. Surely, some patient requests would not be honored, including, for example, a demand for surgery for a simple head cold, since, whatever the patient's values happen to be, they will not be satisfied by this procedure. The professional integrity of the physician is presumably a value that is of considerable social interest, and there do seem to be cases in which patient self-determination either loses its force or is irrelevant to the ultimate course of care.

Another view that might be argued is that beneficence often requires a more flexible view of the physician's appropriate response to such requests, particularly when patients are gravely ill. In this view, it is entirely appropriate for physicians—indeed, it is obligatory—to provide interventions that will not affect the underlying condition but will provide comfort, even if, as in the case of Mrs. Wanglie, only the patient's loved ones are those comforted. Indeed, this has been a traditional role of the physician and was for most of medical history virtually the only role the physician could play in the face of serious illness.

The rejoinder that physicians have traditionally undertaken futile measures for humane reasons may be hard to sustain in some cases. For example, the use of cardiopulmonary resuscitation (CPR) in a dying or incurably ill patient may be perceived as a violent assault, as well as an intervention that does no more than prolong the dying process. Some have argued that the presumption that CPR is part of the standard of care for gravely ill patients should be altered, though it will surely be difficult to change the public perception about resuscitation as an essential, lifesaving intervention.

CPR will be the focus of continuing discussion about the lengths to which physicians must go in the face of conflicts with their reasonable medical judgment. An important part of this discussion should be improved data concerning the conditions under which CPR fails to meet specific clinical goals. The concept of futility must be an evolving standard.

BRAIN DEATH AND ORGAN PROCUREMENT

Medicine has shifted over the past two decades from traditional, cardiopulmonary criteria of death to also include neurologic criteria. Where once the cessation of cardiac and respiratory activity would have been necessary in order for an individual to be pronounced dead, the determination of death can now also rest on cessation of whole brain function, as determined by a combination of careful observation and objective measures of brain function (see Case 11, "A Teenager with Prolonged Unconsciousness"). Thus, often an individual will retain circulatory function, particularly if artificial life support is in place, even though he or she is dead by scientific and legally codified criteria of brain death. Obviously, it can still be determined that an individual is dead according to the traditional cardiopulmonary criteria if instruments to measure neurologic activity are not available. However, those terminal events may occur well after the neurologic ones, and it is only because we are now better able to determine brain death that it is not always necessary to wait for circulatory death to occur.

There are at least two basic pitfalls in applying this relatively new framework. First, what has changed is not the definition of death but the medical criteria for determining death. Death itself has not been changed, so far as anyone now living can tell. Second, the source of many troubles in the clinical setting is the term *brain death*. When one is found brain dead according to the criteria of medical science, one is dead. There is no basis for hope that a brain dead patient will recover, for that patient is dead. On the other hand, to speak of persons in prolonged coma or in the persistent vegetative state as brain dead is also an erroneous and misleading use of a term with a technically precise meaning.

The standard of brain death that has been adopted is, in a sense, a relatively conservative one. What is required is the irreversible cessation of neurologic activity in the entire brain (the cerebral cortex and the brainstem) over a certain period of time. The reason this may be considered conservative is that many would argue in favor of a standard that requires only the irreversible termination of higher brain functions of the neocortex, which is the seat of awareness, the physiologic substratum of consciousness. If a neocortical standard were to be adopted, then patients whose lower brain, or vegetative functions, continued without the possibility of a return to a state of even minimal awareness of their surroundings would be considered dead. Opponents of such a change marshal numerous arguments, including a concern that respect for human life generally would be devalued by such a move, and that in any case the public would not accept treatment of spontaneously respirating human bodies as dead. Proponents of a neocortical standard argue that the public must and would come to understand that, although the human body may continue to function, without the possibility of awareness the person is dead.

Shadowing the debate about the appropriate level of neurologic death, there is a lingering suspicion among many that the shift from a circulatory to a whole brain standard was in the first place motivated by utilitarian factors of a rather gross sort, not any desire for scientific accuracy. The movement for statutory recognition of neurologic criteria of death in the 1970s dovetailed with breakthroughs in organ transplant technology, especially in the development of immunosuppressive drugs that could suppress organ rejection by the host. As organ transplantation became an increasingly viable option for many patients, the shortage of donor organs also became painfully apparent. It happens that many prime potential organ donors are individuals who have suffered devastating neurologic damage but whose other vital organs are intact, with the youthful (and unhelmeted) victim of a motorcycle accident representing perhaps the paradigm case. The opportunity to identify these donors before the breakdown of vital organs such as the heart and kidney created a supply of organs for transplant, although not nearly enough to meet demand. Defenders of the organ donation system heatedly deny any inappropriate connection between the two sets of developments, organ transplantation and determination of death by neurologic criteria, and note the beneficial consequences of organ donation for the donor's survivors as well as for society as a whole.

Candidates for the receipt of solid organs must first be admitted to a waiting list and must then qualify according to two further lexically ordered criteria: severity of illness and length of time on the list. Critics of the current system charge that affluent patients often manage to be placed on more than one list, and that the priority of severity of illness over time on the list means that some organs are "wasted" on patients who are too ill to benefit as much as others who are not as sick. The latter issue is especially salient in cases in which a single patient has received an organ but the graft has failed: How many livers, for example, is one entitled to receive?

For all of these concerns, the underlying problem is the fact that not enough organs are procured for all those who could benefit. Various solutions have been proposed, including substituting the current standard of required request, in which families must be asked to consent to donation after their loved one's death, to a standard of presumed consent, in which families must explicitly decline to donate. Some have advised creating a market for organs, or at the very least allowing incentives for donation, such as permitting payment of funeral expenses. Recently, at least one major center has begun asking dying patients or their families if they are willing to have a respirator removed and would consent to organ donation. This approach, while it may well increase the supply of organs, associates end-of-life treatment with organ procurement in a way that has been thought to be inappropriate.

Finally, the debates about which neurologic standard is suitable for the determination of death, whole brain or higher brain, as well as that about the connection with organ donation are related to a question in infant organ transplantation. During the late 1980s, attempts were made to utilize the organs of anencephalic infants (born without cerebral hemispheres) for transplantation. All such infants are expected to die within a few weeks of birth, and in some cases their parents wish to donate in order to give meaning to their infant's life. At the same time, transplantation in infants is a decidedly underdeveloped procedure with modest chances for success at best, although the potential demand for infant organs is great. The conceptual difficulty is that by whole brain standards anencephalic infants are alive, for they do have a brainstem (some more than others) that sustains a level of cardiopulmonary activity for a time. Nevertheless, they will probably die soon and they lack the minimal necessary physiologic substratum of awareness. By this standard, to remove an anencephalic infant's vital organs for transplant before the complete loss of brainstem activity, indicated by a level (however slight) of spontaneous cardiopulmonary function, is seen by some to be tantamount to infanticide. Advocates of the higher brain standard argued that this sort of case demonstrated the need for a higher brain standard, or perhaps a third category, called *brain absent*. This proposal did not gain wide acceptance, as it appeared to be an ad hoc gambit designed solely to justify the use of anencephalics as organ donors.

Growing pressures on the organ procurement system and improved organ preservation techniques have led to calls to transform the current regional distribution system to a national one. Proponents of such a change argue that it would improve the equitable distribution of organs. Opponents worry that national distribution of donor organs might damage local recruitment efforts and also worry about the viability of local transplant programs forced to compete with large transplant centers. In a larger sense, however, it is hard to see how the gap between supply and demand can be narrowed when more and more sick patients are being added to waiting lists—patients who would not have survived to that point only a few years before. Ultimately the best hope for the organ supply problem may lie in xenotransplants from animals genetically altered for tissue compatibility with human hosts, or in organs grown from human stem cells in vitro. Until that time, however, our sense of justice will be strained by the dilemmas associated with this genuinely scarce resource, as they will, in different and perhaps unforeseeable ways, by the solutions to the organ supply problem.

78   ETHICS IN CLINICAL PRACTICE

REFERENCES

1. J. Arras, "AIDS and Reproductive Decisions: Having Children in Fear and Trembling," *Milbank Memorial Fund* 68 (1990): 353.
2. G. McGee, *The Perfect Baby: A Pragmatic Approach to Genetics* (New York & London: Roman & Littlefield, 1997).
3. In re AC, 539 A.2d 203 (D.C. 1988), *aff'd.*, 573 A.2d 1235 (D.C. 1990).
4. In re Infant Doe, No. GU8204-00 (Cir. Ct., Monroe County, Ind., Apr. 12, 1982).
5. G.J. Annas, "The Baby Doe Regulations: Governmental Intervention in Neonatal Rescue Medicine," *American Journal of Public Health* 74 (1984): 618–620.
6. A.R. Fleischman, K. Nolan, N.N. Dubler, et al., "Caring for Gravely Ill Children," *Pediatrics* 94 (1994): 433–439.
7. R. Bibace and M.E. Walsh, "Children's Conception of Illness," in *Children's Conceptions of Health, Illness and Bodily Functions,* eds. R. Bibace and M.E. Walsh (San Francisco: Jossey-Bass, 1981).
8. C. Levine and C. Zuckerman, "The Trouble with Families: Toward an Ethic of Accommodation," *Annals of Internal Medicine* 130 (1999): 148–152.
9. A. Kleinman, "Anthropology of Medicine" in *Encyclopedia of Bioethics*, Vol. 3, ed. W.T. Reich (New York: Simon & Schuster, MacMillan, 1995), 1667–1674.

5

Assessing the Standard Theory

A CRITIQUE OF THE STANDARD THEORY

Certainly, not everyone subscribes to all of the propositions described as part of the standard theory, and some may think that certain topics covered are not proper parts of the standard theory. In general, however, there is a consensus in the field both about what the standard theory asserts and what topics it covers.

In this chapter, criticisms of and views alternative to the standard theory of clinical ethics are presented. The critique elaborated in this section focuses on problems in the application of the theory, while the alternatives focus on its philosophic limitations as well. Although many aspects of the standard theory are open to criticism, three are especially serious. These three aspects relate to the determination of competence, the ability to achieve an informed consent, and the limits on appropriate treatment.

Competence is a legal term; it is a patient's *capacity* to decide about a particular treatment that is the appropriate moral concern. While a patient's decisional competence or lack of competence is not usually open to serious doubt in a legal sense, the moral requirements are often more stringent. The result is that the clinician can be faced with a conflict between meeting the letter and spirit of the law on one hand and preserving his or her professional integrity on the other. The problem is this: The law normally requires only that a patient understands what treatment he or she is being asked about, but from an ethical standpoint it is generally thought that a patient should appreciate the implications of the decision. The elements of informed consent elaborated previously go considerably further than the law requires.

In practice a clinician is not at great legal risk if, in good faith, he or she insists on a higher level of decisional capacity than merely understanding the question. But how great should that capacity be? In practical terms, just what does it mean to say that a patient should appreciate the implications of his or her decision? The standard theory tends to rely on legal practice, psychiatric expertise, and common sense, but it gives rather little substantive guidance to the clinician who is puzzled by the question of how much capacity to require of a certain patient under given circumstances.

This problem is closely related to assumptions about the extent to which self-determination has practical meaning as the basis of the informed consent doctrine. Particularly when a patient has only recently learned of a serious medical problem, it is not easy to know what are genuine expressions of the patient's deepest wishes and what are expressions of anger and despair. Moreover, many health care settings compromise a patient's sense of self-determination: being bedridden, clothed in hospital garb, subject to the fixed routines of others, and often under medication—all contribute to a feeling (firmly based in reality) of having lost control of one's life and options.

Another factor in the success or failure of a truly informed consent process, and in the patient's decision-making capacity, is the communications skill of the clinician. Rarely in the literature on informed consent—a poor way to describe what is supposed to be an interactive process—is there discussion of the dynamic between the provider of information and its recipient. As well, the setting in which the informed consent process takes place has an important influence on the capacity of the patient, who has already been deprived of many of the visible earmarks of individuality and independence so prized by our society. Then there are also the constraints that some health care organizations have tried to place on clinician-patient communications with regard to services that are not covered by the patient's health plan. In this instance the raw information itself may not be conveyed, quite apart from more abstract elements that condition the informed consent process.

To psychological, sociological, and insurance limits of the received doctrine of informed consent one can also add political naivete. For example, a poor person cannot be self-determining in a health care system that denies access to care or adequate rehabilitative services. When that person is worried that what few assets she has will be eaten up by an expensive hospital stay, this will surely enter into her decision making and compromise her ability to be truly autonomous. Further, consider the subtle social influences on a person's values and preferences. Few people make important decisions without taking account of the views and experiences of others; indeed, we would probably suspect that someone who did not do this had serious psychological problems. The standard theory draws the line at coercion or insidious manipulation by others, but these are not always easy to identify. There is thus good reason to argue that the doctrine of informed consent is politically and sociologically unsophisticated.

Further, there is reason to doubt that the informed consent process usually accomplishes its goals even with a reasonably self-determining patient. What is desired is a collaborative decision-making process, an ongoing partnership between the clinician and patient. Yet there is evidence that very few patients remember most of what they consented to as little as a day after the consent process. This result could be characterized as a problem of recall rather than understanding, but at least it suggests that repeated consent encounters may be required for continuing as an informed patient.

At another level, there is also evidence that surrogate decision makers, such as the spouses of elderly patients, are frequently in error about the patient's wishes concerning life-sustaining treatment. All in all, the chances seem poor that any particular clinician-patient encounter will achieve any but the most modest goals of the informed consent doctrine.

A final sort of problem with the standard theory of clinical ethics recalls again the debate about the futility of certain interventions. That debate arose especially in the context of do-not-resuscitate orders, for in spite of the fact that many attempts at cardiac resuscitation are useless (even in the most narrow sense of reestablishing heart function), and that it is a particularly intrusive procedure, there is general agreement that withholding cardiopulmonary resuscitation requires patient or surrogate approval. There are signs, however, that withdrawing (if not withholding) other medically useless treatment is also being brought under the rubric of an entitlement. Under such conditions not only will reasonable clinical judgment be undermined and patients subjected to unnecessary suffering or indignities, but also vast resources will increasingly be diverted from useful purposes.

This argument, though not terribly different from the earlier discussion of futility (and, for that matter, resource allocation), gains more gravity as part of a general critique of informed consent doctrine, which is the heart of the standard theory of clinical ethics. Further, as the rate of increase of health care costs continues to spiral, and as more Americans find themselves unable to gain access to the health care system, the extent to which patients can be said to have the right to be fully informed about their therapeutic options will be very much open to reconsideration.

The following three sections each address a different alternative theoretical approach to problems in clinical ethics: Casuistry argues for a case-based approach; the care perspective urges listening to patients; and feminism contends that special ethical issues concerning the care of women reflect on the morality of the health care system as a whole. These alternative theories provide important critical perspectives on the standard theory, which will surely continue to undergo modification in light of these and other views.

CASUISTRY

Casuistry was an influential ethical theory in medieval and early modern philosophy. It has recently been revived by a number of major ethicists, including Baruch Brody and Albert R. Jonsen and Stephen Toulmin.[1,2] Rather than concentrate on rules and general principles that may be applied to specific cases, casuists insist that moral judgments must emerge from particular cases, or ideally, from experience with a number of cases that can be compared to one another in various ways. In other words, casuists reject the notion, characteristic of much modern ethical theory, that there is any axiomatic first principle (or principles) of ethics; rather, they regard ethics as a set of practices that arise from human moral experience. To oversimplify, instead of working deductively from generalizations to cases, casuists work inductively, from cases to generalizations.

Casuists contend that moral beliefs arise as the result of particular experiences. These experiences are by no means limited to those of a single individual, but rather embrace those of whole cultures and societies over many years. Certain of these experiences do stand out, however, as paradigmatic. The paradigm cases of ethics function much like the historically important cases in the law in the sense that they provide valuable precedents that can guide us through subsequent situations. There are skill and ingenuity involved in finding the right analogies to our current experience from among the paradigm cases and in analyzing and comparing the fact pattern of the paradigm case to the current case. Just how the facts between the two cases are similar and contrasting will determine how directly applicable the conclusion of the paradigm case will prove to be with regard to the current one.

Gradually, as experience with a number of related cases is accumulated, we become more and more confident that our judgments are correct. Moral rules develop from the elements of these judgments that seem to endure over a range of similar cases. The rules or principles often take the form of bits of folk wisdom or maxims that are so deeply engrained in our moral experience that they begin to appear as self-evident, as in sayings such as "Don't kick a good man when he's down," or, in the realm of clinical ethics, "First, do no harm." That there is some reference to generalization, even in the casuist's method, demonstrates that, as Arras has put it, casuistry is not "theory free" but only "theory poor."[3]

Thus, there is movement over time as our moral experience becomes more and more ramified through our having integrated more and more individual cases. Simultaneously, there is also movement in a logical sense from the clear cases to those that are not so clear. The fact patterns of the paradigm cases are once again compared with those of the new, hard case, and the lessons learned from the paradigm case will apply to the hard one just insofar as they are relevant. Much, if not all, of the hard case's elements can be brought under the ethical rubric that has evolved, so that the classical sources can provide at least some orientation to the otherwise recalcitrant problem. Gradually, the hard case may not appear to be so difficult at all.

As an example of the way that a casuist would interpret advances in clinical ethics, consider the case of Karen Ann Quinlan. The question of withdrawing artificial respiratory support from someone in her condition would, without reference to any other cases, have been quite puzzling to most of us at the time. Yet previous cases of competent patients had helped to reach the settled view that no unwanted touching of a competent adult is permissible, even if it is of beneficent intent. The next step was comparing that sort of case with Quinlan's, and the critical difference seemed to be that she was unable to express her wishes at the time. The problem was then transformed from a purely philosophic one to a far more manageable empiric question: How can we decide what Karen Ann Quinlan would want? Though the court then determined that her parents were appropriate informants, the hard work was already over. That case now serves as a powerful clinical ethics precedent, leading to that of Nancy Cruzan more recently, a case that appears further to have settled our judgment about the removal of any artificial supports once the wishes of the patient are known with an acceptable degree of confidence.

The complex philosophic issues the casuists present in their critique of the standard theory of the practice of clinical ethics cannot be resolved here. It is fair, however, to ask how the casuistic view has affected the approach to this text. In accordance with the standard theory, cases for this book were selected that illustrate important theoretical considerations discussed in Chapters 1 through 6. Further, the cases are developed in a certain order so as to allow rules and principles to be gradually built upon the basis of experience with previous cases, while at the same time weaving in theoretical presentation from this first part of the book. Thus, the book moves back and forth between the standard theory and a more casuistic method, as does much contemporary clinical ethics. To a very great extent, casuistry was already part of clinical ethics before it became self-conscious in the writings of the new casuists; however, this, of course, is precisely their point.

THE CARE PERSPECTIVE

The care perspective also finds fault with the methodology of the standard theory but not only with its deductivism. According to this view, too much emphasis is placed on major philosophic theories and the moral principles that are supposed to flow from them. These principles tend to have rights and duties as their primary conceptual devices and their main reference points for analysis. Instead, proponents of the care perspective contend that the starting point for ethical inquiry should be people's moral experience, in particular the moral experience of care for another human. Technically, an ethics of care begins with narratives by people in their own voices and attends to the moral perceptions and sentiments that are represented in those narratives. Of particular interest in these narratives is the way patients or those close to them manifest their own values and how we all can learn from these manifestations.

Warren T. Reich has elaborated on the important linguistic sources of an ethics of care.[4–6]

The root meaning of the verb *to care* is to feel worry or anxiety, and it is associated with mental distress or mental suffering. This meaning connotes a heavy sense of responsibility. Additional meanings of the word *care* all relate to a moral context: to be concerned about, interested in, or attentive to; to be attentive to a task at hand; to give needed services; to have a liking or attachment for a person or thing.

Reich goes on to cite the two principal meanings of care in the literature of clinical ethics: to take care of (in the sense of rendering services) and to care about (in the sense of exercising an attentive and committed concern). Taking care is directed to the disease that inhabits a body that occupies a bed, while caring about is directed to the human needs of the patient and family as well as the disease. Taking care can be further subdivided into assisting with activities of daily living, attending conscientiously to detail as is normally expected of a professional, and serving the whole person by alleviating and being present for his or her suffering. What gives these meanings of caretaking their dynamism, however, is the caring about that is shown in the context of changing life experience. The persistence of taking care of someone through various life stages manifests that one cares about that person.

An important element of the care perspective, both in its critique of the standard theory and in its own alternative theory, is an orientation to human relations that is often called feminine. Used in this sense, the term does not pertain to women so much as it does to a form of experience that, although usually identified with women, can, and in fact often does, apply to men as well. By contrast, the *command* sensibility of an ethics of rights and duties is commonly attributed to masculine culture. This important feminine aspect of the care perspective does not necessarily lead to the claim that the entire system of health care delivery is systematically distorted and dehumanized by the dominant, masculine view. Thus, the care perspective is a feminine one but not a feminist one.

The feminine element of the care perspective is present in caring itself and in the prerequisite of caring that is called compassion: the "co-feeling" that allows identification with another. Compassion inclines us to be sensitive to the needs of others, but caring goes further in actually providing assistance for those needs. Caring is closely bound up with relationships rather than rules, and thus it is more commonly identified with women than men. Little boys, according to some influential modern psychologists such as Carol Gilligan, define themselves in opposition rather than in cooperative relations with others, as is alleged to be true of little girls.[7] Hence, the former are reported to deal with moral dilemmas by enforcing systems of rules, while the latter reckon as more important the feelings of those involved.

Again, the stories told by people themselves are critical for the insights in the moral sentiments of others that they provide. In one example discussed by Reich, an ethics committee chairperson had recommended that a severely disabled, ventilator-dependent 72-year-old man not be discharged into the care of his daughter at home. Of specific concern to the chairperson was the daughter's statement, "I want to take care of my father; it's my responsibility and I think I'm prepared to do it, but how can I care for him if no one helps me?" Since the means to obtain assistance had been explained to her several times, this remark was interpreted as an excuse not to take on this enormous job. This interpretation was altered, however, when in a lengthy interview, Reich heard the patient's daughter recount a life already accustomed to service, pain, and disappointment. Her son died of cancer at 20 under her care, and her unsupportive husband later slipped into alcoholism, saved only by a support group. Her self-presentation was that of a woman prepared and eager to take care of her father, but also wanting the sort of support her husband received in his crisis. Her statement to the ethics committee chairperson was not an expression of resistance but a wish for the kind of compassion she wished to give her father. To Reich, the salient feature of this case was not a daughter's duties but rather the way this episode appeared in the context of the story of her life.

The care perspective thus focuses on what it is like to experience the world of caring for a particular individual. While decisions about granting authority and responsibility have to be made, legalistic focus on the rights and duties of those involved is not the exclusive background to these decisions, or perhaps even the most appropriate. For example, a typical approach to issues of parental responsibility in the standard theory proceeds from the analysis of what society can legitimately expect of a parent. Such an approach, however, can never hope to comprehend the experience of parenthood, or especially why parents often insist on doing far more for their children than reason could ask of them. The beginning of understanding lies in letting another's story come to light in his or her own way.

FEMINIST ETHICS

Feminist ethics shares with casuistry and the care perspective the view that the standard theory overemphasizes abstract rules outside a human context. In her comprehensive work on feminism in health care, Susan Sherwin cites with approval both of these two alternative movements within bioethics as sympathetic to feminist ethics.[8] She notes that health care ethics has long been more interested in contextual considerations than has the more academic study of ethics; indeed, the given exposition of the standard theory of clinical ethics does not convey the abstract nature of much of the work that feminists criticize.

Nevertheless, feminism is critical not only of the standard theory, but also of casuistry and the care framework. All fail to incorporate an analysis of the political nature of the health care system. For example, functionally, the integration of ethics into curricula and the incorporation of ethics questions on certification examinations serve to mollify public concern about the conduct of health care professionals. Hence, Sherwin suggests, the medical establishment's enthusiastic embrace of medical ethics should itself be cause for suspicion. Applications of the standard theory, especially if accepted as part of the literature, may tend to rationalize existing practices rather than subject them to ongoing criticism.

Of special interest to feminist writers on health care are the masculine origins and orientation of the vast majority of commentators in medical ethics (perhaps as distinguished from nursing ethics). This majority has been notably silent about the patriarchal character of health care practices as systemic rather than as isolated events. Even the classical criticisms of paternalism have been limited to one-on-one doctor-patient encounters rather than used to raise larger questions about health care delivery. Thus, issues having to do with reproductive technologies, while they are commonly analyzed by reference to law, philosophy, and theology, should be placed against the broader background of women in society in terms of current and historic patterns of oppression. Abortion, while increasingly viewed as a conflict between fetal and maternal rights, is framed in feminist ethics in terms of the fundamental relation between woman and fetus, and it is argued that the value accorded the fetus must proceed from that relationship.

Allocation of health care resources also has distinct effects on women as a group, for they tend to be poorer and more socially vulnerable than men, while nevertheless expected to shoulder a disproportionate share of caretaking of the young, poor, and disabled. Women's subordinate social position exposes them to more medical procedures than men, Sherwin points out, while at the same time they are significantly less likely to receive kidney transplants and diagnostic tests for diseases such as lung cancer. Thus, women are overtreated in some respects and undertreated in others, a result that seems to be closely bound up with professionals' stereotypes of female patients as anxious and manipulative. If women's complaints are taken less seriously than those of male patients, they are nevertheless more likely to be recommended for procedures that attempt to change their bodies, such as psychosurgery and cosmetic surgery.

Modern medical research also has an unfortunate history of excluding women from clinical trials, partly due to methodological concerns about controlling for effects of the menstrual cycle, partly due to legal worries about effects on the female reproductive system. Yet most controlled medications are prescribed for women, though they have generally not been tested on women, especially women of reproductive age. Questions about the differences between male and female physiologic responses to substances are thus left as guesswork, which has potentially important implications for clinical management issues such as dosing. Recent policy initiatives by both the National Institutes of Health and the Food and Drug Administration should provide some redress for this problem concerning new drugs but not for older ones already approved for use.[9]

Thus, the agenda of feminist ethics goes beyond that of the mainstream approach. Rather than remaining satisfied with relatively modest reforms of professional conduct, feminism seeks to empower the lay public as active agents rather than passive consumers in accessing health care. For women, a more active role in health care extends beyond allocation issues to redefining the norms of health and illness. Biologically routine functions of a woman's body such as menstruation, reproduction, and menopause have been treated as disease states, and other conditions such as weight are subjected to a medical model according to unexamined values of physical beauty. Ultimately, feminism speaks not only to clinical ethics but also to the epistemology of health and disease; it is an approach that holds out the prospect of profoundly influencing the basic terms of clinical ethics.

REFERENCES

1. B. Brody, *Life and Death Decision Making* (New York: Oxford University Press, 1988).
2. A.R. Jonsen and S. Toulmin, *The Abuse of Casuistry: A History of Moral Reasoning* (Berkeley: University of California Press, 1988).

3. J.D. Arras, "Getting Down to Cases: The Revival of Casuistry in Bioethics," *Journal of Medical Philosophy* 16 (1991): 29–52.

4. W.T. Reich, "The Case: Denny's Story," and "Commentary: Caring as Extraordinary Means," *Second Opinion,* July 1991: 41–56.

5. W.T. Reich, "Caring for Life in the First of It: Moral Paradigms for Perinatal and Neonatal Ethics," *Seminars in Perinatology* 11 (1987): 279–287.

6. W.T. Reich, "Speaking of Suffering: A Moral Account of Compassion," *Soundings* 72 (1989): 83–108.

7. C. Gilligan, *In a Different Voice: Psychological Theory and Women's Development* (Cambridge, MA: Harvard University Press, 1993).

8. S. Sherwin, *No Longer Patient: Feminist Ethics and Health Care* (Philadelphia: Temple University Press, 1992).

9. NIH Guidelines on the Inclusion of Women and Minorities as Subjects in Clinical Research, 59 *Federal Register* 14508 (March 28, 1994).

6

Strategy for a Clinical Ethics Assessment

This chapter outlines some of the key considerations in a clinical ethics assessment. The concrete process itself will depend on a great many factors, including whether the assessment is to be performed by an ethics consultant rather than by the attending physician and, if so, whether the consultation occurs in conjunction with a functioning ethics committee. Alternatively, this outline focuses on strategy rather than tactics, that is, on theoretical aspects that the individual performing the assessment will find useful.

THE ORGANIZATIONAL CLIMATE

A prerequisite to a successful clinical ethics assessment is that the setting in which the care is delivered and in which the putative ethical issue arises must be committed to a fair and open process of ethics consultation and intervention where needed. Ethics consultants and ethics committee members must be supported by management, on the understanding that a process that honors professional discretion and judgment will be best for the organization in the long run. In turn, those responsible for clinical ethics activities must of course be competent and responsible in conducting their sensitive professional role.

The organization's administration should ensure that those identified as clinical ethics consultants or committee members have been trained in the skill areas mentioned in Chapter 1 ("About Clinical Ethics"). The organization should also institute a procedure for dealing with issues involving its own policies when those policies appear to engage ethical issues. One approach is to establish an organizational ethics committee that includes representatives from the entity's various stakeholders, with a liaison from the clinically based ethics committee.

IDENTIFYING THE ETHICAL ISSUES

Just what is an ethical issue? As the celebrated United States Supreme Court justice remarked about pornography, we may not know how to define it, but we know it when we see it—or do we? As was noted in Chapter 1, certain practices that are by general agreement unethical, such as sexual contact with a patient, are not usually within the ambit of clinical ethics proper. These are violations of professional ethics that are not unique to clinical practice and are matters for peer review or the law. What, then, count as issues for clinical ethics?

Issues of special interest to clinical ethics normally involve some sort of conflict about moral values in the course of taking care of a patient. Obviously, many conflicts that arise in the clinical setting are not ethical in nature, rather, they are administrative issues such as interpretations of institutional policy or the law. Others may appear to be ethical conflicts but on investigation turn out to be problems of communication or even personality differences. While administrative issues can usually be identified and distinguished from ethical problems fairly early in the process, problems of communication and personality often do not lend themselves to such ready identification. One very rough approximation of a formula for sorting ethical from nonethical problems is this: When agreement about the facts alone does not settle a disagreement (referring in the clinical setting to the medical facts), the issue may involve a conflict of values.

At times the root disagreement might be about the proper interpretation of the facts. A familiar example is a dispute between a managed care provider and a patient about coverage for a novel treatment, where the organization regards the treatment as experimental. Here, too, the underlying issue is one of values: Considering what is known about the treatment, the patient's needs, and the organization's commitments, how should these factors be balanced?

The management of organizational ethics issues in the clinical setting is a rather new topic, and protocols for dealing with these problems are only now being developed. By contrast, processes for clinical ethics assessments are much more evolved.

COMMON PITFALLS IN ASSESSING DECISIONAL CAPACITY

There are several inappropriate or inadequate criteria for assessing decisional capacity. First among these is the notion that the patient who disagrees with the physician's recommendation must be incompetent. While this may turn out to be true, mere disagreement with a physician or any other professional are not in itself grounds for a finding of decisional incapacity. Second, though it is a less obvious error, the idea that the patient who is unable to pass a formal mental status examination is therefore incompetent is also unsound. The patient who does not know what day of the week it is or even who is president may nonetheless have the ability to make a particular decision about his or her immediate physical condition. Third, even the patient with a classifiable psychiatric disorder often retains the capacity to make a specific decision. This is a common misunderstanding among physicians who ask for a psychiatric consultation; the presence or absence of psychiatric disease is only one factor of the clinical assessment of capacity.[1,2] Put in logical terms, mental illness is neither a necessary nor a sufficient condition to determine incapacity to decide about treatment.

Knowing a patient's status with respect to adequate decisional capacity can have substantial implications for managing the informed consent process. A patient whose understanding is well beyond that minimally required could be informed about sophisticated technical details concerning the available treatment alternatives. On the other hand, a patient whose ability to understand has heretofore been inadequate may be assessed for remedial measures, such as temporizing medications, in order to improve that ability.

This idea is especially pertinent to patient groups who, for one reason or another, possess waxing and waning decisional capabilities or whose capacities are decision-specific. An assessment of decisional capacity of the patient undergoing intensive care must take into account the effects of medication on the decisional capacity of the patient at one time or another. Other patients may be able to make certain specific decisions but not others. The adolescent with terminal cancer may be able to participate in a decision about palliative surgery, or she can be counseled in a way that helps her formulate her wishes. The patient with Alzheimer's disease may be able to achieve an adequate level of clarity and consistency to partici- pate in a decision about long-term care, even if he is unable to consider experimental treatment protocols.

COMMON TYPES OF ETHICAL CONFLICT

It is possible to provide a rough typology that covers most of the ethical conflicts likely to arise in the clinical setting: conflicts between moral prin- ciples, conflicts between interpretations of a patient's best interests, and conflicts between moral principles and administrative policy or the law.

Conflicts between Moral Principles

The most common example of conflict between moral principles is that between autonomy and beneficence or, as described in Chapter 1, patient self-determination and the best interests of the patient. Generally, this sort of conflict requires confirmation of the patient's capacity to make the deci- sion at hand. If the patient has capacity, then the next step is to ensure that the patient understands the nature and consequences of the choice he or she has made. Efforts to dissuade the patient are acceptable, and even morally obligatory in some instances, so long as they are not coercive or manipula- tive. If all this has been done and the patient is steadfast, the most difficult part remains: helping those who are uncomfortable with the patient's choice, including caregivers, family, and friends, to come to respect it.

Another common conflict of moral principles is that between the patient's best interests and justice. The classic example of such a conflict occurs whenever a clinician in charge of admissions to a full intensive care unit is faced with a choice between continuing to care for a patient whose chances for survival are poor and accepting a new patient who may have a better chance to benefit from intensive medical care. Since the intensive care clinicians are already in a professional relationship with the current patient, it is usually thought that they owe him or her their continued ef- forts to promote his or her best interests. Yet in so doing they are arguably engaging in a misallocation of resources. It is generally agreed that even genuinely tragic circumstances such as these do not automatically permit the clinician to reallocate the ICU bed. However, if intensive care practice guidelines are developed and gain wide acceptance, society may have to be prepared to accept a different evaluation of this conflict.

Conflicts between Interpretations of a Patient's Best Interests

Clinicians may disagree with a patient's surrogate or with one another about, for example, the continued treatment of an irreversibly unconscious patient. Collegial disagreements, while usually less fraught with legal complications than conflict with a surrogate, should nonetheless be dealt with expeditiously rather than be allowed to fester, as they may compromise the ability of professionals to work with one another in the care of other patients as well. Moreover, the only instance of a criminal indictment of physicians for letting a patient die, the California case of Drs. Barber and Nadle, which was subsequently dismissed, stemmed from the complaint of another clinician (a nurse) that resulted from a miscommunication.[3] An open discussion of the medical facts and of patient or surrogate wishes can resolve the vast majority of such problems. If substantial difference remains because of conflicts of moral values among clinicians, a discussion moderated by a neutral party (perhaps one who has a background in ethical analysis) can be most constructive; in more extreme cases resort to a hospital ethics committee may be useful.

Conflicts with a surrogate's interpretations of a patient's best interests depend first on the legal status of the surrogate's authority. If the surrogate is court appointed as the health care decision maker for the patient or is authorized by statute to decide for the patient, a negotiated compromise with the surrogate may be the best that can be attained. Otherwise, the only recourse may be a court of law, and experience suggests that such challenges are not likely to succeed unless it can be shown that the surrogate abused or was negligent in the use of his or her authority.

Family members or close friends of the patient without legal authority nevertheless traditionally exert considerable moral suasion on clinicians. This emotional connection with the patient, based on a historical relationship, deserves respect. How much of a voice in decision making these individuals should be given depends on their ability to think in terms of the interests of the patient, whether or not they reach the same conclusions as the clinicians. Ordinarily, the good intentions of family and friends should be presumed and, so far as is possible, these individuals should be made part of the decision process, especially as informants about the patient as a person. Intractable disagreements are infrequent, but when they do occur it is a professional obligation to respect the feelings of those who were close to the patient.

Conflicts between Moral Principles and Institutional Policy or the Law

Occasionally, professionals find themselves in a conflict between their studied moral convictions and institutional policy or the law. Ordinarily, a physician is able to cite an exception of conscience and be relieved of responsibility for the case, but nurses, social workers, and even house officers, who operate under different contractual arrangements with institutions than do attending physicians, often do not have this luxury.

When transferring a case is not a possibility (and even when it is), several factors should be considered. First, the clinician should ensure that his or her understanding of the law or of institutional policies is correct. Often the latter can be more stringent than the former, sometimes due to risk-averse hospital counsel. In that case the institution's regulations may be open to exceptions or modifications. Further, most clinicians have a remarkably poor level of understanding of the law and legal processes among health care professionals, which contributes to misapprehension about what the law actually requires. Accurate information will usually disabuse the clinician of substantial legal concerns, since, as noted repeatedly throughout this book, the law tends to take a minimal position on most questions of clinical ethics. Second, the professional should be quite confident that his or her ethical position is sound and that it takes into account the many factors that usually complicate these problems. Third, if the first two steps do not significantly change the situation, the clinician must determine if the moral violation embodied by law or policy is so great that it demands some form of public protest or even civil disobedience. It goes without saying that such a step can be very serious for the professional, is usually thought to be beyond the call of duty, and should not be undertaken lightly.

Uncertainty

Finally, further complicating all these conflicts is uncertainty. It is difficult to overestimate the importance of this factor in clinical ethics, whether or not it is explicit. In real life, uncertainty can appear in many different ways and often plays a crucial role in the ethical problem. Prognostic uncertainty and uncertainty about the efficacy of one or another proposed therapy are particular instances of the predictive limits inherent in any applied science. In the clinical setting there are still "messier" forms of uncertainty as well, including one's confidence about the patient's capacity to decide, the applicability of an advance directive, the patient's likely wishes, or the best-informed surrogate. Other types of uncertainty arise over the legal implications of one or another possible decision, about the importance of a certain moral principle, or about how to weigh one principle against another. Not uncommonly, real cases may engender uncertainty in several different respects. It is this phenomenon that gives clinical ethics, like any form of intelligent intervention in human affairs that seeks to apply theory, its special character and poignancy.

A PROTOCOL FOR A CLINICAL ETHICS INTERVENTION

The following list summarizes questions to keep in mind when considering what seems to be an ethical problem.

1. What are the facts (medical, social, and legal)?

There is a maxim that states, "good ethics begins with good facts." Clinicians must ask a myriad of questions: Do all parties to the decision understand the medical facts? Do the physicians involved agree on them? Should more diagnostic information be gathered? To what extent is the prognosis uncertain and how does this affect the situation? Is the patient's social situation clear or should more information be gathered? If the problem involves financing the patient's care, are the relevant rules understood? Is there an authoritative statement of the relevant legal requirement or are various theories being thrown around by amateur lawyers? (The latter is not at all a facetious remark; erroneous legal notions are often the source of far more serious problems than the law itself.)

2. Who is confused about what?

Frequently, the apparent difficulty can be settled simply by assembling the involved parties in the same room, sharing information, and facilitating communication. Personality conflicts, whether rooted in historic relationships or as part of relatively recent encounters, should be distinguished from the substantive problem.

3. What ethical principles or moral values are relevant?

Clarity on this point often goes far to settle the issue. Concerns about utilizing an expensive medical technology generally do not in themselves outweigh a legitimate decision maker's preferences, for example. However, this factor in combination with strong doubts about the incapacitated patient's best interests may figure strongly against a surrogate's decision.

4. Is there an ethically acceptable compromise?

Compromise may be ethically acceptable when it preserves the underlying values of the concerned parties. Often a compromise can be short term and turn out to forestall further contention. Agreement to attempt a trial of therapy and to reassess within a specified period of time is a familiar strategy, especially when the issue is clouded by medical uncertainty.

5. If no ethically acceptable compromise is available, how should the alternatives be evaluated?

This, of course, is the $64,000 question of clinical ethics, the so-called hard choice. Rarely, a legal standard will constrain the result, but more commonly, participants will be thrown back on their intellectual resources and those of the clinical ethics field, including the concepts discussed in these first several chapters. Even when it seems that there is such an impasse, it is worthwhile to retrace one's steps through the first four questions.

REFERENCES

1. *Rogers v. Okin*, 478 F. Suppl. 1342 (D. Mass. 1979).
2. *Rennie v. Klein*, 462 F. Suppl. 1131 (D. N.J. 1978), and 476 F. Suppl. 1294 (D. N.J. 1979).
3. *Barber v. Superior Court*, 195 Cal. Rptr. at 488 (1983).

7

Cases

CASE 1

A Religious Objection to a Blood Transfusion

Debra is a 45-year-old multiparous woman who has been healthy all her life. She delivered a healthy 8-pound infant, her fourth child, but shortly afterward she developed severe postpartum hemorrhage and hypotension. Her blood pressure normalized when intravenous saline was given, but the bleeding continued. Her hematocrit is now dangerously low at 18 percent (hemoglobin 6.0 grams per deciliter). Immediate blood transfusions are medically indicated, and it is likely that the bleeding will continue unless surgery is performed.

Before this time, Debra had identified herself as a Jehovah's Witness. She has always been capable of making her own decisions and had stated previously that because of her religious beliefs, she could not receive blood transfusions under any circumstances. The obstetrician explains to Debra and her husband that her life is in danger and he "cannot be responsible" if his "hands are tied" by this prohibition against transfusing blood. Debra's husband says they are aware that there are alternatives to blood transfusions and he hopes the doctor is aware of them.

ISSUES TO CONSIDER

- The principle of self-determination
- The informed consent process
- The place of religious beliefs in the decision-making process

MEDICAL CONSIDERATIONS

1. What are the implications of performing emergency surgery on a critically ill woman who will not accept blood transfusions?

The risks to a patient such as Debra are obvious, but it is important to assess the exact extent of her risk so that she or her decision maker can be fully informed. In short, does she have a chance to survive without transfusions?

As hemoglobin or hematocrit declines, tissue oxygen delivery declines, and if it reaches a critical level, the likelihood of morbidity and mortality increases. However, recent research suggests that this critical level may be lower than previously believed. Hemodilution decreases blood viscosity, which in turn leads to increased blood flow as cardiac output increases, and this improves oxygen consumption as long as euvolemia can be maintained. Hemodilution per se, by decreasing arterial oxygen content, shifts the oxyhemoglobin dissociation curve to the right, improving tissue oxygenation. Experimental use of intentional hemodilution has improved outcome in various types of surgery, illustrating the validity of this physiologic concept (see Question 2, below).

In the present situation, hemodilution is an unintended effect of combined blood loss and infusion of crystalloid to expand volume, and this will only maintain Debra temporarily if she continues to bleed. The critical level of hemoglobin is uncertain, but indications for transfusion have been placed at a threshold level of 7.0 to 8.0 grams per deciliter by professional organizations;[1] overt or occult comorbidity could increase the risk at otherwise tolerated levels of anemia. At the critical level, normal compensatory mechanisms are no longer sufficient, and oxygen consumption outpaces oxygen delivery. The ability to tolerate such a low hematocrit, of course, would depend on the patient's underlying general health. Debra's age and history of good health indicate that she is physiologically fit at baseline and would probably tolerate both the surgery and postoperative anemia. The exact outcome could not be predicted and would depend on her precise physiologic status, the presence or absence of silent coronary insufficiency, the rapidity with which surgery was accomplished, the ability of the operating team to minimize additional blood loss, and the total amount of blood loss that occurred. Certainly, the alternative—not operating—would lead to more dire consequences than operating, unless the bleeding could be stopped with a nonsurgical approach. From a pragmatic point of view, it would be prudent to perform a definitive procedure, such as surgery, without delay, rather than to temporize by convincing Debra and her husband that transfusions are needed.

2. Are there any alternatives to surgery or blood transfusions in this case?

If appropriate technology and personnel are available, there are nonsurgical procedures that can minimize blood loss in this and other states of internal hemorrhage. In Debra's case it might be possible to embolize the uterine artery, for example; however, nonsurgical invasive procedures should not be viewed as solutions if temporizing increases the risk of further blood loss. If they are unsuccessful, valuable time is lost that might have been devoted to a definitive, surgical approach.

In contrast, a number of alternatives exist in nonemergency situations, and some can be applied as adjunctive treatments in the postoperative period of an emergency situation, although not all alternatives are acceptable to Jehovah's Witnesses. For example, autologous blood transfusions, in which the patient predonates blood, is a relatively effective alternative, but is a method generally refused by Jehovah's Witnesses because of the belief that this blood is no longer part of the individual. Moreover, autologous transfusion shares some of the risks of allogenic transfusion, including bacterial contamination, hemolytic transfusion reactions due to administrative error, and volume overload, as well as the risk of producing preoperative anemia and perioperative ischemia. An alternative that is sometimes acceptable is hemodilution, which involves collection of autologous blood during the surgical procedure rather than before. The blood is mixed with appropriate amounts of crystalloid to maintain normovolemia and then reinfused at the end of the surgery. The purpose of this technique, however, is to limit the number of transfusions needed perioperatively in patients whose preoperative hematocrit is above the critical level. Intra- and postoperative recovery of blood is used in certain settings, but the safety and efficacy are controversial.

Since Jehovah's Witnesses do not accept any blood product, cancer patients undergoing chemotherapy would be at high risk. Granulocyte colony stimulating factor (GCSF) is currently used as adjunctive treatment in this setting to delay the duration of neutropenia, but problems remain (see Case 29, "A Religious Objection to a Child's Medical Treatment").

Erythropoietin has been used preoperatively as well as postoperatively to increase blood count and may be effective if iron stores are normal. Several days are generally required before hemoglobin increases, however, limiting its usefulness to the postoperative recovery period or nonemergency procedures. In addition to renal failure, a number of medical conditions have been found to respond to erythropoietin.[2] Erythropoietin preparations contain human albumin as a stabilizing agent and might not be accepted by the patient.

From a purely medical standpoint, it is important to avoid surgical delay in Debra's case. If possible, a method of anesthesia should be selected that will produce the least cardiac compromise. Surgical skill is of paramount importance and hemostasis must be assiduously maintained. In addition to the area of primary hemorrhage, bleeding from all sites entered to the operative site, including the skin, must be minimized, because it is the total amount of blood loss that will be important. While a variety of methods, devices, and topical agents have been employed intraoperatively to maintain hemostasis,[3] meticulous surgical technique is believed to be of utmost importance, and the added utility of newer methods awaits specific testing. Volume expansion using colloid or crystalloid should be continued if the patient loses more blood. Albumin is generally not an acceptable colloid to Jehovah's Witnesses. Alternatives such as synthetic hydroxyethyl starch have been used, but crystalloid such as saline or Ringer's lactate may actually suffice. Currently available blood substitutes that serve as oxygen carriers have questionable utility. The perfluorochemical emulsion Fluosol has only a transient effect and is not believed to improve outcome for surgical patients with severe blood loss. In addition, serious side effects, including bronchospasm, leukopenia, and thrombocytopenia, have been reported. Second generation perfluorochemicals are currently being investigated. A number of new, chemically altered forms of hemoglobin are also under investigation. Even if these are found to be safe and effective, however, some might be unacceptable to Jehovah's Witnesses because of their direct or indirect derivation from human or animal blood. Methods of blood conservation are reviewed in the references.[1]

Erythropoietin, if Debra accepts it, and parenteral iron can be used in order to accelerate normalization of hemoglobin. Diagnostic blood sampling should be kept to a minimum, and pediatric and capillary blood tubes should be used when blood tests are truly essential.

ETHICAL AND LEGAL CONSIDERATIONS

1. On what basis may a patient like Debra refuse a life-sustaining intervention, in this case a blood transfusion?

An adult patient with decisional capacity has the moral and legal right to consent to or refuse any proposed health care intervention. This right is supported by the moral principle of autonomy and has been repeatedly supported through various judicial decisions. The common-law concept of self-determination, as well as state and federal constitutional pronouncements concerning individual liberty, freedom, and privacy, support the right of adults to be the final determiners of the type of health care they receive. The fact that a refusal of care may lead to morbidity or even death does not diminish the strength of this right, so long as the patient understands and accepts the personal consequences of such a refusal.

The concept of individual autonomy allows for the individual patient, like Debra, to factor in whatever values, beliefs, or concerns she wishes in making her decision, even if those elements seem idiosyncratic to her physicians. That Debra may be allowing her religious beliefs to influence her course of care is not only appropriate but also deserving of respect. In the United States, individuals have a constitutional right to religious freedom, although there are limits to the exercise of that freedom (see below). Debra, as a Jehovah's Witness, believes that the acceptance of a blood transfusion would violate her religious tenets, which forbid the eating of blood, of which transfusion is the moral equivalent. She would likely be willing to accept any available alternative medical treatment, but to accept a blood transfusion would cause her to be ostracized from the religious group to which she belongs. If she understands the consequences of her refusal, and accepts its risks, then her choice must be respected.

2. How might one attempt to ensure that Debra understands the consequences of her refusal?

If it is clear that Debra has the ability to make the decision about the recommended treatments, the first priority is to establish that she has been fully informed of all of the important details concerning her condition and care, and of the risks, benefits, and alternatives of the procedure that is being offered. This is known as the informed consent process. The patient must be informed, and, in the physician's judgment, she should be able to understand the information, appreciate her medical situation, appreciate the consequences of consent or refusal of the treatment in question, weigh the risks and benefits, and apply them to her decision. Self-determination can occur only if the patient has at her disposal the information necessary to consider a course of care consistent with her beliefs and wishes. In this way, her consent or refusal will reflect her best interests as she defines them.

In addition to being informed, a choice must also be voluntary; that is, a patient's decision should be made in a supportive and open environment, without coercion or duress. The issue of voluntariness is one that can arise in the context of religious justifications for the refusal of care. In such situations, one must determine if the patient's choice is a reflection of a genuinely held conviction or if perhaps other members of her faith are pressuring her into a choice she might otherwise not have made. This question would most likely arise if a patient chose a course that was unexpected or undesirable, from the perspective of the health care providers. It might also arise if the patient was never allowed to discuss health care choices without other members of her faith present or if her opinion appeared to change depending on who was present for the discussion. Clinicians who are concerned that a patient is being coerced would want to gently explore this issue in a sensitive and supportive manner. At a minimum, they should try to discuss treatment decisions with the patient herself, asking others to temporarily leave the room if necessary. In general, however, the clinician presumes that there is a lack of coercion unless there is evidence to the contrary.

The doctrine of informed consent is equally applicable in the context of refusals. The decision to refuse a suggested course of medical care should be an informed choice, with full understanding of the range of options and the risks and benefits of each option. There is evidence that refusals of treatment are more often reflective of miscommunication or misunderstanding than of any principled choice on the part of the patient.

The refusal of blood should not be viewed as tantamount to a desire to die. In fact, it is likely that the patient does not wish to die; rather, in her hierarchy of priorities, Debra places her religious convictions above saving her life. The proscription against blood transfusion among Jehovah's

Witnesses is also highly specific. People who practice that religion are willing and eager to receive high-quality medical care and are amenable to most if not all other medical alternatives. A decision to risk death rather than receive a transfusion would likely be an uncomfortable choice for physicians to respect, but if made in an informed and voluntary manner, Debra's decision would demand respect in the clinical setting.

3. What are the limitations of Debra's right to be self-determining?

Debra's right to practice the mandates of her religion is not unlimited. She may not, for example, engage in practices that might bring harm to or interfere with the rights and practices of other individuals. Should she try to impose this potentially lethal risk taking on another, for example, insisting that one of her children not receive a blood transfusion, then her religious freedom would be restricted and her authority to direct the course of her child's care would be limited (see Case 29).

However, Debra's choice to refuse a blood transfusion might indirectly harm other individuals. For example, if she were to die as a result of her refusal to be transfused, it could be argued that her actions would harm her husband and children, who would be left without their wife and mother. Courts have considered the possibility that other interests may be so significant in certain situations that they might limit the patient's right to make autonomous health care decisions. Such interests include the sanctity of life, the societal interest in preventing suicide, the integrity of the medical profession, and the interests of innocent third parties, including the children who may be orphaned due to their parent's decision to refuse life-sustaining care. In most cases, while courts of law have found these interests to be important, they have not found the interests to supersede the fundamental right of patients to make autonomous medical decisions. While the interests of children are not insignificant, usually other child care arrangements are possible, so that the needs of the children will be met, while the wishes of the parent are respected. Debra's refusal might deeply affect the lives of her children, but their father would presumably still be available to raise them. These child-centered interests, therefore, do not rise to the level of overriding the fundamental interests of Debra.

4. May the physician refuse to perform surgery in a patient who refuses a blood transfusion?

Although Debra has the right to place restrictions on the type of care she receives, such restrictions do not translate into an automatic obligation on the part of the physician to go along with what he might consider a medically negligent course of care. Although the physician cannot give her the transfusion against her wishes, he may decline to participate in her treatment choice. If it were morally unacceptable to the physician to accede to a patient's wishes, or if he felt he did not have the skill to offer her adequate medical treatment, given her choice, then he would be obligated to arrange for a transfer of care to a physician who would be able to do so. The physician's unwillingness to treat her with the restrictions imposed is another potential risk of Debra's stance on blood transfusions, namely, that it might limit her ability to secure medical treatment in a crisis. It would be important for the physician to inform the patient of his own intentions in this regard, and of her alternatives, prior to a crisis, if possible. Ideally, given Debra's previous expressions of refusal of blood transfusions, her physician should have anticipated this scenario and should have disclosed his discomfort with such a limitation on his ability to care for her. He should also have informed her that even if he was willing to treat her but was unavailable in a crisis, other physicians or institutions might not be so obliging. The obligations of physicians and exceptions to the obligation to treat are discussed further in Case 18 ("Surgery Delay in a Patient Infected with HIV") and Case 20 ("A Difficult Patient and the Limits of Provider Obligations").

REFERENCES

1. L.T. Goodnough et al., "Transfusion Medicine. I. Blood Transfusion; II. Blood Conservation," *New England Journal of Medicine* 340 (1999): 438–447; 525–533.
2. M. Cazzola et al., "Use of Recombinant Human Erythropoietin Outside the Setting of Uremia," *Blood* 89 (1997): 4248–4267.
3. R.K. Spence, "The Status of Bloodless Surgery," *Transfusion Medicine Review* 5 (1991): 274–286.

SUGGESTED READINGS

Applebaum, P.S., and Roth, L.H. 1983. Patients who refuse treatment in medical hospitals. *Journal of the American Medical Association* 250: 1296–1301.

Bennett, D.R., and Shulman, I.A. 1997. Practical issues when confronting the patient who refuses blood transfusion therapy. *American Journal of Clinical Pathology* Supp 1: S23–S27.

Faris, P.M., et al. 1996. The effects of recombinant human erythropoietin on perioperative transfusion requirements in patients having a major orthopedic operation. The American Erythropoietin Study Group. *Journal of Bone and Joint Surgery (Boston)* 878: 62–72.

Kerridge, I., et al. 1997. Clinical and ethical issues in the treatment of a Jehovah's Witness with acute myeloblastic leukemia. *Archives of Internal Medicine* 157: 1753–1757.

Kleinman, I. 1994. Written advance directives refusing blood transfusion: Ethical and legal considerations. *American Journal of Medicine* 96: 563–567.

Malyon, D. 1998. Transfusion-free treatment of Jehovah's Witnesses: Respecting the autonomous patient's rights. *Journal of Medical Ethics* 24: 302–307.

Mann, M.C., et al. 1992. Management of the severely anemic patient who refuses transfusion: Lessons learned during the care of a Jehovah's Witness. *Annals of Internal Medicine* 117: 1042–1048.

Muramoto, O. 1998. Bioethics of the refusal of blood by Jehovah's Witnesses: Part 1. Should bioethical deliberation consider dissidents' views? *Journal of Medical Ethics* 24: 223–230.

Napier, J.A., et al. 1997. Guidelines for autologous transfusion. II. Perioperative haemodilution and cell salvage. *British Journal of Anaesthesia* 78: 768–771.

President's Commission for the Study of Ethical Problems in Medicine and Biomedical and Behavioral Research. 1982. The communication process. In *Making Health Care Decisions*, 69–114. Washington, DC: U.S. Government Printing Office.

Smith, M.L. 1997. Ethical perspectives on Jehovah's Witnesses' refusal of blood. *Cleveland Clinic Journal of Medicine* 64: 475–481.

LEGAL CITATIONS

Case Examples

Application of President and Directors of Georgetown College, 331 F.2d 1000 (1964).
 Blood transfusion ordered despite wishes of Jehovah's Witness patient. The reasoning in this case has been refuted in subsequent cases.

Fosmire v. Nicoleau, 75 N.Y.2d 218, 552 N.Y.S.2d 876, 551 N.E.2d 77 (1990).
 Treatment refusal upheld. Another parent was available to care for dependent child. Limits on refusal of blood because patient was a parent are rejected.

In re Brooks Estate, 32 Ill. 2d 361, 205 N.E.2d 435 (1965).
 One of the first major cases in a state supreme court to uphold the right of a Jehovah's Witness to refuse blood.

In re Fetus Brown, No. 1-96-2316, Ill. App. (Dec. 31, 1997).
 The first appellate court decision in the United States examining and confirming the right of a pregnant Jehovah's Witness patient to refuse an unwanted blood transfusion. This case was decided on appeal after a lower court granted permission to transfuse the patient against her will.

Jehovah's Witnesses of Washington v. King County Hospital, 278 F. Supp. 488, *aff'd* 390 U.S. 598 (1968).

Jehovah's Witness parents could not refuse blood on behalf of their minor child.

Schloendorff v. Society of New York Hospital, 211 N.Y. 127, 105 N.E. 92 (1914).

Seminal right to refuse treatment/self-determination case.

CASE 2

Determining If a Patient Has Decisional Capacity

Harry is a 66-year-old man with hypertension and chronic renal failure. He was recently admitted to a large public hospital where he has undergone a series of diagnostic tests, including a contrast study, for which his consent was obtained. He has end-stage renal disease (ESRD), and despite maximal treatment with medications, his hypertension and hyperkalemia are inadequately controlled. It is apparent that Harry will need long-term hemodialysis in order to survive and to avoid serious symptoms of ESRD, such as vomiting and symptoms related to fluid overload. When approached concerning this new treatment regimen, Harry refused to consent to the dialysis. He stated that he has "had enough" and does not want "any machines."

The patient has a history of alcohol abuse and has no permanent home. He has drifted through a variety of residences over the years and his most recent "home" has been the basement of a small apartment building where he lives in exchange for doing some chores.

On physical examination, Harry is alert and knows that he is "in the county hospital." His blood pressure is 190/90. His complexion is sallow. There are no other pertinent findings.

The medical resident believes that Harry does not fully understand the implications of forgoing dialysis. He tells the intern to "consult psychiatry" to determine if the patient is "competent to refuse dialysis." A psychiatrist interviews Harry and administers a Folstein Mini-Mental Status Examination (MMSE). The patient scores 22 out of a possible 30 points, which the psychiatrist says is "consistent with dementia." The medical intern states that Harry's mental status has not deteriorated discernibly since admission but says that he at times seems confused and is not surprised to hear that he might have dementia.

ISSUES TO CONSIDER

- Determination of decisional capacity
- Informed consent in the presence of diminished decisional capacity
- Competence versus decisional capacity
- Social circumstances as factors affecting patient care delivery
- Palliative care options

MEDICAL CONSIDERATIONS

1. How does Harry's score on the mental status test assist in assessing whether or not he has the decisional capability to refuse dialysis?

Harry's score of 22 on the MMSE is compatible with the diagnosis of dementia, but it is neither diagnostic of dementia nor does it answer the question of whether he lacks the capacity to make this specific decision.

The MMSE, one of a variety of mental status examinations, is commonly used in the evaluation of dementia because it assesses a number of cognitive functions, such as memory, naming ability, attention, language, and higher intellectual function.[1] However, the MMSE and other standard mental status examinations may be falsely positive. A number of factors can modify a patient's performance on the examination; these include educational level, depression, fatigue, aphasia, diminished attention (as in delirium), and language or cultural differences between patient and examiner. Conversely, mental status tests have a high false-negative rate because some aspects of impaired cognition may be too subtle for these examinations to detect. For this reason, many additional factors are taken into account not only when making the diagnosis of specific cognitive disorders, such as dementia, but also when assessing decisional capacity.

Unless a patient's cognitive abilities are obviously poor (as in coma or advanced dementia), the absolute score on formal mental status testing, when taken alone, is usually not a reliable method for assessing decisional capacity. For a patient such as Harry, it is more important to measure functional ability for the specific decision at hand. Some investigators have recommended testing patients by presenting them with hypothetical case scenarios, which might more sensitively assess the ability to understand a clinical situation and make a decision about it. While it seems logical that this form of testing gives more information about the patient's capacities, failing to interpret a hypothetical scenario does not necessarily mean that a patient would be incapable of making a treatment decision about his or her own body.

2. How do cognitive disturbances, such as dementia, affect decisional capacity?

In early dementia, the patient may have a problem with short-term memory, but higher intellectual function may still be intact and adequate for purposes of making an informed decision. This is frequently the case in early Alzheimer's disease. Even when intellectual function is maintained, however, short-term memory deficits may impair the interpretation of information. In more advanced states of dementia, when memory loss is severe or when higher intellectual function is impaired, the patient has little or no ability to make informed decisions. The nature of cognitive impairment in dementia also varies, depending on the etiology of the dementia.

In patients such as Harry, cognitive dysfunction could be multifactorial. If he were suffering from clinical depression, his refusal of dialysis might reflect a wish to die, and the disease itself (depression) might cloud judgment and impair his ability to make a decision. Although it would be unlikely for a patient with psychosis to have decisional capacity, it is nonetheless possible in certain patients with such a history. For example, if a patient with chronic schizophrenia refused surgery for colon cancer because he did not want to be left with a permanent colostomy, this might be considered a reasoned decision, deserving of respect; however, if he refused because voices from another planet told him to refuse, his refusal would be an obvious consequence of decisional incapacity.

3. What sort of treatment exists that might improve Harry's cognitive abilities?

Pharmacologic agents and medical illness, including renal failure, may impair decisional capacity by producing delirium, a confusional state characterized by impaired attention and alteration in consciousness (see Case 4, "Management of Life-Threatening Illness"). In Harry's case, these various aspects of impaired cognition would need to be explored. When there are potentially reversible causes of cognitive impairment, reversing the underlying problem might allow a patient to participate in a more informed manner. In Harry's case, however, attempting to reverse the confusion by performing dialysis would probably require sedating and restraining him, which could perpetuate or even worsen his confusion.

It is possible that Harry has underlying dementia, a disorder of memory loss generally associated with disturbances in executive function. Although reversible forms of dementia exist, most chronic, progressive forms are not reversible. Medication has been approved for the most common cause of dementia, Alzheimer's disease, but as of this writing, the most widely used medication, donezepil (Aricept), has only a minimal effect on cognitive function. Chronic alcoholism has been associated with nonreversible dementia, usually secondary to problems associated with alcoholism, such as thiamine deficiency (Korsakoff's psychosis) or head trauma, or, in late life, unrelated illness such as Alzheimer's disease.

A directed search for reversible causes of dementia should be done,[2] which should include consideration of the patient's medication regimen.

4. What options other than chronic hemodialysis exist?

Peritoneal dialysis, which might be tolerated better than hemodialysis, is an option usually available for patients who can be trained to perform the technical aspects of this treatment on a daily basis or who have caregivers to do it for them. Harry would probably not be a candidate for those reasons, even if he would agree to this or cooperate.

Without dialysis, it is likely that Harry will soon develop symptoms of uremia, which could include confusion, nausea, vomiting, breathing difficulties from fluid overload, and pruritus, and each symptom would need to be addressed as part of a palliative plan of care. Treatment of individual symptoms with medications, such as potent diuretics for pulmonary edema, or antiemetic agents for nausea and vomiting, might reduce or even eliminate symptoms temporarily. Pruritus is a difficult symptom to treat, and uremic pruritus does not always respond to hemodialysis. Emollients, topical corticosteroids, and antihistamines have limited effect in uremic pruritus; a bile acid resin, such as cholestyramine, sometimes reduces symptoms, but the effect is unpredictable, it might not be tolerated if nausea were present, and it can cause severe constipation.

In a patient who might have underlying brain disease, confusion is likely to increase rapidly as uremia worsens. Some symptoms of delirium can be frightening, including confusion, delusions, and hallucinations. Stupor or deep coma might ensue relatively swiftly, however. Deep coma is a sleeplike state, during which a patient is unresponsive to deep painful stimuli and would be unable to experience pain or other physical or psychological symptoms. Deep coma can be induced with sedatives, which are often the only alternative for pain, dyspnea, or other symptoms that do not respond to treatments that preserve consciousness (see Case 3, "Urgent Surgery in a Stuporous Patient").

It is not appropriate to treat hyperkalemia in a dying patient because it does not make the patient uncomfortable, and in fact, might shorten the duration of the dying process by causing sudden death. Metabolic acidosis, on the other hand, can produce dyspnea (Kussmaul respiration). Oxygen might be helpful if it reduces respiratory drive. Treatment of acidosis per se would involve treating the underlying metabolic problem, which might require more complex management than desired. Administration of bicarbonate should generally be avoided because it can worsen fluid overload. If acidosis cannot be reversed sufficiently to palliate symptoms, sedation can be given.

Specific aspects of palliative care are addressed in Case 3, Case 9 ("Withholding Tube Feeding in a Woman with Advanced Dementia"), Case 13 ("A Dispute over DNR Status in a Patient Who Wants Palliative Surgery"), and Case 15 ("Assisted Suicide in a Man with Amyotrophic Lateral Sclerosis").

ETHICAL AND LEGAL CONSIDERATIONS

1. What is decisional capacity and how is it determined in any given clinical situation?

Decisional capacity is the patient's functional ability to consider the factors relevant to a specific decision and to arrive at and communicate an individually appropriate choice. Questions concerning a patient's decision-making abilities most often arise during the informed consent process for a proposed intervention. Only if patients have the ability to consider their options and their personal values will their choices be truly reflective of autonomous decision making.

While the level of decisional capability necessary to consent to or refuse an intervention may vary depending on the individual patient and the nature of the decision to be made, a certain minimum level of cognitive and intellectual skills must be present before the decision can be accepted as a genuine reflection of that patient's interests and desires.

In some patients, decisional incapacity is clear from the patient's status—infants, for example, or those who are comatose. Many situations are much less clear, however, as in the case of Harry, whose physicians are questioning whether he has the ability to make this specific decision. In Harry's case, the dilemma is not about whether he is "incompetent" (a legal categorization, which is discussed below), but, rather, whether he has the capacity to refuse the recommended treatment of dialysis. Does he understand what dialysis is and what it will do for him, and is he willing to accept the likely consequences of his refusal?

Examining capacity in the context of specific circumstances is very different from legal pronouncements of "competency" and "incompetency." All adults at or over the age of majority (the age of 18 in most jurisdictions) are presumed legally competent and are thus empowered to manage their own affairs and to determine the course and nature of their lives. This legal presumption provides a basic level of authority to the individual to take on the fundamental aspects of citizenship (voting, contracting, marrying, etc.) without the undue interference of others. The legal presumption of competency holds fast unless and until a court of law strips away the presumption and disempowers a person, at least for certain aspects of decision making. Only a court can declare an individual incompetent.

Individuals such as Harry are thus legally competent, for no judicial declaration has been made to the contrary (so far as we know in this case). However, this is of little assistance in the clinical reality facing Harry and his physicians. Harry may theoretically still be able to enter a voting booth or marry, but there is a very legitimate concern that he lacks the skills necessary to understand the implications of his refusal of dialysis. This is a specific decision about a specific situation, and there is concern that he lacks decision-specific capacity, or decisional capacity.

To determine this level of capacity in the clinical setting, we must first determine whether or not Harry's spoken choice reflects an informed decision on his part. It should be clear to his physicians that on some basic level he understands the treatment options available in this situation and, in particular, the benefits and risks associated with his specific preference.

The mere fact that Harry may be legally competent does not mean that he has decisional capacity in this situation, and a label of "dementia" or a specific score on a mental status test does not mean that he lacks such capacity. What does matter in the assessment is that he understands the benefits as well as the burdens of dialysis. In order to assess his capacity, the physicians should carefully explain the situation in language he understands, delineate the specific benefits of dialysis—that without it he may die or have severe symptoms and that he will not be "hooked up to a machine" 24 hours a day—as well as its burdens—that it is not a cure and is not without risks and discomforts. They should also explain that he may at any time revoke his consent if he changes his mind. They should then ask Harry to explain to them the specific reasons for his refusal (or consent).

If necessary, this process should be repeated in a few hours to see if his cognition and decision are stable. In patients with waxing and waning mental status (e.g., delirium), this provides the opportunity to assess the patient during a period of lucidity.

If Harry is unable to state the risks of his decision and that he accepts those risks, then it likely that he lacks the capacity necessary to make an informed decision. An alternative process of decision making would then be needed to determine the course of Harry's care (see Cases 3 and 4).

2. Who is qualified to assess Harry's decisional capacity?

The impulse to involve a psychiatrist when a patient refuses a recommended treatment is understandable and even supportable in many ways, but is not always necessary. In many situations the patient's primary care physician, who knows the patient best, may be better able than a new consultant to judge whether or not the patient has decisional capacity. Such a physician will certainly be able to assess decisional impairment in the obvious case of incapacity, such as stupor or coma. He or she will also be able to administer simple questions in order to ascertain that the patient understood the information disclosed; to determine whether other factors, such as religious beliefs, were influencing the patient's choice; and to evaluate and treat delirium, which is a medical rather than a psychiatric illness. It is even possible that some capacity assessments can be performed by nonphysician clinicians who are familiar with the patient.

Nonetheless, psychiatrists are frequently called to rubber stamp this type of workup. In these cases, the consultation may serve more to ease the anxieties of the providers (fear of liability, for example) than to clarify the diagnosis. If, however, the primary care physician lacks experience in determining capacity or if there is evidence of schizophrenia, depression, or other psychiatric illness that can affect judgment, it may be useful to employ the skills of an experienced psychiatrist. This could be important in a patient like Harry, where so many factors could be influencing his capacity.

In cases of refusal, it is not the refusal per se but rather the patient's process of reasoning that must be probed. If problems in this process are identified, it is these rather than the refusal that may lead to the eventual conclusion that the patient lacks decisional capacity. An experienced psychiatrist should be able to discern if there is some flaw or impairment in the patient's reasoning, to assist in determining if this is amenable to correction, or to determine that it is so significant that it impairs his ability to give a consent or refusal.

The psychiatrist would not be called in to declare the patient "incompetent," although in the case of a judicial competency hearing the opinion of a psychiatrist is generally sought. However, it should be emphasized that the presence of a psychiatric disorder does not, by itself, disempower a patient; court rulings have confirmed that even patients involuntarily committed to psychiatric institutions have the right to refuse care, if they understand the consequences of their refusals. For example, in *Rivers v. Katz* (New York), the court upheld the right of involuntarily committed psychiatric patients to refuse medicine that would have helped them.

3. What can be the role in the informed consent process for patients such as Harry who may have some level of decisional impairment?

The fact that a patient has some level of impairment would only indicate that extra caution must be taken to measure his or her abilities in the specific context. Such a person can give informed consent even if some impairment exists, as long as he or she has the capacity in the context of the specific question at hand.

Depending on the type of impairment, its manifestation, and the demands of the decision in question, a patient might be able to participate in certain treatment decisions, yet be unable to participate in others. The determination of a patient's decisional abilities must be decision-specific, and an individual assessment of his or her abilities should be made whenever a major treatment decision is in question. If Harry agrees to dialysis, he might then have to give informed consent to a vascular access, for example, a surgical procedure with significant benefits as well as some risks.

4. Should the same rules have been applied to Harry's earlier consent to treatment?

Harry's consent was sought and apparently obtained for the diagnostic testing performed. It appears that there was no serious inquiry into his decisional skills until he refused a recommended intervention, even though his level of impairment was reportedly the same. How can this apparent discrepancy be explained?

One view of the situation might be that because he agreed with his physicians' recommendations, it was in no one's interests to challenge his choice. While one might argue that capacity should be questioned regardless of whether a patient consents or refuses, especially if there is some indication of decisional impairment, in reality, it is generally only the lack of cooperation that triggers the inquiry into decisional capabilities. Is this wrong?

Certainly, it is reasonable to recommend diagnostic testing if the ultimate goal is to improve symptoms. If Harry agrees with this, does it matter that he may not precisely understand that to which he has consented? Perhaps not, given the limited risks that appropriate diagnostic tests pose in comparison to the benefits. Thus, it may not serve anyone's interest to challenge this "reasonable" decision.

The problem with this sort of reasoning is that it tends to support decisions that coincide with physician preferences at the expense of decisions that do not. If we do not challenge Harry's initial consent because it was "reasonable," this then implies the obligation to challenge decisions when they are "unreasonable," that is, inconsistent with the recommendations of the physicians. This undermines the principle, discussed earlier, that one must judge choices based on the process of arriving at them rather than on the ultimate decision itself. The mere fact that a choice is "unreasonable" does not provide sufficient justification to challenge it, but it may justify further exploration of the patient's reasoning to make certain that he understands the consequences of his decision.

Another view of these discrepancies would take into account the highly specific nature of decisional capacity. Given the relative simplicity of the earlier decisions in comparison to the much weightier and more complex decision regarding long-term dialysis, Harry might have possessed sufficient understanding to consider the proposed diagnostic intervention and to decide that it was acceptable to him. (This, of course, rests on the presumption that Harry participated in an informed consent discussion.) When the later decision concerning dialysis was addressed, even if Harry's abilities had not become more impaired, the demands of the dialysis decision might nonetheless have outpaced Harry's abilities at that point. In essence, the standard for determining decisional capacity becomes more rigorous as the complexity and the risks of the proposed intervention increase. The more that is at stake, the more certain we want to be that the patient truly understands the consequences of his or her choice.

5. What consideration, if any, should be given to the fact that Harry leads a rather unconventional life, disconnected from the mainstream of society?

The fact that Harry has a history of alcohol abuse, and a nomadic and at times homeless existence, will undoubtedly influence the manner in which some providers view him as a patient. It should not be surprising that physicians, just as all other members of society, may harbor biases or prejudices, perhaps fueled by social or class differences, perhaps exacerbated by their often exhaustive efforts for what may seem to them to be little benefit. The crucial issue to consider, however, is whether Harry's social history is relevant to his plan of care.

Clearly, it would be wrong to discriminate against Harry because of his social circumstances. The tradition in medicine has been to studiously avoid blame for what is sometimes considered self-induced illness and, rather, to focus on the fact that a patient is ill and in need of medical care, or at least access to it. Given Harry's isolation and lack of support, as well as the possible impairments that may be affecting his judgment, he may be particularly vulnerable to individual prejudices or biases and he may require more attention and advocacy—rather than less—than a patient with family or other sources of support.

If the circumstances of Harry's life are relevant at all, it may be in the specific aspects of managing his medical care, whether or not the decision to initiate dialysis is implemented. If either Harry or an appropriate surrogate decides in favor of dialysis, then special arrangements may be required to ensure that he is sufficiently connected to a system of support so that he may continue to receive treatment once he leaves the hospital. Likewise, if dialysis is not initiated, Harry's predictable deterioration would have to be addressed and an appropriate palliative care plan implemented. In such a case, he might be an appropriate candidate for hospice care.

REFERENCES

1. M.F. Folstein et al., "Mini-Mental State: A Practical Method for Grading Cognitive State of Patients for the Clinician." *Journal of Psychiatric Research* 12 (1975): 189–198.

2. E.M. Russell and A. Burns, "Presentation and Clinical Management of Dementia" in: *Brocklehurst's Textbook of Geriatric Medicine and Gerontology*, eds. R.C. Tallis, H.M. Fillit, and J.C. Brocklehurst, 5th ed. (Edinburgh: Churchill Livingstone, 1998), 727–740.

SUGGESTED READINGS

American Psychiatric Association. 1994. *Diagnostic and statistical manual of mental disorders (Dementia).* 4th ed. Washington, DC.

Applebaum, P.S., and Grisso, T. 1988. Assessing patients' capacities to consent to treatment. *New England Journal of Medicine* 319: 1635–1638.

Brody, H. et al. 1997. Withdrawing intensive life-sustaining treatment—Recommendations for compassionate clinical management. *New England Journal of Medicine* 336: 652–657.

Buchanan, A., and Brock, D.W. 1986. Deciding for others: Standards for decision-making. *Milbank Quarterly* 64 (Supp. 2): 67–80.

Cohen, L.M. et al. 1995. Dialysis discontinuation: A "good" death? *Archives of Internal Medicine* 155: 42–47.

Crum, R.M. et al. 1993. Population-based norms for the mini-mental state examination by age and educational level. *Journal of the American Medical Association* 269: 2386–2391.

Drane, J.F. 1985. The many faces of competency. *Hastings Center Report* 15: 17–21.

Fellows, LK. 1998. Competency and consent in dementia. *Journal of the American Geriatrics Society* 46: 922–926.

Fitten, L.J. et al. 1990. Assessing treatment decision making capacity in elderly nursing home residents. *Journal of the American Geriatrics Society* 38: 1097–1104.

Golper, T.A. 1997. Peritoneal dialysis. In *Diseases of the Kidney,* eds. R.W. Schrier and C.W. Gottschalk, 2771–2805. 6th ed. Boston: Little, Brown and Company.

The Hastings Center. 1987. Decisionmaking capacity and competence. In *Guidelines on the Termination of Life Sustaining Treatment and Care of the Dying,* 131–133. Bloomington: Indiana University Press.

Kerridge, I. 1995. Competent patients, incompetent decisions. *Annals of Internal Medicine* 123: 878–881.

Lo, B. 1990. Assessing decision-making capacity. *The Journal of Law, Medicine, and Health Care* 18: 193–201.

Malloy, P.F. et al. 1997. Cognitive screening instruments in neuropsychiatry: A report of the Committee on Research of the American Neuropsychiatric Association. *Journal of Neuropsychiatry and Clinical Neurosciences* 9, no. 2: 189–197.

Meisel, A., and Kuczewsk, M. 1996. Legal and ethical myths about informed consent. *Archives of Internal Medicine* 156: 2521–2526.

Miles, A.M., and Friedman, E.A. 1997. Center and home chronic hemodialysis: Outcome and complications. In: *Diseases of the Kidney,* eds. R.W. Schrier and C.W. Gottschalk, 2807–2838. 6th ed. Boston: Little Brown and Company.

President's Commission for the Study of Ethical Problems in Medicine and Biomedical and Behavioral Research. 1982. Decisionmaking capacity and voluntariness. In *Making Health Care Decisions*, 55–68. Washington, DC: U.S. Government Printing Office.

President's Commission for the Study of Ethical Problems in Medicine and Biomedical and Behavioral Research. 1982. The ethical and legal implications of informed consent in the patient-practitioner relationship. In *Making Health Care Decisions*, 381. Washington, DC: U.S. Government Printing Office.

Rogers, S.L. et al. 1998. A 24-week, double-blind, placebo-controlled trial of donezepil in patients with Alzheimer's disease. *Neurology* 50: 136–145.

Sugarman, J. et al. 1998. Getting meaningful informed consent from older adults: A structured literature review of empirical research. *Journal of the American Geriatrics Society* 46: 517–524.

Tobe, S.W., and Senn, J.S. 1996. Forgoing renal dialysis: A case study and review of ethical issues. The End Stage Renal Disease Group. *American Journal of Kidney Disease*; 28: 147–153.

Victor, M. 1994. Alcoholic dementia. *Canadian Journal of Neurological Science* 21: 88–99.

LEGAL CITATIONS

Case Examples

Rivers v. Katz, 67 N.Y.2d 485 (1986).
    A major case supporting the right of involuntarily committed mentally ill patients to refuse antipsychotic medication.

Winters v. Miller, 446 F.2d 65 (2nd Cir.), *cert. denied*, 404 U.S. 985 (1971).
    Case with similar holding to *Rivers*.

CASE 3

Urgent Surgery in a Stuporous Patient: The Use and Limitations of Advance Directives

Nathan is a 78-year-old man hospitalized with inoperable colon cancer and lung metastases. Recently, intestinal obstruction, intractable vomiting, and confusion developed. He is receiving fluids intravenously. A naso-gastric tube has been inserted and connected to suction, in order to decom-press the gastrointestinal tract and provide relief of symptoms. He is stu-porous, and questions regarding his care are addressed to his wife. The attending physician explains to Nathan's wife that it may be necessary to surgically create a colostomy in order to relieve her husband's symptoms. He explains that the colostomy will not be a cure but would make the pa-tient more comfortable. A year earlier, when he was well, Nathan prepared a living will, which stated that he would not want respirator treatment, feeding tubes, surgery, or antibiotics if he were "hopelessly ill" and the treatment would "merely prolong the dying process." On this basis, Nathan's wife tells the physician that she will not consent to surgery, since her husband would certainly "not want to be cut" at this stage of his life.

ISSUES TO CONSIDER

- Decision making for the decisionally incapable
- The use and limitations of living wills
- Other advance directives
- Curative versus palliative aims of care
- Terminal sedation

MEDICAL CONSIDERATIONS

1. Are there any medical alternatives to surgery for relief of Nathan's symptoms?

In many cases, bowel obstruction is intermittent and palliation can be achieved with judicious use of nasogastric suction, antinausea agents, enemas, and intravenous fluids. The efficacy of radiation therapy and chemotherapy depends on the type of tumor and whether these methods had been used previously and to what effect. They are not particularly helpful in adenocarcinoma of the colon, the most common histologic variety. Certainly a reversible, superimposed cause of bowel obstruction should be considered, such as ileus, incarcerated loop of bowel, or fecal impaction superimposed on the tumor. If the patient's symptoms are due to mechanical obstruction from the tumor, surgery provides the most immediate and probably the only reliable relief.

If the surgical solution is not adopted, it is unlikely that antinausea agents would provide sufficient relief in the presence of mechanical obstruction and would only be a temporary solution in any case. Alternatively, the patient could be made comfortable if he were given potent sedation (see Case 2, "Determining If a Patient Has Decisional Capacity"), a mainstay of care for dying patients with intractable symptoms when they are still alert enough to experience these symptoms. Medications used for this purpose include continuous intravenous morphine, benzodiazepines, or barbiturates. The dose is titrated for relief of symptoms, and the dose can be escalated to produce complete anesthesia if necessary. Continuous intravenous sedatives have been used in a variety of clinical situations in the terminally ill (see Suggested Readings).

The term *terminal sedation* has been used in this context, but it has been variously defined. Terminal sedation generally indicates heavy sedation (potentially to unconsciousness) for dying patients in whom symptoms cannot be adequately controlled by other means. Although the use of sedation does not necessarily preclude concurrent treatments, in one view, it is assumed that all other treatments will be stopped, and if death is not imminent it is nonetheless considered acceptable to provide terminal sedation and avoid all other treatments, including intravenous hydration.[1] In this view, terminal sedation is also considered acceptable for patients who do not have intractable physical symptoms. Terminal sedation under those circumstances has been criticized as being tantamount to euthanasia (see Case 15, "Assisted Suicide in a Man with Amyotrophic Lateral Sclerosis") because the physician is allowing a patient to prematurely end his or her life by going under anesthesia for the purpose of starving or dehydrating to death.[2] This would differ from avoiding artificial nutrition and hydration in a patient whose disease prevents adequate intake of food or fluids, as discussed in Case 9 ("Withholding Tube Feeding in a Woman with Advanced Dementia"). Palliative care considerations are discussed further in Case 2, Case 8 ("Withdrawing Mechanical Ventilation at the Request of a Patient with Decisional Capacity"), Case 13 ("A Dispute over DNR Status in a Patient Who Wants Palliative Surgery"), and Case 15 ("Assisted Suicide in a Man with Amyotrophic Lateral Sclerosis").

ETHICAL AND LEGAL CONSIDERATIONS

1. Given the urgency of Nathan's clinical condition and his inability to make decisions for himself, who should be involved in the decision-making process?

Ideally, the goals of treatment at this time would derive from Nathan's own wishes. If he were capable of participating, his providers would be able to find out not only specifically what he wanted regarding the surgery but also his current primary goals. For example, his main concern might have been relief of suffering, or perhaps life prolongation in order to survive for an important family milestone, or even a desire to maintain mental clarity, though it might mean enduring some pain as a consequence.

Given Nathan's current mental status, the question becomes how to arrive at the decision that he would have made, if that is possible. The wishes expressed through his living will provide guidance, but the stipulations on the living will are somewhat ambiguous and perhaps not entirely applicable in the circumstances at hand.

In this case, the physician has made the natural assumption that Nathan's wife will speak on her husband's behalf. By custom, clinicians turn to next of kin to make decisions for patients who cannot decide for themselves, as they assume (though it is not always the case) that they are most familiar with the patient and his values and what his goals of treatment might have been. Knowledge about his personal values, while perhaps not directly relevant to the specific clinical decision to be made, may provide enough of the intangible yet illuminating "essence" of the patient to conjecture what serves the patient's interests, as he defined them. Thus, next of kin will usually be able to make the sort of substituted judgment traditionally sought in these circumstances and decide as the patient would have decided.

There are legal considerations that could diminish or even restrict the decisional authority of Nathan's wife to act as her husband's surrogate. State law may limit the authority of a surrogate, particularly when decisions involve the removal of life-sustaining measures. Not all states permit interpretive, substituted decision making; some require more explicit directions from the now incapacitated patient in order for the surrogate to exercise certain powers. Still other states have made efforts to restrict the types of decisions that can be made. Thus, the exact scope of empowerment of Nathan's wife would depend on the jurisdiction in which Nathan's treatment is being given. The outcome of the decision, however, probably depends most on the ability of the physician and Nathan's wife to reach a mutual understanding of what Nathan's wishes would be in these circumstances.

Whoever is empowered to make decisions on Nathan's behalf must be part of an informed consent discussion, just as the patient would have been if he possessed decisional capacity (see Case 1, "A Religious Objection to a Blood Transfusion").

2. What are the advantages and limitations of the living will in this case?

A living will is a mechanism for documenting, before the onset of decisional incapacity, patient preferences regarding medical treatment. It is only to be used in the event of such incapacity. If a living will is an articulate, well-thought-out expression of the patient's desires, it can be a valuable tool to guide decision making for a now incapacitated patient. A living will can express wishes concerning treatment withholding or withdrawal, as well as wishes concerning treatment that may be desirable or considered obligatory to provide.

The mere fact that Nathan made the effort to execute a living will, and the strength of the wishes that he expressed in the document, illustrate the importance of these wishes to him and thus serve as critical guidance to his wife and physicians. Unfortunately, as the problems in this case illustrate, living wills do have limitations. Nathan describes specific treatment interventions, including surgery, as options he would not wish to employ in the specific circumstance of being "hopelessly ill," and if the treatment would "merely prolong the dying process." At this point, he is certainly gravely ill and arguably in the process of dying. It would therefore appear that he would not want the operation that is now being considered as a treatment option.

Although he is in the process of dying, the proposed operation, ostensibly rejected in the living will, would not merely prolong the dying process but would also provide palliation. If one were to attempt to make the decision merely based on the wording of Nathan's living will, one might conclude that he would be opposed to surgery. Yet should one also assume that he would refuse relief of his symptoms? Wouldn't a reasonable person want to be as free of misery at this point as possible?

This dilemma illustrates the limitations of a living will. Circumstances might arise that have not been addressed by the patient in the context of his living will, and even extraordinary prescience and thorough discussion will not cover every potential occurrence. There are still situations that may require some interpretive process to address the precise options at hand. For example, if he had rejected "tubes" rather than "feeding tubes" in his living will then the nasogastric tube and intravenous line providing symptom relief might also become the subject of dispute. While Nathan's living will does provide guidance as to what was of concern to him, it does not provide the exact answer as to what he would have wanted in this specific circumstance.

It is not known if Nathan prepared this document alone or in consultation with someone. If his physician had assisted him in preparing the document, perhaps he might have alerted him to the possibility of his present situation. Nathan's physician or wife also could have discussed the patient's wishes in greater detail as well as the specific nature of his intentions so they would have felt more certain about his precise wishes in this circumstance. More generally, while the execution of a specific document is helpful, a broader focus on advance care planning, during which the goals of care and the priorities of the patient are fully explored and understood, would help frame and guide the specific, and sometimes unanticipated, treatment choices that can arise.

It is important to emphasize that if a living will or other evidence of a patient's wishes is discovered after treatment is initiated, it can still be used as support for the discontinuation of treatment. Nathan's living will clearly states his wishes regarding life-prolonging treatment and could now stand as support for withdrawing treatments that were already begun.

Patients should also be aware that discussions with their physicians during which they express their wishes for future treatment options can also constitute an advance directive, which would be authoritative if the patient subsequently lost decisional capacity (oral advance directive). In such cases, it is important for the discussion to be as explicit and precise as possible. It is prudent for the physician to thoroughly document the discussion in the patient's medical record and perhaps to have a witness sign the chart note as further evidence of the formality of the patient's directive. In general, patients should be informed about their advance planning options by their health care providers, as part of the providers' obligations to inform patients under the federal Patient Self-Determination Act of 1991. Less formal discussions with family or friends might also provide valuable evidence or insight into how to treat the patient once he has lost decisional capacity.

3. What other advance measures could have been used to address some of the problems identified in this case?

Clearly, if the state permitted such appointment, it would have been helpful for Nathan's wife (or some other surrogate) to have been officially designated as the patient's spokesperson for medical decisions. This would have empowered her to make decisions independent of, or in addition to, those addressed in the living will or to resolve ambiguities regarding his wishes. As not all treatment choices can be anticipated, it is usually very valuable to have an authorized surrogate with the flexibility and discretion to respond to unexpected treatment dilemmas as they arise. Some states might grant Nathan's wife this power even if Nathan himself did not formally make the appointment; others would limit decisions in this case to the precise circumstances addressed in the living will, or would require that Nathan's wife seek judicial intervention to empower her to make decisions. Thus, because of variations in state law, as well as varying institutional policies, the resolution of the situation might take different forms.

The most common appointment, now law in most states, is that of *health care agent,* also known as *proxy, durable power of attorney for health care,* or *medical power of attorney* (Table 7–3.1). The appointment of a loved one or friend as health care agent grants that person tremendous legal authority and responsibility to make decisions on behalf of the patient if the patient can no longer do so. Ideally, agents should have a clear understanding of the values and preferences of the patient and, prior to the exercise of the agent authority, should be comfortable with the role of advocating for those preferences. This type of appointment should not be confused with a power of attorney obtained to make financial transactions for someone who is unavailable to make such transactions himself. An ordinary power of attorney is usually not applicable for health care decisions, although in some states a durable power of attorney can be used for this purpose. If a patient is intending that his financial power of attorney also serve as his health care agent, it would be advisable to discuss this precise empowerment with an attorney.

In most states, forms should be available through the hospital or state health department to make the agent appointment simple. Except in very limited circumstances, such an appointment does not require a court proceeding, and the need for an attorney may not be necessary. State laws governing these appointments are always evolving; it is best to check the state's precise requirements before attempting to execute a health care proxy or living will.

4. How can a palliative care plan be adopted or implemented in an acute care hospital?

The medical treatment option should be selected according to the condition and wishes of the patient and not according to any rigid custom of the institution. The setting of the care should not determine the nature of the care, although clearly some treatment options will not be available in certain treatment settings. The fact that Nathan is in an acute care hospital should not automatically dictate that his care plan include any or all sophisticated treatment options available for his condition. It would be perfectly appropriate to transition from an aggressive treatment plan to a more palliative care plan. For example, surgery could be avoided and palliation could take the form of heavy sedation or complete anesthesia, if this were consistent with the patient's goals. In fact, Nathan's living will makes it apparent that he desired to change the goals of care once his condition deteriorated to a certain level. Although he did not actually state that only

---

Table 7–3.1 Advance Directives

Living will
Durable power of attorney for health care; also called:
- Medical power of attorney
- Health care agent
- Proxy appointment

Other written directive (e.g., a letter or other personal statement)
Oral directive

comfort measures should be provided, he presumably would want to be kept comfortable once it was clear that no curative options were available. A palliative care plan can be implemented in any setting where the proposed treatments or personnel are available—hospital, nursing home, or inpatient or home hospice. Reimbursement realities perhaps more than expertise may drive decisions in this regard. For example, pressures to curtail length of stay would lead to pressure to discharge the patient from the acute care hospital to home hospice, a nursing home, or a palliative care inpatient unit if one existed in his town (see Case 13 and Case 14, "Suicide Risk in a Managed Care Patient").

REFERENCES

1. T.E. Quill et al., "Palliative Options of Last Resort. A Comparison of Voluntary Stopping Eating and Drinking, Terminal Sedation, Physician-Assisted Suicide, and Voluntary Active Euthanasia." *Journal of the American Medical Association* 278 (1997): 2099–2104.
2. D. Orentlicher, "The Supreme Court and Physician-Assisted Suicide. Rejecting Assisted Suicide but Embracing Euthanasia." *New England Journal of Medicine* 337 (1997): 1236–1239.

SUGGESTED READINGS

Berry, S.R., and Singer, P.A. 1998. The cancer specific advance directive. *Cancer* 82: 1570–1577.

Brett, A.S. 1989. Limitations of listing specific medical interventions in advance directives. *Journal of the American Medical Association* 262: 2415–2419.

Choice in Dying. 1998. Maps: State statutes governing living wills and appointment of health care agents. *Right-to-Die Law Digest: A Quarterly Review of Legislative Activity and Case Law,* March.

Committee on Care at the End of Life. 1997. The health care system and the dying patient. In *Approaching Death. Improving Care at the End of Life,* eds. M.J. Field and C.K. Cassel, 87–121. Washington, DC: National Academy Press.

Dubler, N.N. 1995. The doctor-proxy relationship: The neglected connection. *Kennedy Institute of Ethics Journal* 5: 289–306.

Emmanuel, L. 1993. Advance directives: What have we learned so far? *Journal of Clinical Ethics* 4: 8–16.

Green, W.R., and Davis, W.H. 1991. Titrated intravenous barbiturates in the control of symptoms in patients with terminal cancer. *Southern Medical Journal* 84: 332–337.

Gross, M.D. 1998. What do patients express as their preferences in advance directives? *Archives of Internal Medicine* 158: 363–365.

Hammes, B.J., and Rooney, B.L. 1998. Death and end-of-life planning in one midwestern community. *Archives of Internal Medicine* 158: 383–390.

Lambert, P. et al. 1990. The values history: An innovation in surrogate medical decision-making. *The Journal of Law, Medicine and Health Care* 18: 202–212.

Loewy, W.H. 1998. Ethical considerations in executing and implementing advance directives. *Archives of Internal Medicine* 158: 321–324.

Lynn, J. 1991. Why I don't have a living will. *The Journal of Law, Medicine and Health Care* 19: 101–104.

Lynn J. 1998. Terminal sedation. *New England Journal of Medicine* 338: 1230 (letter).

President's Commission for the Study of Ethical Problems in Medicine and Biomedical and Behavioral Research. 1993. Patients who lack decision making capacity. In *Deciding To Forgo Life-Sustaining Treatment,* 136–153. Washington, DC: U.S. Government Printing Office.

Robertson, J.A. 1991. Second thoughts on living wills. *Hastings Center Report* 21: 6–9.

Sulmasy, D.P. et al. 1998. The accuracy of substituted judgments in patients with terminal diagnosis. *Annals of Internal Medicine* 128: 621–629.

Teno, J. et al. 1997. Advance directives for seriously ill hospitalized patients: Effectiveness with the Patient Self-Determination Act and the SUPPORT intervention. *Journal of American Geriatrics Society* 45: 500–507.

Teno, J. et al. 1998. Role of written advance directives in decision making. *Journal of General Internal Medicine* 13: 439–446.

Teno, J.M., and Lynn, J. 1996. Putting advance-care planning into action. *Journal of Clinical Ethics* 7: 205–213.

Truog, R.D. et al. 1992. Barbiturates in the care of the terminally ill. *New England Journal of Medicine* 327: 1678–1682.

LEGAL CITATIONS

Case Example

Cruzan v. Director, Missouri Department of Health, 110 S. Ct. 2841 (1990).
The first U.S. Supreme Court decision to address the withdrawal of life-sustaining treatment from an incompetent patient. The Court stated that states are permitted but not obligated to require clear and convincing evidence of a patient's wishes prior to treatment withdrawal. It also established a Fourteenth Amendment liberty interest to treatment refusals.

Statutory Example

The Patient Self-Determination Act, the Omnibus Budget Reconciliation Act of 1990, Public Law 101-508, §§ 4206,475 1, (OBRA), 42 U.S.C. § 1395 cc (f) (1) and 42 U.S.C. § 1396 a (a) (Supp. 1991).
Federal legislation mandating that patients must be educated as to the advance planning mechanisms available in their states.

CASE 4

Management of Life-Threatening Illness: An Intensive Care Unit Patient with Uncertain Decisional Capacity

Jocelyn is a 40-year-old woman who has had systemic lupus erythematosus (SLE) for 15 years. At age 29 she developed a myocardial infarction and subsequently developed recurrent deep vein thrombosis, which has been attributed to antiphospholipid antibody syndrome, for which she takes warfarin. Two years ago she developed an occlusion of the right middle cerebral artery with left hemiparesis and mild aphasia, but recovered to the extent that she could ambulate with a cane. Carotid angiogram revealed significant bilateral carotid occlusion, and the question of endarterectomy was raised, but this was postponed, as was an earlier plan to evaluate for coronary artery bypass graft, because of concerns over discontinuing anticoagulation for the surgery. Recently she developed depression and headaches, raising the possibility of lupus cerebritis. Prednisone was increased to 60 mg per day, and intravenous Cytoxan was prescribed. Sertraline was given for depression, but Jocelyn developed delusional behavior and the antidepressant was discontinued. MRI revealed multiple punctate white matter lesions, consistent with small vessel disease often seen in central nervous system lupus. After lumbar puncture ruled out an infection, prednisone was increased and the patient improved somewhat.

Jocelyn was doing well until a month ago when she developed shortness of breath and pulmonary edema and was admitted to the hospital. Myocardial infarction was ruled out, but when she failed to respond to intravenous furosemide, endotracheal intubation was performed. A diagnosis of adult respiratory distress syndrome was made. The doctors are unable to wean her from the respirator.

Jocelyn's long-time partner, Nina, visits her daily. Jocelyn and Nina have lived together for 15 years and now own a house together. They have executed estate wills in which they have named each other as the primary beneficiary, and they have taken religious vows as partners in a church service.

Jocelyn's 70-year-old mother, her only living blood relative, is unaware of the precise nature of her daughter's relationship with Nina, whom she speaks of as Jocelyn's "roommate." Jocelyn's mother has been spending virtually all day and night with her daughter, and the doctors direct all their questions to her. It was Jocelyn's mother who consented to a spinal tap, which was done during the admission to rule out an infection of the central nervous system (CNS). Nina was hurt by this but said nothing because she does not want to upset Jocelyn's mother and she and Jocelyn's mother seem to agree on the course to take.

Jocelyn and Nina are both elementary school teachers, but Jocelyn was forced to retire when she had her stroke. Jocelyn and Nina attend a lupus support group together where they have become familiar with many of the manifestations of lupus. They are aware that lupus is associated with accelerated atherosclerosis and that further strokes or heart disease might well be in Jocelyn's future. On several occasions before this most recent event, Jocelyn discussed her fear of a "bad death" with Nina, stating that she did not want to spend her last days on machines "under any circumstances." When it became apparent that Jocelyn could not be weaned from the respirator, Nina asked the physician to administer sedatives, withdraw the respirator, and allow Jocelyn to die, in accordance with what she believed to be her wishes. Jocelyn's mother doesn't think it's time to pull the plug and tells Nina she will not allow the physician to do this. The physicians, conflicted about this, are not yet convinced that Jocelyn cannot make her own decisions, but when they approach her, her views seem inconsistent and uncertain.

An ad hoc meeting of the ethics committee is held. Two designees from the committee, a lawyer from the Department of Risk Management and a psychiatrist not involved in the case, interview Jocelyn. They find that it is difficult to determine if Jocelyn has the capacity to make such a decision: The endotracheal tube prevents her from speaking and she refuses or is unable to communicate by writing. She communicates only by shaking or nodding her head, but her responses are unclear and inconsistent. At times Jocelyn has attempted to dislodge the endotracheal tube and her hands have been placed in restraints.

The attorney states that she feels sorry for Jocelyn and Nina, but that it would be legally inadvisable to discontinue the respirator since the patient's wishes are uncertain and it is impossible to clearly establish if she lacks decisional capacity. Jocelyn's rheumatologist has stated that her prognosis is virtually nil, so the question, he feels, is moot. An internist on the committee thinks the attorney's advice is "outrageous," and that continued use of the respirator amounts to "torturing the patient to death."

ISSUES TO CONSIDER

- The patient whose decisional capacity is uncertain
- The role of health care agents
- The role of nonfamily members as surrogate decision makers
- Best interests
- Ethics committee involvement in clinical decision making
- The place of risk management concerns

MEDICAL CONSIDERATIONS

1. What medical factors might be contributing to Jocelyn's inconsistent responses?

SLE can produce cognitive disorders for a variety of reasons, and Jocelyn's problem could be multifactorial. Antiphospholipid syndrome, which produces a hypercoagulable state, can lead to focal neurologic deficits from thromboembolism, in situ thrombosis, or small vessel disease, all of which could produce a confusional state. Chronic use of high doses of corticosteroids can lead to accelerated atherosclerosis, which can produce chronic confusion when stroke occurs. Lupus cerebritis itself can produce confusion, but high dose prednisone, given for the cerebritis, can worsen confusion by causing psychosis or other cognitive disorders. Immunosuppression increases the risk of infection, including CNS infection.

Jocelyn has had evidence of ongoing cerebrocortical dysfunction, and under those circumstances, she is at high risk of delirium, a confusional state (which is usually but not necessarily acute in onset) characterized by impaired attention and alteration in consciousness. The course tends to fluctuate and the patient may have periods of agitation and psychomotor features such as depressed motor activity or restlessness. Delirium can be caused by a wide variety of medical factors, including, but not limited to, brain lesions, systemic or cerebral infection, metabolic illness, and pharmacologic agents. Delirium is common among patients in intensive care units (ICUs), where factors may include lack of supportive interpersonal interactions and sleep deprivation due to constant noise, around-the-clock lighting, and never-ending invasive maneuvers. The term "ICU psychosis" has sometimes been used to describe delirium that occurs in this setting.

Psychological factors could be contributing to Jocelyn's inconsistent responses, as discussed below under Ethical and Legal Considerations.

2. If Jocelyn cannot be weaned from the respirator, what will her life be like?

A fully conscious patient in Jocelyn's situation is likely to experience a variety of physical discomforts, sleep deprivation, depression, and other severe psychological reactions, including hallucinations. It is not possible to evaluate the specific experiences of a patient with delirium. Physical and psychological symptoms could be reduced or eliminated with deep sedation, as discussed in Case 2 ("Determining If a Patient Has Decisional Capacity") and Case 3 ("Urgent Surgery in a Stuporous Patient"). Sedation would have to be minimized if the respirator were being withdrawn and the patient hoped to recover. The personal experience of an ICU, ventilator-dependent patient, himself a physician, has been vividly described.[1]

ETHICAL AND LEGAL CONSIDERATIONS

1. Considering the prognosis and the patient's previously expressed wishes, why is there hesitation about discontinuing the respirator?

Withdrawal of Jocelyn's respirator support will almost certainly result in her death. When a decision of this magnitude is at issue, it would best serve the patient's interests if she could be actively involved in the decision. From this perspective, it is understandable that her providers would attempt to determine her decisional capacity rather than immediately respond to her companion's request. This path may nonetheless appear counterproductive to others, such as Nina, who may feel that it will subject the patient to the end she most feared or that it is a tactic to postpone a tough decision.

Unfortunately, the determination of Jocelyn's decisional capacity is compromised by many factors. If she does possess any level of decisional capacity, it appears to be waxing and waning. The fluctuating nature of her abilities would not necessarily preclude her involvement if her providers were able to ascertain, at a more lucid moment, what her wishes are at this time.

No one has yet to encounter Jocelyn when it can be determined that she comprehends the situation sufficiently to make a decision or that she is willing to make one. It would have to be clear that Jocelyn understands the gravity of her situation and that removal of the respirator would likely result in her death. Questions would need to be phrased clearly and allow for simple responses that directly addressed the issues. If asked if she "wanted to die," however, it might be quite plausible that she would respond negatively or ambivalently, given her circumstances. She may not want to die, and yet, at the same time, she may not want to continue living in her current circumstances. Thus, an answer to such a question might appear to be inconsistent, although in fact it is quite logical.

The fact that Jocelyn has tried to dislodge the endotracheal tube could mean different things as well. She might be doing this intentionally to demonstrate her wish to discontinue treatment, or she may find the tube physically uncomfortable and may be trying merely to ease her discomfort while not consciously intending to end her life. Her actions could also be involuntary reactions to her discomfort. Unfortunately, unless someone succeeds in communicating with her, any attempt to discern a meaning from this would merely be conjecture.

In cases such as this, the agony of the decision is exacerbated by the pressures and turmoil of the intensive care environment, which neither lend themselves to quiet reflective discussion nor promote the reasoned consideration necessary to make an informed decision.

The ambiguous nature of Jocelyn's decisional capacity creates a dilemma. A decision to err on the side of continuing the respirator would be in direct conflict with her previously stated wishes (oral advance directive) and perhaps her current responses, which do not indicate a desire to continue. Yet, following those previously expressed wishes is an irrevocable decision that will end her life. The irony of this scenario cannot escape notice: As a possibly capable, certainly conscious patient, Jocelyn may experience the type of death she had feared and wished to avoid; yet if she were comatose, and unable to experience any discomfort or anxiety, the decision to end her suffering would probably be more easily made, and her life would come to an earlier but peaceful end.

Another dilemma is that determining her wishes at this time is pure conjecture. Some scholars argue that wishes expressed in advance, whether oral or written, should not determine the outcome of current treatment, for the patient is no longer the person who once conveyed those wishes.[2,3] The current circumstances of the patient are now so radically different from those of her earlier existence that this person's prior preferences can no longer dictate treatment options because she is now a "different" person. As a corollary, others argue that no one can truly decide what they might want until they are actually *in the circumstances* requiring the decision to be made.

Certainly, patients with decisional capacity always have the right to alter or revoke their wishes as described in their advance directive. In this case, however, Jocelyn's ambiguous responses are most likely due to cognitive impairment rather than reconsideration of her wishes. If anything, her attempts to dislodge the tube might even be interpreted as further support of her desire to end the respirator treatment.

2. As she is not technically next of kin, what role should Nina have as the surrogate decision maker?

From our knowledge of their relationship, it seems that Jocelyn and Nina lived together on an intimate basis and shared thoughts and desires as any intimate couple would. The fact that this companion was not a legal spouse should, at least theoretically, have little to do with the substantive factors that help determine how a substituted judgment is made. What may be of concern, however, are the procedural mechanisms in place in this jurisdiction that outline who may serve as a surrogate decision maker for an incapacitated patient and the criteria such a decision maker may employ in order to arrive at a decision.

Jocelyn is now faced with the precise type of "horrible" situation that she used as her marker for the decision to forgo respirator treatment. Therefore, Nina's request to withdraw the respirator seems consistent with the patient's precise, previously expressed wishes. There is nothing to suggest maleficence or a conflict of interest on the part of the companion, any more than there would be with a spouse or next of kin serving in this role. The fact that their relationship is not one that is accepted by all in society has little to do with the fact that Nina is probably the person who knew Jocelyn best and could best transmit her wishes—precisely the type of information that is helpful in this kind of situation.

Because there is no written documentation of Jocelyn's wishes, there might be a problem in jurisdictions that require a high level of evidence of prior wishes before treatment can be withdrawn. That, however, would not be an insurmountable problem if Nina was willing to sign an affidavit swearing to the validity of the statements or if Jocelyn's care providers were willing to accept the companion's verbal assertions without an affi-davit. If the jurisdiction required prior appointment of a formal health care agent, Nina, an informal spokesperson, might have to seek judicial inter-vention. As a practical matter, however, this might not be necessary if all parties agreed on what would be in the patient's best interests.

3. How should a disagreement between Nina and Jocelyn's mother be addressed?

Disagreements among potential surrogates are not uncommon. This may create a unique dilemma when the patient is gay and the disagreement is between a live-in companion and a relative who was unaware of the patient's lifestyle and has emerged at the time of her illness and insists on having the authority to make decisions.

It is understandable that the clinicians in this case looked to Jocelyn's mother. They probably sought some comfort from the technicality that a next of kin agreed with their decision, perhaps thinking this would avoid possible litigation down the road. Yet the most important consideration for this type of surrogate decision would be evidence, as accurate and substan-tive as possible, as to what *Jocelyn would have wanted*, and it seems that Nina, not Jocelyn's mother, is better able to provide that sort of informa-tion.

Another type of disagreement that could arise in this case would be be-tween the health care providers and the surrogate, whether it was the com-panion or the mother. For example, if the doctors believed that the patient had reversible delirium, they might argue that treatment should continue for a while longer. Another situation that could very well provoke dis-agreement would be the decision by a hospital attorney that it would not be worth courting a risk of liability over an "inappropriate" withdrawal of life support. In these circumstances Nina or the hospital might have to seek judicial intervention because neither really has the legal authority to make the decision.

The push to provide treatment in these cases often comes from provider concerns about malpractice, the failure to conform to the appropriate standard of care in a given medical situation and about possible criminal liability. In cases such as this, however, the standard of care is evolving, and the current course of continuing treatment does not necessarily benefit the patient medically. In fact, no judgment of criminal liability has ever been sustained against a physician or institution for discontinuing life support at the behest of a patient or appropriate surrogate. Conversely, doctors have been sued for provision of treatment against the wishes of the patient.[4]

4. If the burdens of the respirator outweigh its benefits, how can the argument to continue it hold any weight?

As the patient's death is likely and continued use of the respirator is tantamount to "torturing the patient to death," it would be hard to say that continuing the respirator would serve the patient's best interests. From a legal perspective, this best-interests standard is applied in situations in which the patient's wishes are not known or in situations in which the patient has never considered such issues, as in the case of a child or mentally retarded adult. In the present case, the patient's previous wishes are known, but it is unclear whether or not they should now be invoked, given the ambiguity of her present mental state. Examining the patient's best interests might help to resolve the dilemma. In contrast to advance directives and substituted judgment, which employ the patient's own wishes or interpretation of those wishes, the best-interests standard attempts to utilize more objective criteria in order to resolve a dilemma.

The best interests of the patient are calculated by weighing the benefits of a treatment against its burdens. If the burdens outweigh the benefits, then the treatment is considered not to be in the patient's best interests. Benefits of a treatment might include saving or prolonging life, alleviation of pain, or restoration to an acceptable level of functioning or quality of life, which might include such individual values as bodily integrity, sentience, dignity, or ability to interact with others. Treatment burdens would include pain, suffering, or the needless prolongation of the dying process. Usually excluded from consideration are such issues as cost of treatment and a patient's "social worth." Cost considerations are becoming more prevalent, however, as society and individual patients struggle to pay the bills for increasingly expensive health care. It is uncertain at this time to what extent cost considerations will alter the allocation of resources in individual cases, although there are clearly situations in which limited or no insurance coverage has influenced clinical options (see Case 14, "Suicide Risk in a Managed Care Patient").

While it is also arguable that continued respirator use in such a case is medically futile, there continues to be much debate in the literature and in clinical practice as to exactly how to determine futility, either using strict physiological criteria or considering the patient's underlying quality of life. While some institutions and organizations have attempted to develop clinically applicable criteria and protocols for determining the futility of such treatment, there is little consensus to date about its use to justify the withdrawal or withholding of life-sustaining treatments such as respirators or feeding tubes (see Case 12, "Resuscitation Decision in a Patient with Lung Cancer").

Although the benefits-burdens analysis is intended to be objective, opinions differ as to which criteria should be considered benefits and burdens or as to the appropriateness of various criteria. Some believe that best interests should be based on what the average reasonable person would want. In this case, the reasonable person might believe that the discomfort, loss of independence, and needless prolongation of the dying process are burdens of the respirator that would outweigh any benefit of life prolongation. Some would reject such quality of life considerations in favor of the "vitalist" view of the sanctity of life, the belief that life is intrinsically the highest good, is always a benefit, and cannot be considered a burden under any circumstances. In the vitalist argument, continuation of life lies heavily on the benefits side of the scale and virtually no treatment could ever be so painful or burdensome as to tip the scale against continued treatment. From a legal perspective, it is unlikely that in any jurisdiction Jocelyn would be forced to continue on the respirator against her will; if Jocelyn wanted to continue this aggressive treatment despite its limited benefit, that, too, probably would be respected. Increasingly, however, physicians are questioning their responsibilities to patients in situations where they consider the intervention to have no medical benefit.

5. What is the appropriate role of an ethics committee in a case such as this?

A hospital ethics committee has no universally mandated role, although hospitals accredited by the Joint Commission for the Accreditation of Healthcare Organizations (JCAHO) are required to have in place an ethics process to deal with ethical issues in the clinical setting.[5] It is not unusual for a committee to become involved in a case such as Jocelyn's, although some might argue with the process and outcome of the particular committee involvement here.

In most institutions, ethics committees are multidisciplinary bodies that provide a forum for an ethical analysis of current or past cases, advise on hospital policies with ethical implications, and serve as a source of information and education on a range of ethical issues. Most members of the committee usually have no special expertise or enhanced moral insight;

rather, they possess an interest in ethical issues and in serving the needs of patients and the hospital. The involvement of an ethics committee in any given case is usually not required, and opinions rendered by the committee are generally considered advisory only, and not a hospital mandate.

The role of a hospital ethics committee is very different from that of the hospital-based risk manager or hospital legal counsel. Risk management is a function of institutional administration that works toward preventing the institution from being exposed to financial loss and legal liability. An important role of risk management is to identify and prevent iatrogenic problems and the malpractice claims that might result. Thus, as traditionally conceived, this department directly serves the interests of the hospital; it indirectly serves the interests of the patient by ensuring that the hospital delivers services consistent with the acceptable standard of care. This role contrasts sharply with that of a neutrally structured ethics committee, which attempts to address ethical dilemmas that affect the patient's care and to directly promote the interests of patients. Thus, a risk management approach to a case might squarely conflict with the ethics committee's mission, as the interest of the risk manager is more to avoid liability than to arrive at the "right" decision. This is not to say that an attorney's viewpoint would not have been valuable, but an attorney who sits on an ethics committee would more appropriately be a volunteer from the community rather than one employed by the hospital, who would bring to the committee the bias that naturally comes with serving as the hospital's legal advocate.

In Jocelyn's case, the viewpoint of risk management is that it is better to avoid the risk of liability that might ensue from an "inappropriate" withdrawal of a respirator than to err on the side of acknowledging her decisional incapacity and rely on her oral advance directive. Such a viewpoint, spawned in an environment targeted with frivolous lawsuits, has nothing to do with the perspective and approach that an ethics committee would utilize in such a case. The role of an ethics committee is not to weigh and consider the hospital's potential for liability, but rather to determine what best serves the interests of the patient, as the patient defined those interests.

Thus, the fact that this committee not only had a representative from risk management on the committee (a controversial appointment in and of itself), but may have allowed a risk management viewpoint to influence the recommendation of the ethics committee, was highly inappropriate. If the hospital itself determines that this risk is not acceptable, that is a decision the administration is empowered to make. For an ethics committee to make that kind of judgment, however, is at odds with its function. An ethics committee should be one forum in an institution disinterested in the liability interests of the facility.

6. How can Jocelyn's situation be resolved?

Jocelyn's physicians, over a series of attempts, have been unable to find a period of time when she clearly possesses decisional capacity. It is likely that she no longer has sufficient abilities to render this sort of decision and her previously expressed wishes should be upheld. One must now investigate her prior wishes in an attempt to decide as she would if she now could. There is nothing in this scenario to lead one to believe that Jocelyn would now revoke or disavow these prior wishes. This is precisely the time to honor her oral advance directive, rather than discard it as not relevant to this "new" incarnation of Jocelyn.

Nina's request that the respirator now be withdrawn should be honored unless some technical, procedural mechanisms in place in this jurisdiction either limit the scope of surrogate decision making or require some more formal proceedings to clarify wishes or oversee the withdrawal of treatment. Caregivers should, however, also facilitate a dialogue with Jocelyn's mother to ensure that her concerns as the mother of the patient are addressed and to make sure that any additional information that she may have about her daughter's wishes are considered in the process. If the decision to withdraw the respirator is ultimately respected, plans must also be developed to provide sufficient medication to ensure the patient's comfort during this process.

REFERENCES

1. E.D. Viner, "Life at the Other End of the Endotracheal Tube: A Physician's Personal View of Critical Illness," *Progress in Critical Care Medicine* 2 (1985): 3–13.
2. R.S. Dresser and J.A. Robertson, "Quality of Life and Nontreatment Decisions for Incompetent Patients," *The Journal of Law, Medicine and Health Care* 17 (1989): 234–244.
3. R.S. Dresser and J.A. Robertson, "Life, Death and Incompetent Patients: Conceptual Infirmities and Hidden Values in the Law," *Arizona Law Review* 28 (1986): 373–412.
4. M.R. Gasner, "Financial Penalties for Failing To Honor Patient Wishes To Refuse Treatment, *St. Louis University Public Law Review* 11 (1992): 499–520.
5. Joint Commission on Accreditation of Healthcare Organizations, "Patient Rights and Organizational Ethics," in *Comprehensive Accreditation Manual for Hospitals: The*

Official Handbook (Oakbrook Terrace, IL: Joint Commission on Accreditation of Healthcare Organizations: 1997), appendix.

SUGGESTED READINGS

Alpers, A. 1998. Criminal act or palliative care? Prosecutions involving the care of the dying. *The Journal of Law, Medicine and Ethics* 26: 308–331.

American Psychiatric Association. 1994. Delirium. In *Diagnostic and statistical manual of mental disorders*, 123–133. 4th ed. Washington, DC.

Boumpas, D.T. et al. 1995. Systemic lupus erythematosus: Emerging concepts. Part 1. Renal, neuropsychiatric, cardiovascular, pulmonary, and hematologic disease. *Annals of Internal Medicine* 122: 940–950.

Boumpas, D.T. et al. 1995. Systemic lupus erythematosus: Emerging concepts. Part 2. Dermatologic and joint disease, the antiphospholipid antibody syndrome, pregnancy and hormonal therapy, morbidity and mortality, and pathogenesis. *Annals of Internal Medicine* 123: 42–53.

Dubler, N.N. 1993. Commentary: Balancing life and death—Proceed with caution. *American Journal of Public Health* 83: 23–25.

Dubler, N.N., and Marcus, L.J. 1994. *Mediating bioethical disputes*. New York: United Hospital Fund.

Easton, C., and MacKenzie, F. 1988. Sensory-perceptual alterations: Delirium in the intensive care unit. *Heart and Lung* 17: 229–237.

Kapp, M.B. 1998. *Our hands are tied: Legal tensions and medical ethics*. Westport, CT: Auburn House.

Krachman, S.L. et al. 1995. Sleep in the intensive care unit. *Chest* 107: 1713–1720.

Luce, J.M. 1997. Making decisions about the forgoing of life-sustaining therapy. *American Journal of Respiratory and Critical Care Medicine* 156: 1715–1718.

Luce, J.M. 1997. Withholding and withdrawal of life support: ethical, legal, and clinical aspects. *New Horizon* 5, no. 1: 30–37.

Prendergast, T.J. et al. 1998. A national survey of end-of-life care for critically ill patients. *American Journal of Respiratory and Critical Care Medicine* 158: 1163–1167.

President's Commission for the Study of Ethical Problems in Medicine and Biomedical and Behavioral Research. 1983. *Deciding to forgo life sustaining treatment*. Washington, DC: U.S. Government Printing Office.

Rhoden, N.K. 1988. Litigating life and death. *Harvard Law Review* 102: 375–446.

Ross, J.W. et al. 1993. *Health care ethics committees: The next generation*. Chicago: American Hospital Publishing.

Solomon, M.Z. et al. 1993. Decisions near the end of life: Professional views on life-sustaining treatments. *American Journal of Public Health* 83: 14–23.

West, S.G. et al. 1995. Neuropsychiatric lupus erythematosus: A 10-year prospective study on the value of diagnostic tests. *American Journal of Medicine* 99: 153–163.

Wolkowitz, O.M. et al. 1997. Glucocorticoid medication, memory and steroid psychosis in medical illness. *Annals of the New York Academy of Science* 823: 81–96.

Zuckerman, C. 1999. *End-of-life care and hospital legal counsel: Current involvement and opportunities for the future.* New York: Milbank Memorial Fund.

LEGAL CITATIONS

Case Examples

Barber v. Superior Court, 147 Cal. App. 3d 1006, 195 Cal. Rptr. 484 (1983), *aff'd People v. Barber,* No. A025586 (Los Angeles Mun. Ct. March 9, 1983).
Criminal charges dismissed in this case involving the withdrawal of treatment.

State of Kansas v. Naramore, Case No. 77,069, Court of Appeals of the State of Kansas (1998).
Criminal charges dismissed on appeal for a Kansas physician charged with murder and attempted murder in a case involving a severely ill patient at the end of life.

CASE 5

"Don't Tell Mother":
Withholding Information
from a Patient

Lillian is an 84-year-old woman who has developed dysphagia. She is not concerned by the symptoms, which she says are mild and occur only if she "eats too fast." Her son is concerned and persuades her to have a medical evaluation. The workup has revealed a mediastinal mass imping-ing on the esophagus. A biopsy is recommended. If, as feared, the patient has cancer, immediate surgery, including laryngectomy and tracheostomy, would be required for obstruction to be avoided. Radiation and chemo-therapy may produce palliation but are not expected to produce a cure. Even with treatment, obstruction is likely to occur, though at a later date.

Lillian appears to be otherwise in good health. She does have severe hearing loss, so that a great deal of time and patience are required to ex-plain matters to her, but she is alert and oriented and appears mentally intact. She lives in an apartment next door to her son and his family and is dependent on them for transportation, but she is able to make decisions concerning activities of daily living, such as shopping and managing her financial affairs. She has not asked many specific questions about her cur-rent situation, to her doctor's relief, since it would take so long to explain to her the intricacies of her workup. Her son asks the doctor not to tell his mother the diagnosis because she will tolerate neither the news nor the disfiguring operation. He says she has a history of depression and has al-ways considered her physical appearance her top priority. He argues that her symptoms are truly mild and do not seem to have progressed signifi-cantly over two years. Perhaps her tumor is so unusual that she may not need radical treatment. Even if it isn't, her son points out, she is 84 years old and may die of an unrelated cause, so that this invasive plan of care would not be appropriate.

ISSUES TO CONSIDER

- Truth telling
- Therapeutic privilege
- Patient delegation of decision-making authority

MEDICAL CONSIDERATIONS

1. How valid is the son's argument that the progress of his mother's tumor eliminates the need for an invasive care plan?

Lillian's son raised a thought-provoking issue that should be factored into the patient's prognosis. The progress of this tumor has been slower than one would expect; her symptoms have not progressed, and the patient has not lost weight. The incidence of cancer increases with age and although a few specific malignancies are more aggressive in older individuals (e.g., Hodgkin's disease) most studies purporting to look at tumors in old age have actually reported on individuals less than 80 years of age. The incidence of cancer continues to increase in the last decades of life, but cancers that appear in the oldest-old tend in general to be less aggressive, nonmetastatic, and less often the underlying cause of death.[1] The reasons for this are not well defined, and if true in some cases it is by no means a universal feature of cancer in late life. Any apparent reduction in cancer aggressiveness may simply represent the greater vulnerability to and higher prevalence of cardiovascular or cerebrovascular disease and propensity to death from such disease.

Another possible factor may be that old age selects for positive biologic characteristics, so that people who have survived into late life may be able to withstand a variety of exogenous insults, including those that initiate and promote carcinogenesis. Very old people who have failed to develop cancer may likewise represent survivors of any heritable tendencies toward the development of cancer. There is evidence from animal studies that at least some cancers tend to grow more slowly in old age; this has been attributed by some to certain aspects of immune senescence, since competent immune cells may stimulate tumor growth factors. From a clinical perspective, all-cause mortality may not be enhanced by treating certain cancers in old age, prostate cancer being an important example.[2,3] Others argue that epidemiologic data are confounded by the existence of a biologic elite or, among cancer victims, by comorbidity, in which the immediate cause of death was a noncancerous condition, even though the presence of cancer might have led more quickly to a noncancer death. Some epidemiologic data show that cancer mortality increases with age, but this, too, may be confounded by the presence of comorbidities, treatment biases, and other confounders.

The controversy over prognosis of cancer among the very old in general remains unresolved. This issue has been reviewed recently.[4] In any case, it is not possible to predict the course of Lillian's tumor.

ETHICAL AND LEGAL CONSIDERATIONS

1. Should Lillian be told her diagnosis?

The physician's primary obligation is to the patient, in this case, Lillian. The principle of self-determination requires that the physician disclose to the patient all reasonable information relevant to her condition and treatment options so that she can make an individually appropriate decision. This discussion would presumably include information that might upset Lillian, and although the physician might need to utilize an especially sensitive approach to deliver the news, this would mean only that the process of disclosure might vary from the typical pattern. The fact that the information is upsetting would not provide a justification to withhold that information from the patient. Presumably, if a dialogue has developed between Lillian and her physician, the patient herself might have given clues as to how much or what type of information she would like to have.

In this case, it appears that little dialogue has actually occurred between Lillian and her physician. Her hearing impairment may have acted as a barrier, however, this could be overcome if the physician took the time to communicate effectively, using written explanations when necessary, or had the son assist in this disclosure either in the doctor's office or privately. This news does not need to be delivered quickly; a gradual process might be adopted as part of a strategy to inform her in a way that she could tolerate emotionally.

Another barrier has been posed by the son's assertion that Lillian will be unable to handle this upsetting news, reinforced by the patient's lack of inquiry. It cannot be concluded, however, that Lillian does not desire information merely because she has not demonstrated an inquisitive nature concerning her illness. As a member of an older generation, she may not feel the need or be aware of a right to know the details or to be so heavily involved in the decision-making process. Alternatively, she may have been reluctant to inquire out of fear concerning her situation. Her physician would have to address this but not by unilaterally deciding to withhold information from her. Clearly, the only way to confirm whether or not Lillian wishes to be shielded from distressing information is to hear her own thoughts through dialogue. There is no evidence that patients in general wish to be protected from distressing information. In fact, evidence from public opinion polls suggests the opposite—that most people want to hear the details of their situation, even if the information is burdensome or devastating.

There may, however, be circumstances in which the cultural or ethnic background of the patient and family influence their preferences for disclosure of information, thereby modifying the decision involvement of third parties from the usual autonomy-based model. Rather than make presumptions or generalizations based upon cultural identity, clinicians should directly inquire as to the particular preferences of individual patients.

The withholding of vital information can deny the patient the opportunity to contemplate and incorporate the *implications* of that bad news. There will be consequences, whether or not the patient is aware of them. In Lillian's case, esophageal or upper airway obstruction is a possibility, and she might want to consider important treatment options while she has decisional capacity. She might want to determine if disfiguring surgery would be preferable to the serious symptoms that might occur if the operation is not performed. If the surgery is not performed, she would need to be informed that she had the option of being sedated if those symptoms were to occur. More broadly, it would be important to know whether Lillian would prefer a palliative approach to care at this point or if she would also be interested in more aggressive, cure-oriented approaches to her condition. Without knowing that these options existed, the patient could not make an informed choice, to infuse her personal quality of life considerations into treatment decisions, or to make appropriate plans concerning her personal affairs.

Lillian still possesses a great deal of independence and authority in her life, despite her physical conditions and the heavy involvement of her son in her affairs. It may be that the patient *desires* to delegate authority to someone else. A competent patient does have the right to waive informed consent; however, before a decision is made to remove Lillian from the decision process, further evidence must be gathered that such removal is in fact in accord with *her* desires.

2. Could a decision be made to withhold information from Lillian based on her son's warning about her emotional state?

There are limited situations in which this would be justified. A physician may be excused from disclosing information to a patient when there is sufficient evidence that the patient is not psychiatrically or emotionally equipped to consider the information or that the disclosure of information itself would pose serious and immediate harm to the patient, for example, by inducing some physiologic response such as a heart attack or prompting suicidal behavior. This is known as the therapeutic exception to the informed consent process. In this limited circumstance, the benefit to be achieved by disclosure is outweighed by the harm induced from the disclosure itself. As a legal principle, the therapeutic exception (also called "therapeutic privilege") is intended to be restricted to few and highly select circumstances. If it is invoked at all, its use should be time limited; attempts must be made to return to the patient as decision maker if her emotional condition changes. It is also intended to be decision-specific; the patient's inability to be involved in one decision does not preclude her ability to tolerate a different, perhaps related decision, so that if additional questions needed to be considered by her, attempts would have to be made to raise them.

In this case, the son seems to believe that this news could actually *harm* Lillian, perhaps causing a deep depression. Given the apparent closeness of his relationship with his mother, one cannot lightly dismiss his concerns. However, it would be important for the physician to further explore Lillian's psychiatric history, values, and current state of mind before concluding that her son was correct.

It is important to remember that fears expressed by family members regarding disclosure of difficult information might reflect their own anxieties and not those of the patient. There is every possibility that her son is distressed about the inevitable loss of this essential person in his life, in addition to his wish to protect her from this burdensome news. Yet those feelings in the son would not support the withholding of information from the mother.

Even if the therapeutic exception were utilized in this case, this would not relieve the physician of the obligation to continually attempt to involve the patient in the decision process and prepare her for problems that may arise.

3. Can it be concluded that Lillian has delegated her decision-making authority to her son?

Clearly, Lillian's son is heavily involved in her medical decision making. He is, after all, the person who convinced her to start down this diagnostic path. The concept of patient autonomy was never meant to imply that patients should and must make decisions about their care in isolation. The fact that a patient would rely on her son for advice and support is natural and even justifiable in view of their close relationship. It is not at all clear, however, that Lillian wishes her son to take her place in the decision-making process. Unspoken delegation of authority may be natural for them, but Lillian's pattern of decision making in other aspects of her life suggests something to the contrary. If she wishes her son to be the primary decision maker, she does have the right to make such a delegation of authority.

Lillian could execute a health care power of attorney or proxy, formalizing her decision to have her son make medical decisions on her behalf. Usually such a formal transfer of authority would not become activated until the patient has lost decisional capacity. It would be unusual, yet perhaps consistent with the wishes of this patient, for a health care agent to make decisions for a patient while the patient still has capacity to participate. Certainly, the pattern here suggests that Lillian's son ought to be the authorized decision maker when and if Lillian does lose decisional capacity.

Such a delegation of decisional authority should be clearly established, however, rather than merely presumed, before the physician acts on it. There is often a tendency to assume that old age alone or physical frailty in an elderly patient reflects an equivalent mental frailty and decisional incapacity and that the patient is therefore in need of protection. This may lead caregivers to treat the elderly as though they are children, in need of others to make decisions on their behalf. The elderly may also be at greater risk of having their freedom of choice constrained because they are less vigorous or assertive or because their comprehension is somewhat slower. Therefore, it may be more important rather than less to take special precautions to ensure that Lillian is fully informed about her situation. Furthermore, physicians whose patients have decisional capacity have no right to discuss the patient's medical care with others unless the patient gives permission for this; this information is confidential and private. The physician should directly ask Lillian whether she wants her son to be involved in the decisions, and to what extent, and whether she would like all or part of the information about her condition disclosed to him.

The physician's primary obligation to the patient does not resolve the dilemma that the son's information has posed. The development of a plan (both as regards treatment and conveying information to the patient) should take time. The son could and probably should be included in this process. The information he has conveyed could well be highly pertinent; furthermore, excluding him outright would alienate him and might disrupt a therapeutic relationship between physician and patient.

REFERENCES

1. K.G. Manton et al., "Cancer Mortality, Aging, and Patterns of Comorbidity in the United States: 1968 to 1986," *Journals of Gerontology* (1991) 46: S225–S234.
2. P.C. Albertsen, "Competing Risk Analysis of Men Aged 55 to 74 Years at Diagnosis Managed Conservatively for Clinically Localized Prostate Cancer," *Journal of the American Medical Association* (1998) 280: 975–980.
3. L.M. Franks, "Latent Carcinoma of the Prostate," *Journal of Pathology and Bacteriology* (1954) 68: 603–616.
4. W.B. Ershler and D.L. Longo, "Aging and Cancer: Issues of Basic and Clinical Science," *Journal of the National Cancer Institute* (1997) 89: 1489–1497.

SUGGESTED READINGS

Buckman, R. 1992. *How to break bad news. A guide for health care professionals.* Baltimore: The Johns Hopkins University Press.

Council on Ethical and Judicial Affairs of the American Medical Association. 1992. Opinion 8.08—Informed consent; Opinion 8.12—Patient information, *Code of Ethics: Annotated Current Opinions*, 69, 72. Chicago: American Medical Association.

Harris, L. et al. 1982. Views of informed consent and decision making: Parallel surveys of physicians and the public. In *Making Health Care Decisions, Vol. 2, Empirical Studies of Informed Consent,* President's Commission for the Study of Ethical Problems in Medicine and Biomedical and Behavioral Research, 17. Washington, DC: U.S. Government Printing Office.

Katz, J. 1984. *The silent world of doctor and patient.* New York: Free Press.

Lidz, C. et al. 1980. Two models of implementing informed consent. *Archives of Internal Medicine* 148: 1385–1389.

MacDonald, M. et al. 1991. *Health care law: A practical guide.* New York: Matthew Bender, Section 18.02 (3)—Consent Exceptions.

Mitchell, J.L. 1998. Cross-cultural issues in the disclosure of cancer. *Cancer Practice* 6: 153–160.

President's Commission for the Study of Ethical Problems in Medicine and Biomedical and Behavioral Research. 1982. The communication process. In *Making Health Care Decisions,* Vol.1, 69–111. Washington, DC: U.S. Government Printing Office.

CASE 6

Alternative Medicine for a Patient with Advanced Cancer

Sally is a 57-year-old woman with advanced rectal cancer. She has undergone two surgical procedures and now has local recurrence of tumor at the skin flap. Following this she has undergone two courses of chemotherapy with limited improvement. The patient is very motivated to "carry on," so her oncologist offers another course of chemotherapy and radiation therapy.

Sally visits her primary care physician, Dr. Wellbing, to discuss her options. She asks him what he thinks about shark cartilage, and mentions Dr. Natrium, a physician who specializes in alternative medicine. Although aware that conventional medicine can't cure Sally's disease, Dr. Wellbing does not want to endorse her going to this doctor, whom some consider a "quack." Besides, he has never heard of shark cartilage.

Dr. Natrium, who was trained in Eastern Europe, has a large patient following, despite his dubious reputation among community physicians. A number of years ago Dr. Natrium treated another cancer patient of Dr. Wellbing with herbal remedies, micronutrients, and Laetrile, and the patient died soon after that.

While pondering Sally's situation, Dr. Wellbing thinks about his cousin, Olga, a 44-year-old nurse with metastatic breast cancer. When spinal metastases appeared three years ago, she received radiation to the spine and chemotherapy, but she has since refused other approved medical treatments, including a bone marrow transplant. Instead, she receives alternative therapies prescribed by Dr. Natrium; these have included micronutrients, selenium, vitamins, pancreatic enzymes, and coffee enemas. He realizes that Olga appears to be in the best of health, and it has been three years since the metastases appeared.

Several other patients have asked Dr. Wellbing his opinion about herbal remedies and nutrients. He has had inquiries about such things as ginkgo, glucosamine, ginseng, and St. John's wort, to name a few, and he generally tells his patients, "We really don't know much about these unproved remedies. You might be wasting your money, or worse."

ISSUES TO CONSIDER

- Complementary/alternative medicine (CAM)
- Methods of ascertaining risks and benefits of CAM
- Physician liability in providing alternative medical treatments
- Provider legal or ethical obligations with regard to other providers who dispense unproven treatments

MEDICAL CONSIDERATIONS

1. What is meant by the term *alternative medicine*?

The term *alternative medicine* generally implies "therapies that . . . replace or substitute for an orthodox treatment." By contrast, *complementary medicine* generally refers to therapy that is used "in tandem with conventional treatments."[1] As terminology and consensus on the classification of these treatments evolves, many use the term *complementary/alternative medicine* (CAM). The boundaries between conventional, alternative, and complementary medicine are gray.

CAM can include approaches that are diverse in terms of their origin, methods, and acceptance compared to the orthodox, biomedical approach that became the prevailing method beginning early in the 20th century. A partial list of CAM therapies is given in Table 7–6.1.

Some approaches are governed by law and licensing requirements in a number of states (see Ethical and Legal Considerations, below), but this does not necessarily guarantee efficacy of the practice in question. For example, acupuncture may be useful in postoperative and chemotherapy nausea and vomiting and in certain types of pain, but more and appropriate study is needed to delineate specific conditions for which efficacy is claimed, such as smoking cessation and depression. Chiropractic involves manipulation and adjustment of the spine, but practitioners sometimes employ other CAM methods in their practice (as do practitioners of orthodox medicine). Although chiropractic manipulation is only infrequently associated with serious problems, neurological compromise and death have occurred. In this regard, it is important to emphasize that orthodox medicine is far from devoid of serious injury.

Table 7–6.1 Categories of Complementary/Alternative Medicine (CAM)

Acupressure	Megavitamins
Acupuncture	Movement therapy
Art therapy	Moxibustion
Ayurveda	Music therapy
Biofeedback	Naturopathy
Chiropractic	Prayer
Herbal medicine	Qi gong
Homeopathy	Relaxation
Hypnotherapy	T'ai chi
Imagery	Therapeutic touch
Macrobiotic diet	Yoga
Massage therapy	

Homeopathy involves administration of microconcentrations of the substance believed to be the etiologic agent of the condition for which it is recommended. Despite its wide acceptance in the United Kingdom and practice acts in a number of states, there is no evidence from controlled trials that homeopathic remedies are effective (other than "tincture of time"). Homeopathic remedies are generally safe, although contamination by heavy metals (as opposed to toxic concentration of intended substances) has been reported.

Naturopathy is variously defined in the states where practice acts exist, but generally emphasizes self-healing, reduction of oxidative stress with nutritional agents, herbal, nutritional, and mind-body approaches, and other CAM practices like homeopathy and acupuncture.

2. What benefits can Sally expect from shark cartilage? Selenium? Coffee enemas?

Shark cartilage contains a protein with antiangiogenic properties that could theoretically inhibit tumor angiogenesis and reduce the growth and metastasis of malignant tumors. Additional theoretical support of efficacy comes from the observation that cartilage is resistant to tumor invasion. There is no information about shark cartilage pharmacokinetics or oral bioavailability, and commercial preparations would be subject to the same problems as other unapproved and minimally regulated substances (see below). One recent uncontrolled trial concluded that shark cartilage had no beneficial effect and mild to moderate toxicity.[2] Like earlier trials of the controversial substance, amygdalin (Laetrile),[3] the shark cartilage trial was conducted in patients with advanced cancer who had failed conventional treatments. Purified antiangiogenic factors are currently a subject of active research.

Selenium is one of many nutrients shown in epidemiologic studies to reduce the risk of a variety of cancers. It is believed to exert an anticarcinogenic effect through antioxidant and immunologic mechanisms. However, the efficacy of selenium and foods high in selenium content in cancer treatment has not been studied.

Coffee and other enemas have been recommended by some CAM practitioners for a variety of ailments for the purposes of "detoxification." Controlled studies have not been done, and frequent coffee enemas, like other enemas, can lead to fluid and electrolyte problems.

3. What benefits can Dr. Wellbing's other patients anticipate from their therapies?

Ginseng (*Panax ginseng*) in its various forms (dried root, leaves, flowers, and other components) has been used for a variety of indications, including lack of energy, infectious disease, cardiac problems, infertility, and others. More than 28 constituents have been identified and these exhibit a range of pharmacologic actions, possibly accounting for scattered reports of a variety of adverse effects. Ginseng has been widely used in China, but research papers are generally not available in English-language journals. Much more information is required before specific actions of available remedies can be delineated.

St. John's wort (*Hypericum perforatum*) is a botanical that may be effective and safe for some mood disorders, such as mild depression.[4] Studies in the United States are in progress. However, animal evidence has been cited to suggest that this agent could harm reproductive cells.[5]

Ginkgo biloba is the leaf of the ginkgo tree. There is some evidence that it improves memory or function in dementia,[6] but it is uncertain if these experimental findings are clinically meaningful. Ginkgo has not been directly compared to approved therapies like donezepil (Aricept) or tacrine (Cognex), both of which have demonstrated the same limited effects, and in the case of tacrine, potentially serious hepatotoxicity. Like St. John's wort, ginkgo may harm reproductive cells.[5]

Glucosamine sulfate has been recommended for osteoarthritis based on its role in the synthesis of cartilage constituents. Limited study suggests that glucosamine is more effective than placebo in reducing pain and stiffness associated with osteoarthritis, and on the short term and (in sharp contrast with nonsteroidal antiinflammatory agents) appears to lack significant side effects. There is no evidence that it cures arthritis, slows the progression, or is equal or superior to standard treatments.

Additional agents are reviewed in Suggested Readings. Unfortunately, some compendia list active ingredients, common indications, or theoretical or observed toxicities, but they provide information that is based largely on anecdotes, opinions, or studies that do not achieve the level of evidence required by contemporary biomedical standards. Published studies of CAM therapies have generally been small, poorly controlled, uncontrolled, or based on anecdote. In some schools of thought, proof of efficacy of alternative medicine is based on observation and often explained by spiritual or psychological factors, what conventional medicine would call the "placebo effect." However, as one commentator has noted with regard to the advent of placebo-controlled trials, "It was no longer sufficient for a therapy to work: it had to be better than placebo."[7] It is also important to note that orthodox medicine therapies are not always based on high levels of evidence but are given just the same,[8] and neither clinical trials nor government approval necessarily guarantee efficacy of a particular remedy.

Other obstacles exist that limit access to information and limit critical review by physicians in the United States. Most clinical trials are not published in English and have not been published in journals listed in Medline. Most trials of herbal remedies have been conducted outside the United States. Efforts are underway by various organizations to review, translate, and compile information contained in those studies. Since the recent establishment of the National Center for Complementary and Alternative Medicine of the National Institutes of Health, increasing numbers of CAM approaches have been subject to critical (evidence-based) review. A partial list of databases and Web sites geared toward evidence-based methods is given in the References,[1] and in Appendix A.

4. What are the potential risks of herbal remedies and nutritionals? How do these risks compare with risks of approved medications and other therapies?

Like approved therapies, unproved and unapproved therapies have been associated with risks. CAM approaches have not been part of standard medical training for most of the twentieth century, so the resulting ignorance on the part of physicians enhances any potential risks. Information that consumers obtain may not be reliable, and their providers are likely not informed enough to clarify any misconceptions or answer questions accurately.[9]

Herbal remedies pose a particular problem in that they are less regulated than traditional medications. Under legislation intended to address consumer interest in using dietary remedies, dietary supplements are not subject to the same pre-market testing requirements as are regular medications (see Ethical and Legal Considerations, below). The definition of dietary supplements was expanded to include herbs and other botanicals prepared to be ingested in pill or liquid form. Unlike morphine, quinine, and digitalis, which are purified extracts of botanicals, and which have been in use for many years, unregulated botanicals may have unexpected effects. Concentrations of active ingredients might vary considerably, depending on the method of preparation and the rigor of the manufacturer. This variability was the case with earlier botanical preparations of quinine, morphine, and digitalis. In addition, reports of dangerous contaminants in herbal remedies are numerous, and include heavy metals, pathogenic bacteria, pharmaceuticals such as steroids and warfarin, and unrelated botanicals not described on the label but that proved to be toxic.[10] Although Dr. Wellbing is aware that certain of his patients are using alternative therapies, large numbers of patients do not inform their doctors about their use of alternative treatments,[11] preventing the recognition of potential adverse effects, which might include interactions with conventional medications. Drug interactions are likely underreported because of physician ignorance of the patient's alternative therapies, as well as lack of available information about their pharmacologic properties.

As Dr. Wellbing notes, patients might be paying for substances that lack efficacy. Although individual over-the-counter remedies might be much less expensive than approved drugs, it is estimated that, nationally, out-of-pocket expenditures for alternative therapies exceed those of conventional therapies.

Clinical trials and government approval do not necessarily guarantee safety. Severe adverse effects are often recognized after a drug is approved by the Food and Drug Administration (FDA), released, and in use; some have been removed from the market after causing fatalities or serious toxicity. This is especially a problem among the elderly, who comprise a very small proportion of subjects in clinical trials but who experience the most adverse drug effects. The problem of adverse effects might be magnified for substances that do not undergo testing in clinical trials.

ETHICAL AND LEGAL CONSIDERATIONS

1. What ethical obligations would a physician have concerning his patient's interest in alternative therapeutic options?

Interest in and use of alternative and complementary modalities of treatment is now commonplace among patients in the United States. Several studies have documented the extensive use of a range of therapeutic options that lie outside of mainstream medicine yet have become integral to the day-to-day health regimens of millions of patients. Moreover, the prevalence of the use of alternative therapies cuts across socioeconomic, ethnic and cultural categories, making it difficult to generalize about the profile of patients who seek out such treatments. Even further complicating the picture is the lack of discussion about patient use of such therapies and the failure of many patients using these alternative options to disclose this to their physicians, as mentioned above. Clearly, conversation about alternative and complementary modalities must become a routine part of the physician-patient dialogue, perhaps even at the initial history-taking stage, no matter what the patient profile or disease entity.

Physicians have the obligation to respect their patients' autonomy, promote their patients' well-being, and prevent harm from befalling the patient due to medical interventions. The question is how to uphold these values in the context of patient interest in alternative therapies. The task is a challenging one, given the extreme range of options, the limited knowledge concerning safety and efficacy of many of these alternative modalities, and the varying motivations that spur patients on to seek out such options. The role of the physician may range from that of educator to facilitator, adviser, supporter, or even protector. Which role is appropriate is very dependent upon the type of treatment sought and the knowledge and expectations of the patient.

At a minimum, education and information would seem to be essential aspects of any conversation about patient usage of alternative therapies. To the extent the physician has limited knowledge or is unaware of the benefits and risks of the proposed treatment, there would be an obligation to admit a lack of knowledge, to become more informed, and to share this information with the patient. It is no longer an option, ethically or legally, in the current health care climate, to shrug off patient interest or give out vague warnings about alternative modalities. Once physician and patient are more informed of the demonstrated benefits and risks of such options, then more informed decision making can occur, and physicians will be better positioned to determine what kind of role to play in facilitating patient use of alternative therapies. To the extent potential harm is identified or possible therapeutic benefits are uncovered, the physician will be better able to advocate in the appropriate direction for the patient.

Determining risks and benefits and helping patients weigh these options, however, is complicated in the context of alternative therapies. First, much of what is known about these treatment options is anecdotal, thus making it difficult to know precise benefits and burdens of particular treatments. To the extent this calculation is not possible, physicians must educate patients about the risks of these uncertainties and how to evaluate the information available to the public. Moreover, many reasons may impel patients to seek out alternative therapies, beyond the benefit they perceive in a particular situation. Commentators have cited many of the characteristics associated with alternative therapies as appealing to a large percentage of the patient population. Such characteristics include an association of what is "natural" with what is safe and appropriate; the linkage made in alternative therapies between the body and the mind, as well as the patient's spiritual self; the sense of control one may be able to exert over one's health; and the individualized approach to care often practiced by alternative practitioners. To the extent these elements are not addressed and discussed with the patient, efforts to dissuade patients from using alternative therapies may be unsuccessful. Some studies have suggested that the extensive use of alternative therapies by millions of patients is not so much a rejection of mainstream medicine so much as a desire to complement or enhance one's health practices with these additional therapies. Few patients exclusively rely on alternative therapies. But many patients seek these out for something more, for something missing from their encounters with the mainstream health system. To the extent these concerns can be identified and addressed, patients and their physicians will be better situated to determine if the benefits they may find in alternative practices are worth the potential risks they may encounter. Such an exploration must, of necessity, result from a shared inquiry and dialogue between physicians and patients.

In this particular case, Dr. Wellbing would be well advised to both investigate whatever is currently known about shark cartilage and explore more broadly with the patient herself what she hopes for in her encounters with Dr. Natrium. For a patient in the late stages of an illness, for whom "nothing more can be done," the desire to seek out therapies beyond the mainstream offerings is understandable and suggests more deep-seated fears, as well as a loss of hope with mainstream options. To the extent that a substance such as shark cartilage offers little benefit but no real harm, the physician may have little role to discourage the patient beyond informing her of what has been studied and what is known of the possible benefits and risks of the treatment. The greater the potential risk of harm of the alternative option, the stronger would be the educational and advocacy role of the physician. Certainly patients are entitled to seek out whatever treatments they wish, but Dr. Wellbing, to the extent possible, should at least try to ensure that the patient doesn't suffer further as a result of her treatment strategies, especially if no benefit is likely to be gained.

2. What is the role of the government in regulating the use of alternative therapies or the prescribing of nontraditional substances for therapeutic effect? Can patients at least be assured of some regulatory oversight and safety of these options?

Unlike the practice of mainstream medicine, in which physicians, nurses, and other clinical staff are licensed and regulated, and whose drugs, medications, and devices are regulated by the FDA, regulation of alternative and complementary health practices is less standardized and often varies significantly from one state to another and from one practice to another. Some alternative therapies have reached the point of integration into mainstream health practices to the extent that their practitioners are fully licensed akin to physicians (e.g., chiropractors) whereas others, such as homeopaths, are governed by state practice acts in certain states yet not in others. As well, substances "prescribed" for various ailments or health problems by alternative practitioners may or may not be under scrutiny of regulatory bodies, so that the ingredients and degree of purity of any particular substance may vary by brand and manufacturer, leaving patients in a potentially vulnerable situation concerning the risks of ingesting such substances.

There are several levels of state governmental oversight that can apply to various practitioners of alternative and complementary medicine. The most rigorous oversight is that of licensing, which defines and restricts the scope of practice of the practitioner and which makes it illegal for unlicensed individuals to offer the same service. The purpose of licensing is to set and sustain criteria intended to ensure the safety, efficacy, and propriety of the health service. For example, in all 50 states, chiropractors are licensed, thus ensuring a certain level of quality of services provided and creating the opportunity for state boards to discipline or remove the licenses of those chiropractors whose quality of services falls below a set professional standard. Licensing also mandates a certain level of education and training and is usually a prerequisite for insurance reimbursement of such services. In 42 states, health insurance coverage for chiropractic services has been mandated by state law. Currently, 27 states license acupuncturists, 23 states license massage therapists, and 3 states license homeopathic doctors.

A less rigorous method of state oversight is certification, through which certain standards regarding education, exam scores, and experiences are set and which grant the title of "certified" to those individuals meeting such criteria. The least rigorous method of oversight is registration, which merely requires the practitioner to file his or her name with a state agency but which does not mandate a certain level of skill or educational attainment per se. Various arguments can be mounted to support or oppose these state-imposed requirements on alternative and complementary practitioners. To a great extent, requiring certain levels of expertise and education provides a level of assurance to the public regarding the safety and quality of the individual practitioner. It may also, then, allow them to seek insurance reimbursement for the services. Alternatively, some argue that this type of oversight does not neatly fit with many alternative therapies, whose individualized approaches defy standardization. As well, the more government oversight and scrutiny, the more likely the costs of the service will need to incorporate those additional costs as part of the service fee.

Regarding the various substances used as a part of alternative and complementary medicine, much activity has occurred on the federal level in recent years to determine the level of government oversight necessary and to set standards for claims that can be made by various products and manufacturers. In 1938, the original Food Drug and Cosmetic Act was passed by Congress, in response to the tragic deaths of almost 100 individuals as a result of ingesting elixir of sulfanilamide. This original act was intended to put the manufacturing and marketing of various drugs and other therapeutic substances under the oversight of the federal government. A 1962 amendment to this act, known as the Kefauver-Harris Act, further required manufacturers to provide proof of the safety and efficacy of the product to the FDA prior to marketing the drug. This amendment was prompted by the early 1960s tragedies involving thalidomide. Interestingly, the 1938 passage of the original act exempts homeopathic remedies from FDA regulation, an exemption that remains in effect today.

Meeting the safety and efficacy standards set by the FDA can be a time-consuming and expensive process for manufacturers, involving three different phases of testing for safety and efficacy under carefully controlled experiments. Such experimental trials can take years and require extraordinary financial investment on the part of the manufacturer, with no clear guarantee that the end result will be a profitable product that can be offered to the public. Moreover, further surveillance is also required after FDA approval. This process, while attempting to ensure a certain level of safety and efficacy for the public, also contributes to the extraordinary costs associated with many common pharmaceutical products. For practitioners and consumers of alternative and complementary practices, such a rigorous process would probably mean that many of the currently employed products would no longer be available or affordable.

A groundswell of various political interests aligned in 1994 to spearhead the passage of the federal Dietary Supplement Health and Education Act, which was directly intended to address consumer use of nontraditional, alternative products. In essence, under the passage of this legislation, many of the substances commonly used and recommended as a part of alternative health practices are exempt from the stringent regulation of the FDA. The Act was specifically intended to address the use of substances ingested as a "dietary supplement." Under the regulations of the Act, substances that are intended to supplement the diet, rather than directly treat, cure, or mitigate a specific disease, fall under this FDA exemption. Such substances are likely to contain vitamins, minerals, botanicals, or herbal products and would include such commonly used substances as ginseng, garlic, or various fish oils.

Exemption from FDA regulation has meant, however, that the packaging and promotion of these substances is restricted regarding claims that can be made about their health benefits. Products that fall under the 1994 Dietary Supplement Health and Education Act cannot be marketed with the claim that they will aid in the prevention or treatment of illness. Their labels can make no claims concerning the ability to treat, cure, or mitigate disease. Furthermore, the label must make clear that the product has not been approved by the FDA. The labels and advertising are permitted to claim that they help affect or maintain a structure or function of the body. Such subtle distinctions, however, may clearly escape the notice of average consumers, many of whom clearly believe that the use of such products will, in fact, help treat their various illnesses or cure their diseases. This is especially worrisome given the lack of regulatory scrutiny over the exact ingredients and production of these products. It is possible, for example, that a patient purchasing two different brands of ginseng will in fact be purchasing very different products, with different ingredients, leading to different results. Harm resulting from such products can only be addressed after the fact, as the FDA may only intervene in the manufacturing and marketing of such products after they have been sold to the public, if harm results. Patients, therefore, are at potential risk of either purchasing ineffective products or, even worse, putting themselves at risk from the unknown by ingesting various substances contained in such products.

3. Do physicians risk any liability in supporting their patients' use of alternative or complementary health options?

Physician liability for the use of or referral to alternative or complementary treatment modalities is a new area of malpractice concern for physicians. To date, there has been little litigation for malpractice directly aimed at alternative care providers (such as chiropractors, massage therapists, or acupuncturists) and even less involving mainstream physicians whose patients brought suit against them following the use of alternative modalities of treatment. This limited litigation to date is likely the result of a number of factors: The burgeoning use of such alternative methods is relatively recent; the invasiveness of many of these procedures is limited, thus suggesting fewer harmful outcomes that might lead to malpractice litigation; and the types of relationships patients often have with alternative practitioners is likely to be very individualized, leaving patients less likely to use litigation as a means to resolve disputes or address poor outcomes. While the risks of many of these procedures and substances is unknown (thus leaving open the possibility of real harm and subsequent litigation), to date this has been a limited area of malpractice litigation.

Despite the lack of precedent, for mainstream physicians who wish to support their patients' choices involving interventions and options outside of mainstream medicine, there are some concerns with regard to theoretical possibilities of liability. First, if a physician were to incorporate any of these nonstandard practices into her own practice, she would need to be fully informed about the existing risks and benefits of such treatments, and she should be prepared to both inform and justify to patients why such a nontraditional alternative might be appropriate for the particular patient. If the physician were to have direct responsibility or oversight for the delivery of such services (for example, if the physician employed a massage therapist as a part of her practice), then, due to her supervisory position, she could be held accountable for the actions of this employee and could be held responsible for poor outcomes in the patient. For example, there have been malpractice cases brought against physicians for the negligent actions of allied health professionals under their supervision.

Another possible area of liability would arise from the physician's referral of the patient to an alternative health practitioner. For example, if the physician referred the patient to a local chiropractor to help with back pain, or referred the patient to a local acupuncturist for help with pain management, such referrals ought to be done with care and in an informed manner. Certainly in such cases the physician should do all she can to ensure that the referral practitioner is a licensed professional (to the extent that is possible within the state), in good standing, and whose treatment is known to be efficacious and safe, to the extent such knowledge is available. What would be of particular concern is if physician and referral practitioner were jointly managing the patient, such that the physician might be held accountable for actions of the referral practitioner. This concern underscores the necessity of being familiar with the scope and quality of services of the referral practitioner, just as the physician would do in cases of referring the patient to other specialist physicians. In this particular case, Dr. Wellbing would be well advised to more carefully explore or understand Dr. Natrium's training, licensing status, and scope of practice before endorsing the patient's seeking out such help or before cooperating in a collaborative way with this other physician's practices.

In general, physicians are obligated to provide patients with treatment options that fall within the acceptable standard of care, and to inform patients of the risks and benefits of each option so that the patient can make an informed choice. They must also ensure that the quality of the care they provide meets the prevailing standard of care. To the extent that a physician and patient begin to explore options outside of the usual standard of care for the patient's particular situation, they must be sure that the patient is fully cognizant of the benefits, risks, and uncertainties of such a path. In addition, the patient must be made aware of the more mainstream approaches to the condition (and the risks and benefits of these interventions), so that whatever the patient's choice, it is both informed and voluntary. Critical to this process is open and ongoing communication that is responsive to the fears and concerns of the patient. Open communication and a relationship of trust and honesty are critical factors in developing a strong physician-patient relationship and also critical factors in lessening the likelihood of litigation should a poor outcome arise.

Finally, as stated earlier, the majority of patients using alternative therapies do not disclose this fact to their primary physician, and, in fact, most use of alternative or complementary options is done so without the supervisory input of a physician or other professional expert. To the extent that such alternative practices, in combination with more mainstream options, could lead to potential harm to patients (for example, toxic interactions between prescribed pharmaceuticals and patient use of various herbal remedies) the physician would be well advised to become familiar with possibly negative interactions and to inquire about patient use of such substances prior to prescribing such recommendations to the patient.

REFERENCES

1. J.W. Spencer and J.J. Jacobs, *Complementary/Alternative Medicine. An Evidence-Based Approach.* (St. Louis: Mosby, 1999).
2. D.R. Miller et al., "Phase I/II Trial of the Safety and Efficacy of Shark Cartilage in the Treatment of Advanced Cancer," *Journal of Clinical Oncology* 16 (1998): 3649–3655.
3. C.G. Moertel et al., "A Clinical Trial of Amygdalin (Laetrile) in the Treatment of Human Cancer," *New England Journal of Medicine* 306 (1982): 201–206.
4. K. Linde et al., "St. John's Wort for Depression—An Overview and Meta-Analysis of Randomized Clinical Trials," *British Medical Journal* 313 (1996): 253–258.
5. R.R. Ondrizek et al., "An Alternative Medicine Study of Herbal Effects on the Penetration of Zona-Free Hamster Oocytes and the Integrity of Sperm Deoxyribonucleic Acid," *Fertility and Sterility* 71 (1999): 517–522.
6. B.S. Oken et al., "The Efficacy of Ginkgo Biloba on Cognitive Function in Alzheimer Disease," *Archives of Neurology* 55 (1998): 1409–1415.
7. T.J. Kaptchuk, "Powerful Placebo: The Dark Side of the Randomized Controlled Trial," *Lancet* 351 (1998): 1722–1725.
8. R. Smith, "Where Is the Wisdom...? The Poverty of Medical Evidence," *British Medical Journal* 303 (1991): 798–799.
9. J. Borkan et al., "Referrals for Alternative Therapies," *Journal of Family Practice* 39 (1994): 545–550.

10. N.R. Slifman et al., "Contamination of Botanical Dietary Supplements by *Digitalis lanata*," *New England Journal of Medicine* 339 (1998): 806–811.
11. D.M. Eisenberg et al., "Trends in Alternative Medicine Use in the United States, 1990–1997: Results of a Follow-Up National Survey," *Journal of the American Medical Association* 280 (1998): 1569–1575.

SUGGESTED READINGS

Angell, M., and Kassirer, J.P. 1998. Alternative medicine—The risks of untested and unregulated remedies. *New England Journal of Medicine* 339: 839–840.

Assendelft, W.J. et al. 1995. The relationship between methodological quality and conclusions in reviews of spinal manipulation. *Journal of the American Medical Association* 274: 1942–1948.

Astin, J.A. 1998. Why patients use alternative medicine. Results of a national study. *Journal of the American Medical Association* 279: 1548–1553.

Blumenthal, M., ed. 1998. *The complete German Commission E monographs—A therapeutic guide to herbal medicine.* Integrative Medicine Communications, Newton, MA.

Brzezinski, A. 1997. Melatonin in humans. *New England Journal of Medicine* 336: 186–195.

Cohen, M.J. 1998. *Complementary and alternative medicine; Legal boundaries and regulatory perspectives.* Baltimore: The Johns Hopkins University Press.

da Camara, C.C., and Dowless, G.V. 1998. Glucosamine sulfate for osteoarthritis. *Annals of Pharmacotherapy* 32: 580–587.

Davidoff, F. 1998. Weighing the alternatives: Lessons from the paradoxes of alternative medicine. *Annals of Internal Medicine* 129: 1068–1070.

Eisenberg, D.M. 1997. Advising patients who seek alternative medical therapies. *Annals of Internal Medicine* 127: 61–69.

Eisenberg, D.M. et al. 1993. "Unconventional" medicine in the United States: Prevalence, costs, and patterns of use. *New England Journal of Medicine* 328: 246–252.

Ernst, E. 1997. Complementary AIDS therapies: The good, the bad and the ugly. *International Journal of STD and AIDS* 8: 281–285.

Ernst, E., and Cassileth, B.R. 1998. The prevalence of complementary/alternative medicine in cancer: A systematic review. *Cancer* 83: 777–782.

Hensrud, D.D. et al. 1999. Underreporting the use of dietary supplements and nonprescription medications among patients undergoing a periodic health examination. *Mayo Clinic Proceedings* 74: 443–447.

Kaptchuk, T.J. et al. 1998. Chiropractic. *Archives of Internal Medicine* 158: 2215–2224.

Kaptchuk, T.J., and Eisenberg, D.M. 1998. The persuasive appeal of alternative medicine. *Annals of Internal Medicine* 129: 1061–1065.

Lerner, M. 1996. *Choices in healing.* Cambridge, MA: MIT Press.

Linde, K. et al. 1997. Are the clinical effects of homeopathy placebo effects? A meta-analysis of placebo-controlled trials. *Lancet* 350: 834–943.

National Institutes of Health. 1997. *NIH Consensus Statement (Acupuncture)* 15(5): 1–34.

Milbank Memorial Fund. 1998. *Enhancing the accountability of alternative medicine.* New York: Milbank Memorial Fund.

Miller, L.G. 1998. Herbal medicinals. Selected clinical considerations focusing on known or potential drug-herb interactions. *Archives of Internal Medicine* 158: 2200–2211.

PDR for herbal medicine. 1998. 1st ed. Montvale, NJ: Medical Economics Company.

Sale, D.M. 1994. *Overview of legislative development concerning alternative health care in the United States.* Kalamazoo, MI: John E. Fetzer Institute.

Simmons, C., and Simmons, M. 1998. Drugs and dietary supplements: Ramifications of the Food, Drug, and Cosmetic Act and the Dietary Supplement Health and Education Act. *West Virginia Journal of Law and Technology* 2: 3–19.

Studdert, D.M. et al. 1998. Medical malpractice implications of alternative medicine. *Journal of the American Medical Association* 280: 1610–1615.

Sugarman, J., and Burk, L. 1998. Physicians' ethical obligations regarding alternative medicine. *Journal of the American Medical Association* 280: 1623–1625.

Wilt, T.J. et al. 1998. Saw palmetto extracts for treatment of benign prostatic hyperplasia: A systematic review. *Journal of the American Medical Association* 280: 1604–1609.

LEGAL CITATIONS

Statutory Examples

Colorado General Statute 12-36-117 (enacted August, 1997): Unprofessional Conduct: (3a).
State statute providing that the practice of alternative medicine by itself is not sufficient grounds to take disciplinary actions against a physician. Physicians who practice alternative medicine must inform patients in writing, at the first visit, of the physician's education, experience, and credentials related to the alternative medicine practiced by that physician.

Dietary Supplement Health and Education Act of 1994 (Public Law 103-417).
Federal law that exempts dietary supplements from regulation by the Food and Drug Administration.

CASE 7

Painful Treatment for a Severely Retarded Man

Bill is a profoundly retarded man who has lived in a state hospital for many years. He has no contact with family members, and he has become a ward of the state. At the age of 58, Bill developed acute myelogenous leukemia (AML). Chemotherapy has been recommended, but its appropriateness was questioned on the basis that Bill would not understand the uncomfortable and prolonged treatment of a disease with such an uncertain prognosis. His physicians wonder if they should forgo attempts at treatment and instead adopt a palliative care plan.

ISSUES TO CONSIDER

- Medical decision making in adults who have never had decisional capacity
- State interests in treatment decision making
- Treatments with a limited chance of success: balancing benefits and burdens and establishing goals of care

MEDICAL CONSIDERATIONS

1. What factors should enter into the decision regarding chemotherapy or other treatments?

Acute myelogenous leukemia has a limited prognosis. Disease-free and overall survival have improved with advances in treatment protocols, so that approximately 70 to 80 percent of patients under the age of 60 who are well enough to undergo chemotherapy achieve a complete remission following induction chemotherapy. Their five-year survival, however, which may involve continued treatments for relapse or complications, still remains under 40 percent and is probably closer to 25 percent for someone

Bill's age. The prognosis for patients over age 60 is poor, largely due to treatment-related mortality.

In order to achieve and sustain remission, Bill would need to undergo induction chemotherapy, an intensive hospital-based regimen of three to four weeks, followed by an intensive course of postremission chemotherapy. Both the initial and postremission therapy would be expected to produce toxicity and would require frequent blood tests and intravenous treatments. Although the problem of venous access can be simplified by a subcutaneously lying, central venous (Hickman) catheter, special vigilance would be needed to ensure that Bill would not attempt to dislodge it. Induction chemotherapy would be expected to produce alopecia, anorexia, nausea, vomiting, and bone marrow toxicity, with its attendant complications and need for further treatments and hospitalizations. A variety of other, less common drug-related toxicities, such as oral mucous membrane ulceration, abdominal pain, cholestasis, fever, myalgia, and rash can occur. Neurotoxicity occurs with greater frequency in patients over the age of 50. Bill might also experience complications of the disease itself, including painful leukemic cell infiltration of the bone marrow and involvement of other organ systems. Because he is incapable of understanding the disease and the reasons for the treatment interventions, the recurrent physical symptoms and the side effects of the treatment regimen are likely to be complicated by anxiety and fear.

Without bone marrow transplant, only about 20 percent of patients diagnosed with AML experience permanent remission, and this success rate depends on age and presence of cytogenetic abnormalities in leukemic cell line, conferring a poor prognosis. The likelihood of such abnormalities increases with age. New chemotherapy regimens (e.g., high-dose cytarabine) may produce better overall five-year survival than even allogeneic bone marrow transplant.[1] Overall, a few affected adults, most of these relatively young, achieve a prolonged disease-free survival.

Treatment decisions may be guided by cytogenetic studies. If the predicted prognosis were favorable, the treating physician might recommend a less toxic course of chemotherapy in a patient like Bill, although this decision would be based on practical or humanistic considerations rather than known outcomes.

2. Considering the fact that bone marrow transplant (BMT) offers the best hope of cure for this disease, should it be considered for this patient?

Allogeneic BMT from a immunologically matched relative offers the best hope for a cure. Among those who survive five years after treatment, relapse is rare, and survival rates from unrelated donors may approximate those from matched relatives. Unfortunately, the risk of acute graft-versus-host disease (GVHD) is approximately 30 to 60 percent, even when the donor is a fully matched sibling. Chronic GVHD, a debilitating illness that may last for years, occurs in approximately 50 percent of patients. The incidence of GVHD is higher when the donor is matched or partly matched, but unrelated, and increases with the age of the recipient. For this reason, allogeneic BMT for patients beyond 50 or 60 years of age is controversial. Autologous (autogeneic) transplant of stem cells from the patient is sometimes offered when no matched marrow donor can be found, but this carries a risk of reintroducing leukemic cells that were not apparent when the harvest occurred. Bone marrow harvest (whether autologous or allogeneic donor) involves an approximately two-hour procedure in which a series of needle aspirates are transplanted under regional or general anesthesia, followed by transfusions to counteract anemia caused by extraction of sufficient marrow. Postoperative pain is common.

Quality of life would be a particularly important consideration in a patient unable to comprehend the procedure or its consequences. Many patients die during the peritransplant period. Early death or serious morbidity can be due to the high-dose chemotherapy regimens given to patients expected to undergo BMT, the transplant itself, acute GVHD, relapse of leukemia, or other complications. Allogeneic transplant requires from one to two years of treatment with immunosuppressive agents, which increase the risk of opportunistic infections, and require prophylaxis with several antimicrobial agents. Neurologic problems are a known complication of allogeneic transplant, including encephalopathy, seizures, and psychiatric symptoms. Overall, patients in their first complete remission who have allogeneic or autologous bone marrow transplant experience worse quality of life from an array of symptoms and recurrent medical problems than those who received only intensive consolidation chemotherapy.[2]

3. Can a patient who is mentally retarded have the ability to participate in medical decision making?

The hallmark of mental retardation is impairment of intellectual function that has become manifest in the developmental period, that is, in childhood. This contrasts with cognitive disabilities that do not become manifest until adulthood, such as dementia (see Case 2, "Determining If a

Patient Has Decisional Capacity"). Like those with adult-onset cognitive dysfunction, patients with mental retardation have varying abilities. Some classifications have only two categories, mild and severe, while traditional systems include intermediate categories. Both systems base the grading on standard IQ tests,[3] with those with mental retardation having an IQ more than two standard deviations below the mean. This type of classification has been criticized because it does not take into account functional abilities or other aspects of a person's cognition and personality that foster the ability to adapt and perform activities of daily living. Classifications based solely on IQ have also been criticized because they do not take into account the many patients who are educable or trainable. The ability to perform activities of daily living, however, or even to engage in productive employment, does not necessarily mean a patient has the capacity to make an informed decision about medical treatment.

Bill's cognitive abilities are profoundly impaired, and there is no question that he lacks the ability to participate in the formal decision-making process. It is likely that most patients with mental retardation, except those with the mildest cognitive disabilities, lack the intellectual function to weigh risks and benefits of complex treatment interventions. Capacity is decision-specific, however, and some decisions would be amenable to the participation of certain patients with milder degrees of mental retardation. The elements of decisional capacity are discussed more fully in Case 2.

ETHICAL AND LEGAL CONSIDERATIONS

1. Who may make treatment decisions for a patient who never possessed decisional capacity?

Patients such as Bill are in a unique, and particularly vulnerable, situation. Given that this patient never possessed decisional capacity and perhaps not even a significant level of cognitive function, it is not possible to resort to the usual methods of surrogate decision making—reference to the previous wishes of the patient or the patient's previously held values. There can be no substituted judgment for someone who has never possessed judgment skills. Thus, any decision made on Bill's behalf would have to examine the proposed treatment in terms of promoting Bill's best interests. (It is possible that with patients with milder forms of retardation, they might have the capacity to consider at least some treatment options and perhaps to even execute an advance directive.)

Bill also lacks the sort of surrogates who normally are consulted when treatment decisions must be made on behalf of incapacitated patients. There is no one in a natural position of advocating for Bill, such as family or friends, who could serve as a wellspring of good intentions. His lack of a natural advocate makes him susceptible to the sort of value judgments and biases that might lead physicians to either overtreat, because of perceived legal obligations, or undertreat, because of biased evaluations concerning the quality of life or "value" of someone like Bill.

For individuals whose degree of mental retardation renders them decisionally incapable, it is not uncommon for their natural parents to become their legally appointed guardians once they reach the age of majority, that is, 18 years. In the normal transition from adolescent to adult, the legal presumption of competency empowers an individual when that person reaches majority. For mentally retarded persons such a legal presumption is not appropriate, as their level of impairment is such that even when reaching 18, they likely still do not possess the abilities necessary to conduct their life's affairs. Even though now technically adults, in the eyes of the law, they still retain the status of children. Thus, if important decisions needed to be made, such adults would require the appointment of a legal guardian to make decisions throughout their lives. Parents must in fact bring a formal judicial hearing to gain authority as the legal guardians for their retarded adult children. Such guardians, often the natural parents, would in most circumstances be empowered to make any and all decisions for the person, just as a parent would for a child, in accord with what the guardian perceives to be in that person's best interests. Of course, given the range of abilities and skills among the mentally retarded, it is possible that some such persons may be able to take on some activities of adult living without oversight or approval, either independently or with a guardian's assistance.

Bill has neither a natural parent as guardian nor any partial abilities that might permit him some involvement in the conduct of his life. He is a ward of the state, which means the state has the obligation, through the exercise of its officials, to look after him and support his well-being and welfare. There is a common-law principle, embodied in state statutes and regulations governing persons such as Bill, that the state has the obligation to oversee and support the well-being of those vulnerable persons in society who cannot look after themselves. This is known as the *parens patriae* power of the state, and it is the same authority that allows the state to intervene in family circumstances when the well-being of children is at stake, for example. The state's historical responsibility to oversee the well-being of persons such as Bill is reflected by the existence of state-run institutions, such as the one in which Bill resides.

The most likely resolution of this type of situation would be for the institution to seek judicial appointment of a guardian for the purpose of empowering someone, separate and apart from the institution, to make decisions for Bill. In a judicial hearing, a *guardian ad litem* would be appointed, whose job it would be to investigate the precise circumstances of Bill's condition and his physician's recommendations concerning treatment and then report this information back to the court. The judge would rely heavily on the *guardian ad litem*'s report and recommendations and would then rule on the appointment of a separate guardian in accord with the way the judge believes this case should proceed. The guardian would be legally empowered and required to make all subsequent health care decisions for Bill. Such decisions probably would be guided by whatever pronouncement the court made concerning the direction Bill's care should take, as well as the guardian's assessment of what serves Bill's best interests.

It should be noted that if a guardian already existed for Bill, whether a parent or some other involved person, resort to a court of law might not be necessary, although that would depend on the specific jurisdiction in which this occurred. It should also be noted that a court might appoint an organization, such as the Association for Retarded Citizens, to be the guardian for someone such as Bill, rather than a specific individual.

Separate from the procedural issue concerning who should make decisions for Bill, there would also be a question concerning the substantive criteria to be used in the decision-making process. As discussed previously, the standard of substituted judgment is not useful here, as this patient never possessed decisional capacity or a set of values that could guide the current decisions.

Despite a legal and ethical consensus that the substituted judgment standard does not apply in such a case, in the seminal *Saikewicz* case, the court purported to utilize this standard in reaching its decision. The *Saikewicz* case in Massachusetts involved circumstances essentially the same as Bill's, and the patient, Joseph Saikewicz, faced the same poor prognosis although with perhaps fewer treatment options. The Massachusetts Supreme Court stated that in the case of Mr. Saikewicz, the standard for surrogate decision making would be "one which will yield a decision which would be made by the incompetent person, if that person were competent, but taking into account the present and future incompetency as one of the factors which would necessarily enter into the decision making process of the competent person."

Although this early decision to allow the patient to forgo treatment has been hailed for its sensitivity, the reasoning has been soundly criticized as a contorted attempt to fit Mr. Saikewicz's situation into a scenario that defies both logic and reality. The *Saikewicz* case was one of the first high court decisions involving the forgoing of medical treatment, and as such, the court perhaps was reluctant to say that society could make a judgment to allow for the withholding of treatment. Instead, it appealed to the reasoning that a mentally retarded adult would have utilized if he could magically have been transformed into a decisionally capable person. While the logic of this line of reasoning is questionable, most of the considerations raised by the court in *Saikewicz* would be incorporated into a best-interests analysis. Thus, though couched in a substituted judgment approach, in essence the court was utilizing a best-interests standard, and the case has been admired for its sensitivity and comprehensive assessment of the factors and interests to be accounted for when such a decision is made.

Interestingly, a similar case in New York generated a decision diametrically opposed to *Saikewicz*. In the 1981 case, *In re Eichner (Storar)*, the New York Court of Appeals ruled that treatment for a retarded man, whose mother asked that such treatment be withheld, must nonetheless be given. The patient, John Storar, suffered from bladder cancer, and the treatment in question was the provision of blood transfusions. In such a case, the court stated, as there could never be evidence of what the patient would have wanted, and thus the decision would rest on the patient's best interests, it would be unacceptable to consider withholding life-prolonging treatment as being in the patient's best interests. In New York, the ability to withhold or withdraw life-sustaining treatment from incapacitated patients is significantly limited if such patients did not previously appoint a health care agent. If no such agent exists, then in the State of New York such care could only be withheld or withdrawn if clear and convincing evidence (such as a written or oral advance directive) exists of the patient's prior wishes (see Case 9, "Withholding Tube Feeding in a Woman with

Advanced Dementia"), something impossible to produce for a patient such as Bill.

The *Storar* case probably represents an unusual resolution to the scenario confronting Bill and his caregivers. The decision arrived at in *Storar* represents an early, conservative resolution in a state that chose and has frequently chosen since that time to err on the side of maintaining the patient's life. In most states, this type of problem is probably resolved without resort to a judicial proceeding. Interestingly, the *Saikewicz* decision is noted also for its insistence that all cases of withholding or withdrawing care in the state of Massachusetts would be appropriate for judicial intervention. Subsequent court decisions have modified this position somewhat so that most cases in Massachusetts no longer require judicial involvement.

2. What interests of the state might be invoked that could influence or restrict decisions to withdraw or withhold care?

Several cases, including *Saikewicz*, have articulated several interests of the state that might influence decisions to withhold or withdraw care in certain situations. Interests that have been invoked include the interest in the sanctity of life, the interest in the prevention of suicide, the integrity of the medical profession, and the interests of vulnerable third parties affected by the treatment decision.

In Bill's case, the concern regarding suicide is obviously not relevant because he is not capable of forming the intent to commit suicide. Moreover, courts of law and commentators have rigorously distinguished intentional acts of self-destruction from cases of withdrawing and withholding life-prolonging treatment.[4] In this case, there are also no vulnerable third parties affected by a decision for Bill. This concern is sometimes generated in cases in which a parent wishes to forgo life-sustaining treatment, leaving behind minor children who will then lack a caregiver. In such cases, the interests of the minors are not usually held to trump the self-determination of the patient, unless the children will truly be abandoned, with no available caretakers to step in (see Case 1, "A Religious Objection to a Blood Transfusion").

Bill's case, however, does raise the issue of the sanctity of life and the integrity of professionals who might be involved in his treatment. The *Saikewicz* court dealt directly with these two concerns. Regarding the sanctity of life, the court in *Saikewicz* made clear that the focus should not be merely on the length of the person's life, but also on the suffering and dignity of the individual whose life is in question. For a person such as Bill, who would experience significant additional suffering if treatment were initiated, the fact that his life *may* be extended is not enough reason by itself to administer the treatment. What must also be considered is the quality of that life, to the patient, in the context of the treatment intervention. For a patient such as Bill, who would not understand the pain and burdens he was made to suffer, concern over the sanctity of his life would not be sufficient to trump other considerations of the quality of that perhaps briefly extended life.

Regarding the integrity of the involved health care professionals, the *Saikewicz* court underscored the notion that the prevailing medical ethic does not require the provision of treatment in all circumstances. As the *Saikewicz* court asserted, "the prevailing ethical practice seems to be to recognize that the dying are more often in need of comfort than treatment." Likewise, for patients with decisional capacity who wish to forgo life-prolonging treatment, the prevailing ethical consensus also requires physicians to respect the wishes of the patient, as part of their obligations as health care professionals. *Not* honoring a patient's wish to forgo treatment would violate professional integrity. This notion has been consistently upheld by courts of law and supported by medical organizations and commentators in the field of bioethics.

Thus, in most cases in which these state interests are raised in decisions regarding life-prolonging treatment, such interests have not been found sufficiently weighty to counterbalance other legitimate interests of the patient.

3. What is the significance of the limited probability of the proposed treatment's success?

When determining what interests of Bill's are at stake and how those interests might best be served, the likelihood of a poor outcome would be significant in the balance. As discussed in Case 4 ("Management of Life-Threatening Illness"), the best-interests standard would require an examination of such issues as pain and suffering; diagnosis and prognosis, with and without treatment; and the quality of life, for that patient, if the treatment were initiated. More broadly, the benefits of the treatment for Bill ought to outweigh the burdens he would experience if the treatment were rendered.

The pain and suffering that Bill would be put through for a low likelihood of success would greatly influence the direction of the decision. In fact, the quality of his life would be paramount, not because as a retarded person his life is less valuable, but, because of his retardation and, thus, inability to understand what pain might be worth bearing for what possible benefits, his pain and suffering might be more significant than for a cognitively normal person in the same situation. The burdens of treatment must be examined in the context of the specific case. In Bill's case, these would be difficult to justify given the strong possibility of very limited benefit.

These factors would arguably lead a best-interests analysis to conclude that treatment for someone such as Bill could ethically be withheld. In place of treatment, providers would be obligated to do their utmost to keep him comfortable and free of pain and suffering as his physical condition deteriorated. While palliative care should always be a goal, in a case such as Bill's, relief of pain and suffering, rather than attempts to cure, should be the *primary* goal of care.

REFERENCES

1. P.A. Cassileth et al., "Chemotherapy Compared with Autologous or Allogeneic Bone Marrow Transplantation in the Management of Acute Myeloid Leukemia in First Remission," *New England Journal of Medicine* 339 (1998): 1649–1656.
2. R. Zittoun et al., "Quality of Life in Patients with Acute Myelogenous Leukemia in Prolonged First Complete Remission after Bone Marrow Transplantation (Allogeneic or Autologous) or Chemotherapy: A Cross-Sectional Study in the FORTC-GIMEMA AML 8A trial," *Bone Marrow Transplant* 20 (1997): 307–315.
3. E. Cipani, "Educational Classification and Placement," in *Handbook of Mental Retardation,* eds. J.L. Matson and J.A. Mulick. 2nd ed. (Elmsford, NY: Pergamon Press, 1991), 181–191.
4. *Vacco v. Quill,* 117 S. Ct. 2293 (1997).

SUGGESTED READINGS

Antonini, G. et al. 1998. Early neurologic complications following allogeneic bone marrow transplant for leukemia: A prospective study. *Neurology* 50, no. 5: 1441–1445.

Armitage, J.O. 1994. Bone marrow transplantation. *New England Journal of Medicine* 330: 827–838.

Buchanan, A.E. 1979. Medical paternalism or legal imperialism: Not the only alternatives for handling Saikewicz-type cases. *American Journal of Law and Medicine* 5: 97–117.

Friedman, R.I. 1998. Use of advance directives: Facilitating health care decisions by adults with mental retardation and their families. *Mental Retardation* 36: 444–456.

Kusnierz-Glaz, C.R. et al. 1997. Influence of age on the outcome of 500 autologous bone marrow transplant procedures for hematologic malignancies. *Journal of Clinical Oncology* 15: 18–25.

McKnight, D.K., and Bellis, M. 1992. Forgoing life-sustaining treatment for adult, developmentally disabled, public wards: A proposed statute. *American Journal of Law and Medicine* 18: 203–232.

Miller, T.E. et al. 1997. Treatment decisions for patients without surrogates: Rethinking policies for a vulnerable population. *Journal of the American Geriatrics Society* 45: 369–374.

Quill, T.E. 1991. Death and dignity: A case of individualized decision making. *New England Journal of Medicine* 324: 691–694.

Scheinberg, D.A. et al. Acute leukemias. In: *Cancer. Principles and practice of oncology.* eds. V.T. DeVita, S. Hellman, and S.A. Rosenberg, 2293–2321. 5th ed. Philadelphia: Lippincott-Raven.

LEGAL CITATIONS

Case Examples

In re Eichner (In re Storar), 52 N.Y. 363, 420 N.E.2d 64, 438 N.Y.S.2d 266, *cert. denied,* 454 U.S. 858 (1981).
Court refused to permit mother of profoundly retarded man to refuse life-prolonging measures on her son's behalf.

In re Guardianship of L.W., 167 Wisc. 2d 53, 482 N.W.2d 60 (1992).
Wisconsin Supreme Court ruled that a guardian has the authority to consent to the withholding of all life-sustaining medical treatment, including artificial nutrition and hydration, for a patient who never had capacity, provided there is a determination that such withholding or withdrawal of treatment is in the patient's best interests.

Superintendent of Belchertown State School v. Saikewicz, 373 Mass. 728, 370 N.E.2d 417 (1977).
State case that permits the withholding of life-prolonging treatment from a severely retarded man who is a ward of the state.

Massachusetts cases, post-*Saikewicz*, that step back from the requirement of obligatory state involvement in cases of withdrawing or withholding life-prolonging measures:

In re Dinnerstein, 6 Mass. App. 466, 380 N.E.2d 134 (1978).

In re Spring, 380 Mass. 629, 405 N.E.2d 115 (1980).

Custody of a Minor, 385 Mass. 698, 434 N.E.2d 115 (1982).

In re Beth, 412 Mass. 188, 587 N.E.2d 1377 (1992).

Vacco v. Quill, 117 S. Ct. 2293 (1997).

United States Supreme Court case finding a fudamental distinction between physician-assisted suicide and decisions to withhold or withdraw life-sustaining treatments.

CASE 8

Withdrawing Mechanical Ventilation at the Request of a Patient with Decisional Capacity

Catherine, a 70-year-old woman with severe emphysema, was found unresponsive at home. Her husband called for emergency assistance and an ambulance soon arrived. Emergency medical service (EMS) personnel performed endotracheal intubation and resuscitated her. She was admitted to the hospital, where she was treated for pneumonia and respiratory failure. Catherine is now alert and oriented, but her physician has been unable to wean her from the respirator.

There is no question as to Catherine's decisional capacity. She is able to communicate her wishes by using head signals and by writing notes. After several weeks of treatment, Catherine asks that the respirator be discontinued and that she be allowed to die. She asserts emphatically that it would not have been her choice to be resuscitated in the first place, although she never executed an advance directive or discussed these specific wishes with anyone in the past.

ISSUES TO CONSIDER

- Withdrawing life-sustaining treatment
- Community-based planning for emergency circumstances
- The provision of sufficient pain medication and the principle of double effect

MEDICAL CONSIDERATIONS

1. If Catherine's physicians respect her decision to discontinue mechanical ventilation, what provisions can be made for her comfort during this process of withdrawal?

In patients with obstructive lung disease who are maintained on respirators, the PCO_2 is maintained at an artificially low level. If respirator support is then withdrawn, it is common for the patient to experience severe dyspnea before the onset of CO_2 narcosis. Although in some situations, the ensuing respiratory failure rapidly leads to CO_2 narcosis, which may produce a peaceful, sleeplike state, in other cases, the patient may suffer severe symptoms and anxiety prior to coma and death.

Even when CO_2 narcosis occurs swiftly, the anticipation of the withdrawal of treatment could be sufficiently terrifying to produce suffering even in the most stalwart patient. For this reason, experienced physicians generally advocate the administration of sufficient sedation during this process to reduce the attendant anxiety and dyspnea that are likely to occur in a patient who is conscious.

Although small doses of sedatives such as morphine may have a central effect to reduce dyspnea without significantly depressing respiration, it is theoretically possible that any dose would hasten the patient's inevitable death, and it is not possible to precisely predict what dose will be required in any case. Conversely, one could also argue that by reducing anxiety, the sedative could delay death. While it is impossible to prove that the sedative has moved the expected death to an earlier moment, many health professionals are concerned that administering a potent sedative would amount to actually causing the patient's death, rather than merely relieving suffering. This thinking has led to reluctance on the part of many physicians and nurses to administer sufficient sedation to produce relief of symptoms. Ethical justifications and legal support for this practice are discussed in the following section.

An alternative would be to adjust the respirator setting to allow CO_2 to accumulate naturally, but it is not possible to know in advance if this would be less comfortable for the patient than the administration of a sedative. Also, like sedation, oxygen would produce respiratory depression and lead to CO_2 narcosis, although it would be a less reliable means of controlling symptoms than administration of a sedative. Anything that might produce respiratory depression, whether sedative, oxygen, or adjustment of the respirator, is subject to the same moral argument, but the sedative is likely to have the most reliable palliative effect. Approaches to terminal weaning are suggested in the references.[1,2]

2. Are there any alternatives to Catherine's current method of treatment?

Noninvasive positive pressure ventilation is a method of providing mechanical ventilation without an endotracheal tube. A face mask is used and various concentrations of oxygen are forced into the lungs under pressure. Because no tube is needed, this process might be more comfortable for the patient. Unfortunately, the process is not associated with better long-term outcomes for patients with irreversible lung disease. Other problems include the need to insert a nasogastric tube to decompress the stomach if too much air enters the esophagus. Likewise, the patient's ability to communicate and move about is hampered by the apparatus.

ETHICAL AND LEGAL CONSIDERATIONS

1. Are there ethical or legal concerns when treatment already in place is withdrawn, as compared to being withheld from the outset?

The prevailing consensus among ethicists, with support from various courts of law, consistently maintains that there is no difference between a decision not to initiate treatment and a decision to withdraw treatment already begun. That is, legal and moral justifications that support one action should be equally applicable to support the other type of decision. Criteria that would be used to justify either action would include the wishes of the decisionally capable patient, an advance directive, surrogate decisions on behalf of the patient, evaluation of the patient's best interests (see previous case discussions), or a determination that the treatment is medically futile, that is, of no medical benefit to the patient, given the patient's medical condition (see Case 12, "Resuscitation Decision in a Patient with Lung Cancer"). Any of these criteria might ethically and legally justify either withholding or withdrawing treatment. It should be noted, however, that the determination of medical futility is an evolving and somewhat disputed concept.

It is not uncommon for physicians to be reluctant to initiate life-sustaining treatment in certain cases, for fear that once begun, it could not be terminated even if it became clear that it was not achieving its goals. This reluctance might stem from the feeling on the part of individual physicians that withdrawing life-sustaining treatment amounts to actively killing the patient and is therefore morally unacceptable. However, commentators on medical ethics view the disease as the ultimate explanation of the patient's death under such circumstances. Legal concerns are also unfounded, and life-sustaining treatment can be withdrawn under the circumstances noted above. Reluctance to initiate life support could deprive the patient of the chance to try a potentially useful treatment. For example, many patients who develop acute respiratory failure can be weaned from a respirator and go on to live a life that is acceptable to them, once the immediate cause has been reversed. If the potential medical benefits seem to outweigh the potential burdens, and if the patient or an appropriate surrogate agrees to the treatment, then there is no reason to hesitate to initiate a trial.

A case such as this illustrates the utility of discussing such therapeutic possibilities with patients in advance. In such a discussion, the patient should be informed not only of her right to refuse the intervention but also of her right to have a trial of treatment and her right to have unsuccessful or burdensome treatment subsequently withdrawn. Such advance discussions will help ascertain the wishes that the patient or the surrogate may have concerning trial interventions. They may also help to lessen the guilt or reluctance experienced by a surrogate who may believe that by agreeing to a treatment's withdrawal he or she is somehow responsible for the patient's death. If the patient plans to utilize a living will, it would be important to include this specific decision in the document.

In Catherine's situation, because there was no advance knowledge of what she would have wanted, and considering that this was an emergency, it was appropriate to presume that she would have wanted to be resuscitated (see Case 13, "A Dispute over DNR Status in a Patient Who Wants Palliative Surgery"). Simply because the intervention has been initiated, however, does not necessitate that it be continued. Once her physicians feel comfortable that Catherine possesses decisional capacity and understands her options and their consequences, then the patient's choice should be respected. This is so regardless of the fact that she wishes treatment to be withdrawn, rather than withheld, and that her death is likely to follow the withdrawal. The fact that she is going to die does not lessen the authority of her choice. Catherine understands and accepts the likelihood that her death will follow the ventilator withdrawal. For her, the burdens accompanying the permanent reliance on a respirator outweigh any benefits she receives in continued life.

If Catherine lacked decisional capacity, treatment might also be withdrawn at the request of an authorized surrogate (likely to be her husband) acting on her behalf.

2. Given Catherine's assertion that she would never have agreed to be resuscitated initially, what kind of community planning could have prevented this scenario?

Catherine was a seriously ill woman even before the onset of this crisis, and there was a good possibility that she might at some point develop respiratory failure. It would have been extremely helpful for her community-based physician or a physician from a previous hospitalization to have informed her, prior to this crisis, about problems that might occur and options to consider in the event of such a crisis. If she had been informed that she might develop respiratory failure and coma, she might have been able to consider at that time whether or not she would want to undergo a therapeutic trial, and what might happen if such a trial should fail. If she elected not to take that route, she could have requested a do-not-resuscitate (DNR) order, which could have been placed in her medical records. Along with her doctors and her husband, she could have developed a plan of action to be implemented in the event of a crisis at home. For example, the support and services of a home hospice program might have been very valuable for Catherine and her husband, particularly given the likelihood of a life-threatening crisis and the desire not to have life-prolonging treatment administered.

Thirty-five states now have legislation outlining the legal mechanism to be employed in order to implement a community-based DNR order.[3] Even in the absence of such legislation, a plan of action can be developed. For example, with counseling and support, Catherine's husband might have avoided contacting emergency service personnel, which resulted in her intubation and resuscitation, as EMS workers are not permitted to use discretion in deciding when to intervene, or to desist once they initiate their efforts.

3. Why might a physician be reluctant to administer sedation to Catherine during the process of withdrawing the respirator?

It is not uncommon for physicians or nurses to be reluctant to administer sufficient pain medication for patients during their final moments of life. Some of this reluctance is due to insufficient training. Physicians may be reluctant to provide opioid analgesia chronically because of fears of producing addiction in the patient, although medicinal use of these drugs rarely produces true addiction. Patients themselves might be reluctant to receive chronic opioid analgesia for similar reasons. In short, many societal norms mitigate against the use of certain drugs even in the therapeutic setting.

At the end of life, there has been concern that administration of medications such as strong opioids or intravenous barbiturates intended to provide relief of symptoms may hasten or even cause the patient's death. This act of intending one consequence (symptom control), although such efforts might also bring about another, unintended consequence (hastened death), is known as the double effect. The doctrine of double effect, which is derived from Catholic theology, holds that while more than one effect may result from an individual's actions, the morality of the act is determined through an examination of the intent of the actor. Thus, if the physician's intent is to reduce Catherine's fears and discomfort during the process of respirator withdrawal, yet he suspects that such medication might have a second, unintended effect of depressing respiration and hastening her death by moments or hours, the appropriateness of the physician's actions will be determined by the specific intent. The physician intended that the patient experience maximal symptom relief during the process of dying but did not intend to actively bring about the patient's death. The risk of hastening death is considered morally acceptable if withholding the medication would cause the patient to suffer.

Strong legal support, including a recent Supreme Court decision, exists to support the practice of administering adequate symptom control to patients in the terminal phases of their conditions. The prevailing consensus among ethicists supports the administration of sufficient pain medication to bring about maximum comfort to patients in their final hours. A number of medical organizations support this practice as well.

High doses of medication for control of symptoms and the double effect differ ethically and legally from performing an intervention to intentionally cause a patient's death, which would constitute active euthanasia (see Case 15, "Assisted Suicide in a Man with Amyotrophic Lateral Sclerosis").

REFERENCES

1. H. Brody et al., "Withdrawing Intensive Life-Sustaining Treatment—Recommendations for Compassionate Clinical Management," *New England Journal of Medicine* 336 (1997): 652–657.

2. B.J. Daly et al., "Withdrawal of Mechanical Ventilation: Ethical Principles and Guidelines for Terminal Weaning," *American Journal of Critical Care* 2 (1993): 217–223.

3. "Choice in Dying. Map: State Statutes Governing Nonhospital Do-Not-Resuscitate Orders," *Right to Die Law Digest,* September 1998.

SUGGESTED READINGS

Allard, P. et al. 1999. How effective are supplementary doses of opioids for dyspnea in terminally ill cancer patients? A randomized continuous sequential trial. *Journal of Pain and Symptom Management* 17: 256–265.

Bruera, E. et al. 1993. Subcutaneous morphine for dyspnea in cancer patients. *Annals of Internal Medicine* 119: 906–907.

Cohen, M.H. et al. 1992. Treatment of intractable dyspnea: Clinical and ethical issues. *Cancer Investigation* 10: 317–321.

Council on Ethical and Judicial Affairs of the American Medical Association. 1992. Opinion 2.20—Withholding or withdrawing life-prolonging medical treatment; Opinion 2.21—Withholding and withdrawing life-prolonging medical treatment—Patients' preferences. *Code of Ethics: Annotated Current Opinions.* Chicago: American Medical Association.

Farncombe, M., and Chater, S. 1994. Clinical application of nebulized opioids for treatment of dyspnoea in patients with malignant disease. *Supportive Care in Cancer* 2: 184–187.

Hillberg, R.E., and Johnson, D.C. 1997. Noninvasive ventilation. *New England Journal of Medicine* 337: 1746–1752.

Manning, H., and Schwartzstein, R. 1995. Pathophysiology of dyspnea. *New England Journal of Medicine* 333: 1547–1553.

President's Commission for the Study of Ethical Problems in Medicine and Biomedical and Behavioral Research. 1982. Withholding versus withdrawing treatment. In *Deciding To Forgo Life-Sustaining Treatment,* 73–77. Washington, DC: U.S. Government Printing Office.

Truog, R.D. et al. 1991. Sedation before ventilator withdrawal: Medical and legal considerations. *Journal of Clinical Ethics* 2: 127–129.

Truog, R.D. et al. 1992. Barbiturates in the care of the terminally ill. *New England Journal of Medicine* 327: 1678–1682.

Wilson, W.C. et al. 1992. Ordering and administration of sedatives and analgesics during the withholding and withdrawal of life support from critically ill patients. *Journal of the American Medical Association* 267: 949–953.

LEGAL CITATIONS

Case Examples

Washington v. Glucksberg, 117 S. Ct. 2258 (1997).
    Supreme Court decision that held that state criminalization of assisted suicide is not unconstitutional, but which also underscored the legality of, and indeed obligation for, aggressive pain management for patients at the end of life.

Statutory Examples

State statutes addressing intractable pain relief:

Michigan Compiled Laws Section 5658 (1997).
A physician who prescribes a Schedule 2 to 5 narcotic as part of a medical treatment plan for a terminally ill patient is immune from administrative and civil liability if the prescription was written in good faith and with the intention to treat the patient or alleviate the patient's pain.

Oklahoma Statutes Annotated Title 63, Section 2-551 (1998).
A physician may prescribe a high dosage of controlled dangerous drugs if the benefit of the relief outweighs the risk of the high dosage, even if its use may increase the risk of death.

CASE 9

Withholding Tube Feeding
in a Woman with Advanced Dementia

Vivian is an 88-year-old woman with advanced dementia, who lives in a nursing home. As her dementia progressed she was able to take less and less food by mouth and percutaneous endoscopic gastrostomy (PEG) was performed for the provision of total enteral nutrition and hydration. Vivian is now mute, bedridden, incontinent, and completely dependent. She moans at times, occasionally scratches herself, and pulls at her feeding tube. Wrist restraints have been applied periodically to prevent her from dislodging the tube.

Vivian was diagnosed with Alzheimer's disease nine years ago. Except for mild hypertension and intermittent pressure sores, she currently has no other illnesses. In the past three years, however, she has been hospitalized with pneumonia on four occasions, but she improved rapidly with systemic antibiotics.

Although Vivian's niece originally authorized the feeding tube, she is distressed at her aunt's condition and now requests that tube feeding be discontinued, but the nursing home refuses. The niece insists, stating that her aunt had once said, "If I ever get senile, I hope they shoot me," and that she would never have wanted this type of treatment in her condition. The nursing home rejects the notion that this is "treatment" at all; they believe that the feeding tube is basic care that should be provided, and have a "conscience objection" to forgoing artificial nutrition and hydration. The physician says that not to do so would amount to "starving the patient to death." What's more, the physician points out, the patient has hypoalbuminemia, pressure ulcers, and a susceptibility to aspiration pneumonia, making the feeding tube "strongly indicated."

ISSUES TO CONSIDER

- Benefits and burdens of artificial nutrition and hydration (tube feeding)

- Terminal dehydration
- The legal and moral aspects of tube feeding
- Withholding versus withdrawing life-sustaining treatment
- Advanced dementia versus persistent vegetative state
- Vulnerable nursing home patients
- Do-not-hospitalize orders

MEDICAL CONSIDERATIONS

1. What methods could be used to provide nutrition and hydration to a patient such as Vivian, other than long-term tube feeding?

Oral feeding is often the most appropriate alternative. Progressive dementia is associated with a variety of abnormal feeding behaviors without frank abnormalities in swallowing mechanisms or digestive function. Such patients are able to eat when fed, but may take in only small amounts at a time or must be fed very slowly, sometimes requiring frequent small feedings throughout the day. In nursing homes, the time required may be greater than existing staff can provide, and a common solution is to insert a feeding tube.

In some cases, certain strategies can improve food intake. Addressing a patient's food preferences, including ethnic favorites, sometimes causes a dramatic reversal of "anorexia." Sometimes patients stop eating temporarily because of intercurrent illness and may not have been given an adequate trial of oral feeding before long-term tube feeding is instituted. In such cases, intravenous hydration can be maintained while the amount of oral food and fluids are increased as tolerated until the patient returns to baseline. Patients receiving PEG feedings may take in food by mouth if tube feeding is stopped for several hours to maximize intake of food. The potential benefits of such supplementation include enjoyment for the patient and, occasionally, abandonment of tube feeding if oral feeding returns to normal. The latter situation would not be expected to occur in patients in the latest stages of dementia. However, a trial of spoon feeding does not require removal of the gastrostomy tube.

In the latest stages of dementia, patients develop oropharyngeal dysphagia, a feeding dyspraxia or apraxia,[1] related to progressive cerebrocortical failure. At that stage, the patient is unable to eat when fed and will die of dehydration unless provided with enteral or parenteral hydration. The usual method is coadministration of nutrition and hydration by enteral tube feeding, via the nasogastric, gastrostomy, or jejunostomy route.

2. What impact has tube feeding had on Vivian's tendency to get pneumonia? Hypoalbuminemia? Pressure ulcers?

There is no evidence that enteral tube feeding reduces the risk of pneumonia, even though it is commonly recommended for that purpose, as is happening in Vivian's situation. Pneumonia in neurologically impaired elderly can occur as the result of extrinsic bacterial or viral infection, as in other patients. Aspiration pneumonia, when it occurs, can be due to aspiration of oropharyngeal secretions or microaspiration of gastric contents, including enteral feed. The risk of pneumonia in general is higher in such patients on account of immobility, failure to clear secretions, failure to cough, age-related changes in the mucosal clearing mechanisms in the tracheobronchial tree, and decline in humoral or cellular immunity. Aspiration of large amounts of gastric contents with chemical pneumonitis is unusual in patients who eat only small amounts and theoretically would be increased rather than decreased by large volumes of feed provided by tube.

It is generally difficult if not impossible to know if pneumonia is actually due to aspiration. Many patients aspirate without developing pneumonia, while others have recurrent pneumonia without documented aspiration of food. The incidence of pneumonia is roughly comparable among patients whether fed by nasogastric, gastric, or jejunal route, and there is no evidence that any kind of tube reduces the risk of pneumonia or aspiration in patients with depressed consciousness or other neurological impairments. Likewise, swallowing studies, including videofluoroscopic ones, do not predict which patients would benefit from tube feeding, even if they demonstrate aspiration. These studies are sometimes abnormal in people who are clinically well, and the laboratory environment of the swallowing evaluation does not duplicate the natural situation.[2]

In late life, serum albumin can decline quickly in the setting of illness, because protein synthesis, muscle mass, and protein reserves decline. Hypoalbuminemia itself is nonspecific and can occur as the result of inflammation (such as a pressure ulcer or cellulitis). This is thought to be mediated by cytokines, which reduce hepatocellular protein synthesis.[3] Under these circumstances, a high protein diet would not be expected to correct serum albumin completely, if at all. Hypoalbuminemia per se may be asymptomatic and need not be treated unless it leads to edema or anasarca. Pressure ulcers are due to pressure, not to hypoalbuminemia, and will respond to meticulous nursing care. Although healing would be theoretically faster if protein stores were adequate, attention to the pressure sore must come from another source. In fact, tube feeding might reduce nursing vigilance.

3. What impact does the tube feeding have on Vivian's comfort level?

Tube feeding is more likely to reduce her comfort than to increase it. Nasogastric or nasointestinal feeding can be very uncomfortable for patients and is less often used today since the advent of PEG, which permits gastrostomy feeding after a surgical procedure that can be performed in the endoscopy suite. Although small-bore nasal feeding tubes are less uncomfortable than large-bore tubes, nasal tubes are easy for patients to dislodge, thus leading to the imposition of mechanical restraints. Gastrostomy and jejunostomy feeding avoid the nasal route and are thus less intrusive and more comfortable and do not produce erosions in the esophagus, oropharynx, or nasopharynx. In addition, these forms of tube feeding, by being less noticeable to the patient, are less likely to lead to the imposition of restraints, allowing the patient more physical freedom and producing less agitation. Despite this, Vivian has been given wrist restraints. A simple alternative is to cover the PEG site and tube with a soft pad or bandage, which usually prevents dislodgement, but does not eliminate any potential discomfort the patient experiences.

Although safer and simpler than surgical gastrostomy, PEG is an invasive procedure, and has occasionally been associated with serious morbidity. In addition, the tubes can produce erosions of the gastrointestinal mucosa and, like all forms of enteral feeding, are associated with diarrhea, bloating, and regurgitation. Jejunostomy tubes are associated with a higher incidence of diarrhea, owing to entry of feed into the jejunum, but otherwise have approximately the same spectrum of side effects as PEG tubes.

Tube feeding is a passive process, based on calculation of nutritional and fluid requirements, rather than a patient's level of hunger or thirst, and feeding continues despite the possibility that the patient feels full or has nausea. This in turn could contribute to the gastrointestinal symptoms often associated with tube feeding. This contrasts with the cognitively intact patient fed by tube, who would be able to report any symptoms and could help guide the provider in accurately assessing the volume and speed of the feed. Unlike eating and drinking, tube feeding lacks a sensory and potentially pleasurable component.

Vivian, who has late stage dementia, will not become stronger with tube feeding, nor will cognition be restored by tube feeding. There is no evidence that tube feeding contributes to comfort in such a patient, and would be more likely to reduce comfort. The "myths" about tube feeding have recently been critically reviewed.[4]

4. What physical symptoms would Vivian experience if tube feeding were discontinued?

If Vivian takes in no food by mouth and intravenous fluids are not given, then dehydration will occur rapidly. Death occurs within 3 to 14 days, and the immediate cause of death is likely to be infection, usually pneumonia. Because of Vivian's advanced age and debility, death would be likely to occur in less than a week.

A question often posed by patients or their surrogates, and not infrequently by health professionals, is whether terminal dehydration produces a painful death. Vivian's niece would need to have information about this, because the doctor has told her that Vivian would die by starvation. Used in the context of terminal dehydration—a physiologic process that occurs during natural death—the term "starvation" is imprecise and carries emotional overtones, implying the physically uncomfortable process and the spectrum of physical changes that healthy and hungry persons undergo if they are involuntarily deprived of food.

There is no evidence that terminal dehydration is a painful process and there is substantial indirect evidence that it is not. Although the inability to obtain water in response to thirst is unpleasant, thirst is a normal physiologic response of healthy people, and might be quite diminished in the sick and dying. In acute illness, it is common, and may be physiologic, to reject food and water. Thirst is impaired in response to dehydration under experimental conditions in healthy and alert elderly subjects. This may be a partial explanation for the rapid development of severe dehydration among previously healthy patients, and particularly among debilitated elderly patients in whom acute illness such as diabetes or infection develops. In patients with overt or subclinical neurologic impairments, hypodipsia may occur, and such patients may become rapidly dehydrated because they fail to seek fluid replacement. Hypernatremia and hyperosmolarity can set in rapidly, which further impairs mental status and can lead to coma. While central mechanisms impairing thirst may be partly responsible, this situation is probably exacerbated by disturbed renal concentrating ability, which is a common and age-related physiologic change.

For Vivian, discontinuing enteral feeding without fluid replacement would most likely lead to the rapid development of hyperosmolarity and coma. Comatose, the patient would not be able to experience pain or suffering. There is no direct evidence of what a conscious but neurologically impaired patient might actually experience, but substantial indirect evidence suggests that Vivian would not experience pain or discomfort if allowed to die without tube feeding. Direct evidence comes from competent hospice patients, who eat and drink very little in their last weeks or days of life, but who report that what hunger, thirst, or dry mouth they experience is adequately satisfied by small amounts of food and water given ad lib.[5] In contrast, forced feeding of a patient whose physiologic state leads to meager intake, might theoretically produce more discomfort than not feeding.

5. How does Vivian's condition differ from the persistent vegetative state?

In the persistent vegetative state (PVS), a chronic form of eyes-open unconsciousness characterized by sleep-wake cycles, higher cortical function is absent but brainstem function is present. By definition, the patient cannot experience sensory input, including pain, and does not exhibit any voluntary behavior.

The persistent vegetative state can represent the most advanced form of brain damage in survivors of coma (see Case 11, "A Teenager with Prolonged Unconsciousness"), whatever the cause. It is likely that it occasionally occurs as the end stage of neurodegenerative diseases, such as Alzheimer's dementia, but clinical assessments may differ. It may be difficult to differentiate between far-advanced dementia, as seen in the present patient, and true PVS, since the neurologic deterioration is a continuum rather than an all-or-none phenomenon, and the difference grows slight as the dementing illness progresses. Most patients with advanced dementia do not have PVS, and physicians and nurses should assume they are able to experience pain. This would be important when deciding if painful diagnostic or therapeutic interventions should be undertaken, including decisions about tube feeding.

Terminal dehydration would produce essentially the same clinical picture for Vivian at this time as it would in the future, if she were to survive until PVS developed. In PVS, Vivian would be incapable of experiencing discomfort or anxiety from the tube itself.

6. What are the medical differences, if any, between withholding and withdrawing the tube?

A patient in whom tube feeding is considered, but not instituted, may be in a somewhat different clinical state than one who had been receiving tube feeding only to have it subsequently withdrawn. Having been tube fed, the patient might be more alert (but no less demented) than a neurologically similar patient who was now in a state of dehydration, but the advanced neurologic disease would make it unlikely that the patient would crave food or fluids, whether the issue were the withholding or the withdrawal of the feed.

Withdrawal of tube feeding differs markedly from the situation with the respirator (see Case 8, "Withdrawing Mechanical Ventilation at the Request of a Patient with Decisional Capacity"). A conscious patient might experience severe anxiety and air hunger on abrupt discontinuation of respirator support. If that same patient had been comatose prior to respirator treatment, withholding the respirator would not be uncomfortable or frightening. The cognitively unimpaired patient is aware that death is near and experiences additional anxiety for that reason. Cessation of tube feeding in a conscious patient would not impose the same type of burden as cessation of respirator support, and in fact might actually enhance comfort.

The ethical and legal aspects of withholding versus withdrawing life-sustaining treatment have been discussed in Case 8 in connection with mechanical ventilation. The ethical and legal arguments surrounding tube feeding are similar and are discussed in the following section.

ETHICAL AND LEGAL CONSIDERATIONS

1. What ethical and legal differences exist, if any, between tube feeding and other medical treatments?

The provision of nutritional and hydrational support through such mechanical means as nasogastric or gastrostomy tubes involves skill and expertise. The amount and type of feed provided must be carefully calculated and monitored; various degrees of invasiveness are involved, and morbidity may occur. As such, virtually all courts of law that have ruled on this question have categorized the provision of tube feeding as a "medical intervention," thus subject to the same sorts of analyses utilized when considering the use or withdrawal of other medical interventions, such as respirators or dialysis. In every jurisdiction, patients with decisional capacity have the right to forgo tube feeding as long as they understand the consequences of such a decision. This fundamental right of competent patients was underscored by the United States Supreme Court in the *Cruzan* case, when it stated that a competent person would have a "constitutionally protected right to refuse lifesaving hydration and nutrition." The competent patient's legal right to refuse is based on the Fourteenth Amendment liberty interest, and the ability to refuse tube feeding is based on the court's determination that it is a medical treatment. In support of this same notion, a number of medical organizations have declared that the use of artificial nutrition and hydration constitutes medical treatment, thus susceptible to the same choices of refusal or withdrawal as other treatment options.

This legal and ethical consensus has come about only after much debate. For many people, tube feeding constitutes basic caring and compassion, owed to any patient and encompassed within basic obligations that providers owe to their patients. For some, this is a religiously based belief; for others, there is an elementary sense that food and fluid are basic components of comfort care, like the provision of warmth and cleanliness. This contrasts with the medical position that artificial or forced feeding is not necessarily a palliative procedure.

Since the Supreme Court *Cruzan* ruling, state law regarding the withholding or withdrawal of artificial nutrition and hydration has evolved to reflect this consensus in virtually every state.[6] Through either case law or legislation, states have now granted authorized surrogates or health care agents the authority to permit the withholding or withdrawal of such a treatment, akin to their authority over other medical interventions such as dialysis or cardiopulmonary resuscitation.

The *Cruzan* decision, however, did permit individual states to set specific evidentiary standards for the withholding or withdrawal of treatment for patients without decisional capacity. The patient in question, Nancy Cruzan, was a Missouri woman in a persistent vegetative state, and her parents sought to have her long-term tube feeding discontinued. The Missouri courts upheld the state's mandate that there must be "clear and convincing evidence" of the patient's previously expressed wishes regarding the question at hand. The U.S. Supreme Court, in this first review of a right-to-die case, upheld the right of the state to restrict the withholding or withdrawal of life-sustaining treatment for the incompetent patient. A few states currently mandate such a high evidentiary standard, but, according to Cruzan, they are empowered to do so. Thus, it is important for providers to ascertain any specific restrictions on the ability of surrogates to make decisions about tube feeding or other life-prolonging treatments in their specific state.

From a general legal perspective, then, patients with decisional capacity have the right to refuse tube feeding as part of their fundamental right to refuse or consent to any medical intervention. In fact, although it is not commonly sought, the consent of a patient, or of a patient's authorized surrogate, should be obtained before the initiation of any method of artificial nutrition and hydration, including nasogastric tubes. Such consent is usually presumed as part of the general consent to treatment that patients sign on admission to the facility, for such things as the administration of medication, blood drawing, or X-rays. Tube feeding, however, carries with it different meaning for some people that should be specifically addressed with the patient or surrogate prior to its initiation. Provision of tube feeding should be the result of a conscientious decision by the patient or surrogate, rather than presumed under a blanket consent to treatment.

2. Would it be possible to initiate artificial nutrition and hydration, and subsequently decide to withdraw it?

There should always be the ability to initiate an intervention to assess the possible benefits for the patient. If a treatment is instituted, however, and after some time it is apparent that there is no meaningful benefit or the burdens of the treatment outweigh the benefits, then there is no justification for not withdrawing treatment, just as it might have been withheld for the same reason. In fact, if more stringent requirements were created for withdrawing treatment rather than withholding it, physicians might feel reluctant to initiate treatment trials, thus preventing patients from obtaining the potential benefits that such treatments might hold.

In the case of a patient such as Vivian, explicit discussion of the risks and benefits of tube feeding should have occurred when the tube feeding was instituted. In this way, it could have been determined if such a choice would have been acceptable to the patient and in keeping with her goals of care, had she been able to choose for herself. The fact that it was not discussed does not mean that tube feeding must or ought to continue.

3. What accommodation exists for providers who hold a specific moral objection to withholding or withdrawing tube feeding?

As discussed earlier, for many people, the provision of food and fluids is influenced by religious beliefs or other strongly held personal values. For institutions with religious affiliation, this perspective may influence the facility's tube feeding policy. Facilities sometimes have explicit policies prohibiting the withholding or withdrawal of food and fluids. This sort of "conscience objection" to the legal consensus is usually accommodated, but not at the cost of trumping basic rights of patients. The State of New York, in fact, has recognized this in the context of a judicial decision on the matter of withholding artificial nutrition and hydration. In *Elbaum*, the New York State Appellate Court held that the patient's nursing home, which had objected to removing the patient's feeding tube, did not have to honor the withdrawal request if it was able to find an alternative institution that would do so within 10 days of the court ruling. Thus, if a facility had such a policy, it would be mandatory that this be made clear to patients and families who were considering entrance into the facility. In this way, patients and families could consider this restriction when selecting a place of residence for long-term care. For residents of such a facility who then chose to forgo such treatment, the facility would be obligated to assist the patient or family in seeking an alternate facility where their request would be honored. This accommodates the "conscience objection" of individual providers or institutions but not at the cost of preventing the patient from exercising her fundamental right to make choices for herself.

4. What legal protections exist for dependent institutionalized patients and how might they affect decisions for Vivian?

Patients such as Vivian who are mentally incapacitated and reside in long-term care facilities constitute an extremely vulnerable patient population. A large proportion are unable to advocate for themselves, may lack relatives or friends to look after their welfare, and are thus unable to direct or control the course of their treatment. Decisions made for them by nursing home owners, administrators, doctors, and nurses may at times be influenced by factors other than the best interests of the patient, such as convenience for staff or financial considerations. In the heyday of for-profit nursing homes, a series of highly publicized scandals illustrated such things to the public and led to a series of actions by citizens' groups, regulatory agencies, and politicians. This culminated in the Nursing Home Reform Amendments of the federal Omnibus Budget Reconciliation Act of 1987 (OBRA), in which certain principles were laid out to improve the quality of care in nursing homes. The Health Care Financing Administration was empowered to set specific regulations and guidelines delineating the survey process that must be employed in order to achieve these goals.

The general intent of the nursing home amendments was to orient nursing homes concerning patient autonomy and to limit the influence of administrative concerns in clinical decision making. Specific areas of concern addressed under OBRA were the need to involve patients or designated surrogates in treatment decisions, reduction in the use of mechanical restraints and "chemical restraints" (sedatives), periodic assessment of patients' functional capacity and medical status, and the rights of nursing home residents to live in a dignified way and to make decisions regarding daily life wherever possible.

Mechanical and chemical restraints in nursing homes have a long and checkered history. There has been significant evidence that restraints were employed as much to serve the administrative interests of the facilities, such as the shortage of staff or concerns about liability from falls, as to serve the interests of the patients. Published reports have documented that mechanical restraints are associated with an array of morbidity, including but not limited to agitation, depression, pressure sores, and even strangulation. The adverse effects of chemical restraints have been well documented, and there is evidence that in many cases these medications are not indicated. Thus, under the rubric of empowering patients and protecting them from abuse or neglect, OBRA drastically limited the justification for the use of mechanical and chemical restraints in the long-term care setting. Under OBRA, Vivian's wrist restraints might come under question. Current regulations, regardless of the state in which Vivian lives, would not allow her to be restrained unless other measures had been taken and found to be inadequate for her safety and well-being, and they would have to allow her to maintain her highest possible function.

5. What kind of planning could have been undertaken for Vivian in the event that she became acutely ill, requiring hospitalization?

Nursing home patients are frequently transferred to hospitals for the treatment of acute illness, since nursing homes generally lack monitoring devices, sophisticated equipment, and equipment and personnel to conduct cardiopulmonary resuscitation. Unfortunately, such patients often return to the facility in a more deteriorated state, having acquired pressure sores, nosocomial infections, and severe deconditioning. The ratio of nonregistered nursing staff-to-patient tends to be much higher in skilled nursing facilities than in acute hospitals, where needs such as toileting, turning, feeding, monitoring of mental status, assistance in ambulation, and others have a lower priority than treatment of acute illness. Hospitalization has been associated with many hazards for elderly patients.[7]

Another problem with hospitalization is that once the patient is in the acute care setting, most decisions are, not surprisingly, made with an eye toward aggressive cure, and the use of technology may go unquestioned. Nursing home residents or their families are reluctant to allow a transfer to this environment with its hazards. For many in long-term care facilities, the institution is more than just the setting in which they receive their medical care; it is also their home. Such patients may in fact prefer to die quietly in the facility, with familiar caregivers and in a familiar setting.

To address this concern, many nursing homes have implemented do-not-hospitalize (DNH) orders, although there are no laws governing such orders. The purpose of such an order would be to decide, before the time of a crisis, if transfer to an acute care hospital would be desirable for such a patient. Like a do-not-resuscitate order or a living will, a do-not-hospitalize order is a form of advance planning to be used in the event of a crisis. Patients in such facilities have the right to refuse transfer to a hospital, preferably in advance of loss of decisional capacity, but an authorized surrogate may be able to make the same sort of decision on the patient's behalf if the facility and state law permit such surrogate decision making. Advance planning in accordance with state law would satisfy administrative concerns about the occurrence of patient deaths in a facility, since this would prevent a DNH order from being interpreted as denying the patient life-sustaining treatment. At times, the death of a resident can cause regulatory investigation and potential problems for a facility, even if good justification can be put forth for not transferring the patient to a hospital. Advance planning would also allow thorough discussion as to whether a blanket order not to hospitalize might impede wanted treatment of an intercurrent illness. For patients, families, and providers who, in advance of crisis, agree that no justification exists for such a transfer, it would be important to document in the patient's chart the reasoning for such a decision, the patient's involvement in this decision if possible, and the integrity and quality that went into such a decision. The best support for such a decision would stem from the patient's wishes.

REFERENCES

1. G. Blandford et al., "Assessing Abnormal Feeding Behavior in Dementia: A Taxonomy and Initial Findings," *Research and Practice in Alzheimer's Disease* 1 (Suppl) (1998): 47–64.

2. M.J. Feinberg, "Radiographic Techniques and Interpretation of Abnormal Swallowing in Adult and Elderly Patients," *Dysphagia* 8 (1993): 356–358.

3. A.J. Rosenthal et al., "Is Malnutrition Overdiagnosed in Older Hospitalized Patients? Association between the Soluble Interleukin-2 Receptor and Serum Markers of Malnutrition," *Journals of Gerontology* 53A (1998): M81–M86.

4. J.C. Ahronheim, "Artificial Nutrition and Hydration in Terminal Illness," *Clinics in Geriatric Medicine* 12 (1996): 379–391.

5. R.M. McCann et al., "Comfort Care for Terminally Ill Patients: The Appropriate Use of Nutrition and Hydration," *Journal of the American Medical Association* 272 (1994): 1263–1266.

6. "Choice in Dying," *Right To Die Law Digest* (September 1998).

7. M.D. Creditor, "Hazards of Hospitalization," *Annals of Internal Medicine* 118 (1993): 219–223.

SUGGESTED READINGS

Arras, J. 1988. The severely demented, minimally functional patient: An ethical analysis. *Journal of the American Geriatrics Society* 36: 938–944.

Castle, N.G. et al. 1997. Risk factors for physical restraint use in nursing homes: Pre- and postimplementation of the Nursing Home Reform Act. *The Gerontologist* 37: 737–747.

Ciocon, J.O. et al. 1988. Tube feedings in elderly patients: Indications, benefits, and complications. *Archives of Internal Medicine* 148: 429–433.

Council on Ethical and Judicial Affairs of the American Medical Association. 1992. Opinion 2.20—Withholding or withdrawing life-prolonging medical treatment; 8.18—Use of Restraints. In *Code of Ethics: Annotated Current Opinions*. Chicago: American Medical Association.

Derr, P.G. 1986. Why food and fluids can never be denied. *Hastings Center Report*. 16 (Pt. 1): 28–30.

Ditesheim, J.A. et al. 1989. Fatal and disastrous complications following percutaneous endoscopic gastrostomy. *American Surgeon* 55: 92–96.

Fabiszewski, K.J. 1990. Effect of antibiotic treatment in outcome of fevers in institutionalized Alzheimer's patients. *Journal of the American Medical Association* 263: 3168–3172.

Finucane, T.E., and Bynum, J.P.W. 1996. Use of tube feeding to prevent aspiration pneumonia. *Lancet* 348: 1421–1424.

The Hastings Center. 1987. Guidelines on medical procedures for supplying nutrition and hydration; Guidelines on antibiotics and other life-sustaining medication. In *Guidelines on the Termination of Life Sustaining Treatment and the Care of the Dying,* 57–64. Bloomington: Indiana University Press.

Kapp, M.B. 1999. Restraint reduction and legal risk management. *Journal of the American Geriatrics Society* 47: 375–376.

Mion, L.C. et al. 1996. Physical restraint use in the hospital setting: Unresolved issues and directions for research. *Milbank Quarterly* 74: 411–433.

Phillips, P.A. et al. 1984. Reduced thirst after water deprivation in healthy elderly men. *New England Journal of Medicine* 311: 753–759.

Siegler, M., and Weisbard, A. 1985. Against the emerging stream: Should fluid and nutritional support be discontinued? *Archives of Internal Medicine* 145: 129–131.

Steiner, N., and Bruera, E. 1998. Methods of hydration in palliative care patients. *Journal of Palliative Care* 14, no. 2: 6–13.

Volicer, L. 1997. Persistent vegetative state in Alzheimer disease. Does it exist? *Archives of Neurology* 54: 1382–1384.

LEGAL CITATIONS

Case Examples

Barber v. Superior Court, 147 Cal. App. 3d 1006, 195 Cal. Rptr. 484 (1982).
This was the first reported state case to raise the question of the withdrawal of artificial nutrition and hydration.

In re Browning, 568 So. 2d 4 (Fla. 1990).
A Florida case in which a patient's surrogate sought to have the patient's feeding tube withdrawn, in accord with the patient's living will, despite the state's natural death act, which prohibited such treatment withdrawal; the surrogate was ultimately successful in court under a common-law right to self-determination.

In re Conroy, 98 N.J. 321, 486 A.2d 1209 (1985).
Nephew of severely demented patient given court permission to have aunt's feeding tube withdrawn in accord with what he believed her wishes to be; considered to be one of the major state court cases involving the termination of artificial nutrition and hydration.

Cruzan v. Director, Missouri Department of Health, 110 S. Ct. 2841 (1990).
The first "right to die" case to be taken up by the United States Supreme Court in which the fundamental liberty interests of competent individuals to refuse life-prolonging measures were enunciated.

Elbaum v. Grace Plaza of Great Neck, Inc., 148 A.D.2d 244, 544 N.Y.S.2d 840 (1989).
State case in which the ability of a facility to raise a conscience objection to a request for the withdrawal of artificial nutrition and hydration was addressed.

Gilmore v. Annaburg Manor Nursing Home, Chancerry No. 44386,Va. S. Ct. (1998).
The Virginia Supreme Court granted permission to terminate the artificial nutrition and hydration of a patient in a permanent vegetative state.

In re Jobes, 108 N.J. 394, 529 A.2d 434 (1987).
Facility obligated to comply with a surrogate request to withdraw artificial nutrition and hydration from an incompetent patient in a persistent vegetative state unless a voluntary transfer of the patient can be arranged.

Rasmussen v. Flemming, 154 Ariz. 207, 741 P.2d. (1987).
Case addressing treatment decisions for a nursing home patient, including a Do-Not-Hospitalize order.

Statutory Examples

New York Pub. Health Law Sect. 2928 to 2994 (McKinney 1993 and Supp. 1998).
Health care agent must have "reasonable knowledge" of the incompetent patient's wishes in order for artificial nutrition or hydration to be withheld or withdrawn from such a patient.

States whose living will statutes permit the withholding or withdrawal of artificial nutrition and hydration through a living will include:

Connecticut Removal of Life Support Systems Act, Conn. Gen. Stat. Ann., Sec. 19a-570 to 19a-580 (West 1997).

Colorado Medical Treatment Decision Act, Col. Rev. Stat. Sec. 15-18-101 to 15-18-113 (1997).

See also, Choice in Dying, *Right To Die Law Digest* (June 1998): Maps: Artificial Nutrition and Hydration in Statutes Authorizing Health Care Agents; Artificial Nutrition and Hydration in Living Will Statutes.

Omnibus Budget Reconciliation Act of 1987 (OBRA), Pub. Law No. 100-203, 101 Stat. 1330.
Landmark federal legislation addressing the rights of nursing home patients and the need of nursing home reforms, including significant limits on the use of restraints in the nursing home setting.

CASE 10

A Religious Objection to the Determination of Brain Death

David, a 20-year-old previously healthy man, was injured in an automobile accident. He sustained severe head trauma and at the accident scene was unresponsive and without spontaneous respiration. He was rushed to the local hospital and was resuscitated in the emergency room. Heartbeat and blood pressure were restored, but after 24 hours of exhaustive treatment, the doctors reached the conclusion that he was brain dead.

David appears to be a potential candidate for organ donation, although no organ donor card was found among his possessions. The hospital's transplant procurement team has been notified. In the meantime, David is being maintained on artificial life support and a neurologist has been consulted in order to confirm the diagnosis of brain death.

The nurse from the transplant procurement team tells the doctors that she understands the patient is Jewish and that there might be a religious objection to the brain death diagnosis. A physician who has been taking care of David says that they have been attempting to notify the family, but he expresses surprise that religious factors could affect a diagnosis. "If a patient is brain dead, he's legally dead," he says, adding that he is not even obliged to continue life support at that point. While awaiting family contact, the doctors continue full life support measures.

ISSUES TO CONSIDER

- Declaration of death using the whole brain death standard
- Religious objections to the declaration of death
- Protocol for obtaining organs for donation

MEDICAL CONSIDERATIONS

1. What are the clinical criteria for the determination of death and how have they been determined?

Physiologically, someone is dead when it has been demonstrated that irreversible cessation of circulatory and respiratory function, or of the whole brain, has occurred. Cardiorespiratory criteria for death are determined by a clinical examination that reveals the absence of responsiveness, heartbeat, and respiratory effort. An electrocardiogram (EKG) can confirm the absence of cardiac function if there is doubt, such as in cardiac tamponade, which can lead to electromechanical dissociation. Irreversibility is determined by observing the patient using these or other appropriate methods for an amount of time that would vary, depending on the history and the clinical situation.

When cardiorespiratory death occurs, brain death follows within minutes, unless circulation is maintained artificially. The irreversible cessation of brain function (brain death) can occur before cessation of circulation, as is suspected in David's case. The diagnosis of brain death can be made when it has been demonstrated that cerebral as well as brainstem functions are irreversibly absent. In brain death the patient is unresponsive to all painful and other sensory stimuli, and spontaneous respiration and cephalic reflexes, including pupillary light, corneal, oculocephalic, and oculovestibular reflexes, are absent. Spinal cord reflexes do not rule out the diagnosis of whole brain death, since these functions operate independently of the brain and may persist or even increase after the death of the brain. A spinal cord reflex, such as withdrawal of a limb after a noxious stimulus, should not be confused with true decerebrate or decorticate posturing, which are abnormal motor responses most often seen in severe, acute brain disease.

Without mechanical ventilation, heartbeat may persist for 10 to 30 minutes following brain death. With full life support systems, heartbeat and other signs of peripheral circulation may continue for hours or even days. However, there are numerous, well-documented cases of patients diagnosed as brain dead, using clinical as well as laboratory confirmatory testing, who remain alive for weeks or even months, with various degrees of life support.[1] The longest reported survival is a case of a 4-year-old who has survived over 14 years following the diagnosis of whole brain death (as opposed to cortical death or persistent vegetative state, concepts discussed in Case 11, "A Teenager with Prolonged Unconsciousness"). Prolonged survival is more often (but not invariably) seen in young patients and those with brain pathology in the absence of apparent somatic pathology. These cases have recently called into question long held assumptions that loss of brain integrity inevitably leads to death of the organism (the somatic disintegration hypothesis) and have renewed philosophical debate about the validity of brain death.[2,3] The diagnosis of brain death in the youngest age group is discussed in Case 28 ("Determination of Death in a Newborn").

2. How can the diagnosis of brain death be made with certainty?

It is important to rule out potentially reversible conditions that can resemble brain death on clinical examination or even in confirmatory testing, including electroencephalogram (EEG), and occasionally, somatosensory evoked potentials. Conditions include hypothermia, drug intoxication, neuromuscular blockade, shock, and unusual problems such as brainstem encephalitis. Even in the presence of head trauma, as in David's case, it is possible to be misled by the superficial clinical situation. Drugs, alcohol, or other central nervous system depressants are often contributing factors in motor vehicle accidents. A directed toxicology screen should be done. Drugs that can produce profound central nervous system depression or apnea can result in a clinical situation mimicking brain death, may fail to produce physical signs outside of the central nervous system, and may not produce specific laboratory abnormalities. These substances include alcohol, barbiturates, anticonvulsants, carbon monoxide, major and minor tranquilizers, hypnotics, and antidepressants.

Body temperature should be evaluated with a special thermometer that can measure core body temperatures below 95°F. Although not the diagnosis in this particular case, hypothermia is sometimes overlooked.

The apnea test should be used to test central respiratory centers. The principle of the test is to allow sufficient carbon dioxide accumulation to stimulate respiratory effort. An accepted version of the apnea test is as follows: While the patient is connected to the respirator, and in order to prevent dangerous hypoxia that could damage the brain, 100 percent oxygen is administered for 10 to 30 minutes, with the duration depending on the clinical situation. The respirator is then disconnected, arterial blood gas (ABG) determination is made, and 100 percent oxygen is given via cannula in the endotracheal or tracheostomy tube. The patient is observed for spontaneous respiration, sigh, cough, or hiccup. After 10 minutes, the ABG is repeated and respirator support is resumed. If PCO_2 has reached 60 mm Hg and there is no spontaneous respiratory effort, the patient is considered to have apnea. If PCO_2 is below 60 mm Hg, the procedure should be repeated and the duration off the respirator lengthened. There is some debate as to whether PCO_2 needs to be raised as high as 60 mm Hg—with attendant risk to vital organs—to confirm the diagnosis of brain death. Apnea testing should not be performed in patients with chronic obstructive pulmonary disease and related illnesses; in these individuals, raising PCO_2 would fail to stimulate respiration because of lung rather than brain pathology.

The diagnosis of brain death is made by clinical examination, but in many cases of presumptive brain death, confirmatory objective tests are indicated. Traditionally, an EEG showing electrocerebral silence (a flat or isoelectric EEG) was considered a key confirmatory test for brain death determination, but false positives as well as false negatives may occur. An alternative to an EEG is measurement of intracranial blood flow, the absence of which indicates that the brain parenchyma has undergone destruction (autolysis) and death. The four-vessel (carotid and vertebral) angiogram is considered the most sensitive and specific test of intracranial blood flow, but it is invasive and cumbersome and exposes organs intended for transplant to potentially toxic contrast material. Intravenous radionuclide cerebral angiography is a sensitive method of confirming brain death, but it can be falsely positive or negative.[4] The technique does not measure vertebral blood flow and hence cannot give definitive information on brainstem function, which would have to depend on clinical examination or additional objective testing, such as brainstem evoked potentials. These and other confirmatory techniques, along with guidelines for brain death determination in adults, have been reviewed in detail.[5]

Even exhaustive testing does not take into account isolated residual groups of functioning neurons or evidence of persistent endocrinologic activity of the organism. Current brain death standards do not take into account this residual activity because it does not contribute to the functioning of the brain or the organism as a whole. However, this residual functioning has been the source of debate as to the precise timing of death from a philosophic point of view.

3. If the declaration of death were delayed because of a religious objection, how would this affect the suitability of David's organs for transplant?

In order for highly perfused (vital) organs to remain viable for transplant, circulation needs to be maintained, and this requires close monitoring of blood pressure and fluid status, and often administration of vasopressors, and other agents. Vital organs, including the kidney, liver, heart, lungs, and pancreas, are highly sensitive to oxygen concentrations and would undergo necrosis in the absence of adequate circulation. Since an organ cannot ethically or legally be removed before death, vital organs would have to be removed after brain death but before cessation of circulation.

Recently, however, a study of kidney transplantation has demonstrated that organ viability is well maintained when kidneys are harvested from donors whose hearts had stopped beating (average time from cessation of warm blood perfusion to start of preservation of the organ was 14 minutes), although the need for dialysis during the first week post transplant is greater.[6] Further study will be needed to identify which kidneys obtained under such circumstances are likely to malfunction and to determine if function of other vital organs can be maintained after cessation of heartbeat.

In contrast, nonvital organs, or tissues, such as the cornea, skin, bone, and heart valves, can be harvested several hours after cessation of circulation. From a medical point of view, David could still serve as a tissue donor as long as he met standard medical criteria.

ETHICAL AND LEGAL CONSIDERATIONS

1. If brain death is confirmed, will David in fact be legally dead?

Once a physician makes a declaration of death, that declaration constitutes the legal determination of death, triggering a range of consequences and potential actions. The physician may make that determination using either cardiorespiratory or neurologic criteria.

The advent of advanced life-sustaining technology and the resulting ethical dilemmas led to the replacement of traditional criteria for the determination of death with dual (cardiorespiratory and brain death) criteria. The movement to codify and legitimize dual standards gained momentum in 1968, when the Harvard Ad Hoc Committee on the Definition of Death set forth a standard definition of death. Further refinements of the "Harvard Criteria" led to a proposed Uniform Determination of Death Act (UDDA) in 1981.[7] This proposal has served as a model for state legislatures in crafting law for their own jurisdictions. It states, "An individual who has sustained either (1) irreversible cessation of circulatory and respiratory functions, or (2) irreversible cessation of all functions of the entire brain, including the brainstem, is dead. A determination of death must be made in accordance with accepted medical standards."

The language in this model statute specifies only that there are two ways to determine death, by cardiorespiratory criteria and by brain death criteria. This represents a change over traditional criteria that defined death as the cessation of all vital functions. The UDDA does not set out specific tests or methods to determine brain death, since science and technology are expected to continually advance.

While not all states have ratified this exact language in their own jurisdictions, most have adopted the concept that whole brain death constitutes death for legal purposes. In some states, this has been accomplished by legislation, and in others, through judicial decisions or government regulations. Because the language in force may vary slightly from state to state, practitioners need to be fully knowledgeable of their own state's law in this area before discontinuing treatment of a patient who meets the medical standard for whole brain death.

The legal determination of death ends any obligation the physician may have to provide medical treatment, and life support can be terminated without permission of a surrogate. At that point, the patient has the status of a corpse and is thus owed the respect and dignity given to dead bodies in the course of preparation for burial or cremation. Moreover, regulations in some states specifically address objections that may be raised (see below).

While a declaration of death based on whole brain death criteria is legally valid, all required steps necessary to confirm such a declaration must be performed in accordance with accepted medical standards before such a declaration would be legally binding. For example, family members may have standing to challenge such a declaration of death—not because they object to the declaration on spiritual or philosophic grounds, but because they may assert that accepted medical practices have not been employed in their particular circumstance (see Case 28).

2. In addition to organ donation, what practical issues are addressed by the dual criteria for brain death?

Among the issues that gave impetus to the establishment of brain death criteria was that with the advent of advanced life support technology, grief-stricken relatives were led to believe that hope existed for their loved one, when in fact it did not. In other cases, physicians and hospitals may have felt obligated to expend limited medical resources on patients whose conditions were inconsistent with life. An additional impetus that led some states to adopt the brain death standard was a number of troubling homicide cases in which it became important to establish the precise moment of death. If the patient was brain dead but was not legally dead until the doctors discontinued life support, it was sometimes argued that the defendant could not be tried for murder but only for attempted murder.

Also, the exact time of death may carry important consequences concerning rights of inheritance for surviving kin, or rights under medical or life insurance policies. For example, a third-party payer might refuse to pay for health care once a determination of death is made; thus, if David were declared brain dead at a certain time and this time were stated on his death certificate, there might be no reimbursement for the medical services rendered subsequent to that time. If David had been fatally injured in an accident along with a beneficiary of his life insurance, payment of benefits would be determined on the basis of whether David or his named beneficiary died first. These same issues might arise if the two individuals stood to inherit each other's estate; inheritance rights are contingent on the timing and the order of the deaths of the beneficiaries.

3. If David is legally dead, what authority do religious objections carry?

As the diagnosis of brain death is a medical determination that carries the weight of law if properly determined, a family's objection to such a determination would not constitute a legally valid exception to the law. Thus, family members could not insist that David was still alive if he met the legally valid definition of death in his jurisdiction—namely, brain death. In this case, the physician would be correct in saying that family permission was not necessary for him to discontinue life support, since it was not necessary for the legal determination of death using the brain death standard. Such objections and claims of exceptions to the law could lead to a perverse and inequitable system in which two individuals with identical clinical circumstances could be treated very differently: one dead, with treatment withdrawn and, perhaps, organs removed, and the other "alive" and on full life support.

The fact that religious objections to brain death may not prohibit a legal declaration of death, however, does not mean that such assertions should be ignored. In fact, certain states have formally addressed this issue through regulations that exhort hospitals to work with families and temporarily accommodate their concerns, usually religious ones, until an amicable closure can be attained. This need to accommodate religious concerns recognizes the heterogeneous nature of our society and the need to be sensitive to varying perspectives. One state, New Jersey, has specifically adopted a statutory religious exemption for brain death determinations. From a very practical point of view, when there is a strong objection to a declaration of brain death, it is prudent for a hospital to temporarily address and accommodate family wishes, so as not to create undue ill will or community hostility. In most cases, this should not be a major concern for the hospital, given the fact that respiratory and circulatory functions in a brain dead patient will shortly cease.

Accommodation of a religious objection to withdrawal of treatment differs from upholding a religious objection to the provision of treatment, as in the case of a Jehovah's Witness patient who refuses blood transfusions (see Case 1, "A Religious Objection to a Blood Transfusion"). The refusal of treatment based on religious views does carry the force of law under the common-law concept of self-determination and constitutional liberty interests of the patient. Such refusals stand in marked contrast to demands for treatment based on a religious objection to the declaration of brain death. No one has a legally supportable right to any special treatment other than the right to expect that whatever care is rendered is given according to accepted medical standards. The determination of whole brain death is now an accepted medical standard. Despite religious objections to this, a demand to opt out of the accepted standard of care has no legal authority and is thus not legally actionable. Nevertheless, failure to accommodate the objection in a heterogeneous society could theoretically lead to a lawsuit, especially in a jurisdiction that adopted regulations governing this accommodation, as in David's state. Such a regulation is a public policy statement that reflects public support for such accommodations. If David's physician, who has now been made aware of this policy, chooses to blatantly ignore it, a religious family might have cause to bring suit because of the physician's refusal to recognize the public policy. If, however, the physician continues in his effort to notify the family, and if he addresses any family objections before acting on a brain death determination, there would not appear to be cause for legal action.

4. Who is authorized to give consent for organ donation?

Individuals over the age of 18 may decide before death that they wish to donate their organs for transplant. The Uniform Anatomical Gift Act of 1968, a model law adopted in some form in every state, permits such predeath decisions to donate, along with determinations to donate one's body for research or teaching purposes. When there is no next of kin, such decisions made by the patient prior to death carry full legal validity and empower the facilities to act accordingly.

When next of kin have been involved or are present, theoretically the wishes of the now deceased patient concerning organ donation should still prevail. Families have no ownership right, per se, to the body of their next of kin, but in practice there is usually an attempt to obtain the next of kin's consent to donation, even when the previously expressed wishes of the patient are clear. While a family has no legal ownership claim, it does have a common-law interest in how the body is treated once death has been declared. Family members may even have cause to bring legal action against providers for emotional or mental distress if they believe the body of their loved one has not been appropriately handled or if they have had trouble obtaining the body for burial or cremation.

Just as sensitivity is often demonstrated in cases of religious objections to brain death, the wishes and interests of family members are usually given recognition if they wish to override a patient's desire to donate organs. If a family objects to organ donation, it is highly unlikely that a facility would remove the donor organs, even if the patient had a donor card. While such an action might not be technically illegal, it would nonetheless violate a commonly accepted family interest and would certainly invite the kind of ill will that institutions wish to avoid.

5. What ethical and legal concerns arise in the attempt to procure organs for donation?

At present, the demand for donated organs far outpaces their availability. A system of rationing these scarce resources is in place, with potential recipients often dying before their turn is called on the queue or before a medically suitable organ is available. In order to enhance availability, Congress passed legislation in 1986 requiring all hospitals receiving Medicare or Medicaid funds to set up protocols for the identification of potential organ donors. Almost all states have passed their own "required request" laws, requiring doctors to ask if the patient has an organ donor card and to offer organ donation to families of potential donors. There really are no penalties for failing to make the request, however, and, of course, patients or their families are not required to accede to such requests. Currently, only an estimated 20 percent of Americans have organ donor cards and fewer than 2 to 3 percent of donors have actually been found to carry them. The purpose of the donor card is to inform the facility of a patient's intent.

Because it would be imprudent to act against the wishes of an angry and distraught family, wishes on a donor card would likely not be honored if they conflicted with the wishes of the surviving family. In short, the effect of the legislative system is little more than a public policy statement that the community endorses organ donation and wishes to encourage it. By contrast, in France and Spain, a system is in place that presumes consent for donation unless a patient or a family specifically refuses. Such a movement has been resisted in this country because of concerns that the rush to retrieve organs might in some way compromise the care of the patient, or even lead to organ retrieval before the patient's death.

Despite these concerns, there is no evidence that the presumed donation system has led to such behavior.[8] Nonetheless, concern that interest in donor organs might lead to a conflict of interest on the part of a patient's provider has led to a nearly universal system in which those in charge of organ donation requests and retrievals are totally separate from those who provide clinical care to the patient. Such separation of functions is intended to avoid both the appearance, and the reality, of conflicted motives in the clinical setting. Thus, the physician who declares a patient brain dead should not be the same person who approaches the family regarding organ donation once the determination of death has been established (for additional information concerning organ donation and distribution, see Case 22, "A Man with Alcoholic Cirrhosis Wants a Liver Transplant").

REFERENCES

1. D.A. Shewmon, "Chronic 'Brain Death.' Meta-analysis and Conceptual Consequences," *Neurology* 51 (1998): 1538–1545.

2. J.L. Bernat, "A Defense of the Whole-Brain Concept of Death," *Hastings Center Report* 28, no. 2 (1998): 14–23.

3. R.D. Truog, "Is It Time To Abandon Brain Death? *Hastings Center Report* 27, no. 1 (1997): 29–37.

4. W.M. Flowers and B.R. Patel, "Radionuclide Angiography as a Confirmatory Test for Brain Death: A Review of 229 Studies in 219 Patients," *Southern Medical Journal* 90 (1997): 1091–1096.

5. E.F.M. Wijdicks, "Determining Brain Death in Adults," *Neurology* 45 (1995): 1003–1011.

6. Y.W. Cho et al., "Transplantation of Kidneys from Donors Whose Hearts Have Stopped Beating," *New England Journal of Medicine* 338 (1998): 221–225.
7. "Guidelines for the Determination of Death: Report of the Medical Consultants on the Diagnosis of Death to the President's Commission for the Study of Ethical Problems in Medicine and Biomedical and Behavioral Research," *Journal of the American Medical Association* 246 (1981): 2184–2186.
8. B. Merz, "The Organ Procurement Problem: Many Causes, No Easy Solutions," *Journal of the American Medical Association* 254 (1985): 3285–3288.

SUGGESTED READINGS

Choice in Dying. 1998. Maps: State laws concerning brain death. *Right To Die Law Digest*, March.

Ebrahim, A.F. 1998. Islamic jurisprudence and the end of human life. *Medical Law* 17: 189–196.

Ikes, C. 1997. Kidney failure and transplantation in China. *Social Science and Medicine* 44: 1271–1283.

Kirkland, L. 1992. Family refusal to accept brain death and termination of life support: To whom is the physician responsible. *Journal of Clinical Ethics* 3: 78.

The Hastings Center. 1987. Part 4—Declaring death. In *Guidelines on the termination of life sustaining treatment and care of the dying*, 86–98. Bloomington: Indiana University Press.

New York Academy of Medicine. 1994. *The end of life: guidelines for health professionals concerning death certificates, autopsies and organ and tissue donations.* 6th edition.

Olick, R.S. 1991. Brain death, religious freedom and public policy: New Jersey's landmark legislative initiative. *Kennedy Institute of Ethics Journal* 1: 275–288.

Peters, T.G. et al. 1996. Organ donors and nondonors: An American dilemma. *Archives of Internal Medicine* 156: 2419–2424.

President's Commission for the Study of Ethical Problems in Medicine and Biomedical and Behavioral Research. 1981. *Defining Death: Medical, Legal and Ethical Issues in the Determination of Death.* Washington, DC: U.S. Government Printing Office.

Rosner, F. 1995. Jewish medical ethics. *Journal of Clinical Ethics* 6, no. 3: 202–217.

Spike, J., and Greenlaw, J. 1995. Ethics consultation: Persistent brain death and religion: Must a person believe in death to die? *The Journal of Law, Medicine and Ethics* 23, no 3: 291–294.

Truog, R. D., and Fackler, J. C. 1992. Is it reasonable to reject the diagnosis of brain death? *Journal of Clinical Ethics* 3, no. 1: 80–81.

LEGAL CITATIONS

Case Examples

In re Long Island Jewish Medical Center, N.Y. Supp. 2nd Ser., 641: 989–992 (Feb. 28, 1996).
Litigation involving a hospital's attempts to withdraw life support from an infant determined to be brain dead, over the religious objections of the patient's family.

Massey v. Duke University, N.C. Ct. App., No. 95 CVS 05592 (Aug. 1998).
Litigation initiated by a distressed family for infliction of emotional distress following the unauthorized removal of a deceased relative's eyes during autopsy.

Statutory Examples

New Jersey Declaration of Death Act (West, 1996). *New Jersey Statutes Annotated.* Title 26, Sec. 6A-I to 6A-8.
State regulation permitting religious exemptions to brain death declarations.

New York Codes, Rules and Regulations, 1997. Title 10, Sec. 400.16. Pub. Law 99-509, Sec. 9318, 1986.
State legislation governing the definition of death and requiring hospitals to develop policies that reasonably accommodate religious or moral objections to brain death criteria.

CASE 11

A Teenager with Prolonged Unconsciousness

Mike is a 17-year-old boy who has sustained serious head trauma in a motor vehicle accident. He has been unconscious for three months. On his initial admission to the hospital, Mike was stuporous and was found to have an epidural and multiple intracerebral hematomas. He had several fractures but no significant internal injuries. Mike has been unconscious since surgery when the epidermal hematoma was evacuated. He is fed by gastrostomy tube. Although he breathes on his own, he has a tracheostomy and is intubated, with humidified air delivered by T-tube. The physician has informed Mike's parents that his prognosis for full recovery is poor. Even with recovery, there is a good chance that he will be left with residual neurologic damage, such as paralysis and defects in speech, memory, and intellect. The patient is the oldest of four children. His parents, though married to each other, have been devastated by the accident and are bitterly divided as to how they should proceed. Mike's mother wishes to cling to whatever hope there is and has virtually abandoned all other aspects of her life. Mike's father, fatigued and resigned to his son's fate, wishes to move on with his life and the lives of the rest of his family. He does not wish to continue under the strains of the emotional and financial pressures from this situation and wants nothing further to be done to promote any "recovery" in his son. In fact, he frequently hints that he hopes nature takes its course and that his son will soon pass away.

ISSUES TO CONSIDER

- Prognostication in coma
- Determination of best interests in a patient with prolonged unconsciousness
- Family interests in the decision-making and caregiving process
- Conflicts among surrogate decision makers
- Quality of life

- Institutional conflict resolution
- Persistent vegetative state compared to coma

MEDICAL CONSIDERATIONS

1. What is coma and how is the prognosis determined?

Coma is a state of unarousable unconsciousness in which the patient lies with the eyes closed in a sleeplike state. It is uncertain if Mike's condition is true coma or another form of prolonged unconsciousness (see below). In any case, it will be difficult to predict the outcome. In coma, there are no absolute guidelines that can predict with certainty if an individual patient will survive or for how long or what the extent of residual brain damage will be in the event of survival.

A number of studies have shown that early neurologic signs indicating depth of unconsciousness and extent of neurologic damage, the cause and duration of coma, age of the patient, and laboratory evaluations assist in prediction of outcome (see Figures 7–11.1 and 7–11.2).

Head-injured patients who are not awake or arousable, that is, who are comatose, have at best a 50 percent chance of survival. The vast majority of deaths occur within the first few hours or days of injury. Among those who survive this early critical phase, recovery ranges from good (return to previous level of function) to poor (severe neurologic damage and dependence).

Nontraumatic coma is associated with 75 percent mortality in the first month, depending on the specific cause of coma and the general overall condition of the patient. In contrast, head trauma patients with coma generally have a better prognosis than this. However, these patients, especially those whose trauma was incurred in a serious motor vehicle accident, frequently have attendant internal injuries that may have produced hypotension or cardiac arrest, leading to anoxic encephalopathy. Anoxic insult to the brain significantly worsens prognosis. In general, from five to seven minutes of oxygen deprivation or circulatory failure is the maximum that can be sustained without severe brain damage. The exact duration tolerated depends on attendant factors, including the overall medical condition of the patient.

Certain neurologic signs at presentation or occurring sometime during the course may assist in prognostication. Determining level of arousal may be helpful in predicting outcome. For example, failure to respond to verbal or noxious stimuli or predominantly abnormal responses (decerebrate or decorticate posturing) or signs of brainstem dysfunction such as absent pupillary or oculocephalic response are generally predictive of a poor outcome, defined as death or severe disability and dependency. A variety of scales, including the widely used Glasgow Coma Scale, is helpful in predicting survival and extreme degrees of recovery, but these scales are less reliable in prolonged coma or in predicting intermediate states of recovery (see Suggested Readings).

It is particularly difficult to predict outcome in young patients like Mike. Good recovery is common when consciousness returns within 12 to 24 hours. For people over the age of 50, survival after six days of coma is rare, while for those under the age of 20, survival with good return of function is common even after several weeks of coma. Because prolonged coma is rare, there is little data on which to predict outcome in a case such as Mike's. In general, the longer the duration of coma, the worse the chances of complete recovery, even among children. The chances that Mike will recover are very slim.

Laboratory methods such as electroencephalography (EEG) and somatosensory evoked potentials are not believed to be more accurate than clinical examination in predicting outcome, but when used together with clinical examination early on, they may enhance reliability of the prediction.[1] Although the findings of a mass lesion may be associated with poor outcome after head trauma, imaging studies such as CT scan and magnetic resonance imaging (MRI) do not generally add much in terms of predictive value. Overall, however, it is difficult to avoid false positives—that is, to identify patients who are expected to have a poor outcome, but who do in fact recover.

The age of the patient has some predictive value. Mortality after head injury is lower in children than in adults, but age-related mortality begins to climb in adolescence. The increased mortality among teenagers may be due partly to the severity of head trauma sustained in motor vehicle accidents, which are a far more common cause of head injury in this group than in very young children. Mortality continues to increase with age, although in late life falls become the predominant cause of head trauma. Children are in general expected to have a better prognosis for functional recovery than adults, however, the duration of coma is generally shorter for children than for adults, and it is this shorter duration of coma that may be a predictor for a better recovery. Some studies have shown that children under five years of age did worse than older children, but this could be related to the mechanism of trauma. In adolescence, the likelihood of functional recovery begins to approximate that of adults.

The better prognosis for children has been attributed to the "plasticity" of the youthful nervous system. Recent studies suggest that the preadolescent nervous system may actually be more vulnerable than the adolescent or adult brain to subtle damage such as memory deficits or learning disabilities; however, these data may be confounded by the preexistence of behavioral disorders in children who are prone to trauma. In Mike's case, age is in his favor, but the duration of his unconsciousness is not.

The best methods fail to predict outcome with much specificity. It is easier to predict extremes (good recovery or death) than intermediate outcomes. The best predictors also fail to identify a very small number (5 to 8 percent) of patients who are predicted early on to have a poor outcome but who actually recover, or, conversely those expected to recover who do not. Thus, while Mike is expected to have a poor outcome, it is not possible to predict this with absolute certainty. Early brain resuscitation in an effort to improve outcome is the focus of intensive research.[2]

2. What are the best and worst predicted outcomes for Mike if he awakens from coma?

Complete neurologic recovery is nearly but not entirely impossible. Approximately 50 to 60 percent of patients, regardless of age, who remain in coma for more than two weeks and do not die awaken to severe neurologic impairments and dependency. The prognosis in prolonged states of unconsciousness is uncertain because of a lack of data, but published experience suggests it is far worse.

Worsening prognosis

Head injury
Medical illness
   Metabolic
   Infection
   Drug overdose
Subarachnoid hemorrhage
Pure anoxia (e.g., carbon monoxide poisoning)
Anoxic encephalopathy (e.g., post–cardiac arrest)

Figure 7–11.1 Prognosis in Coma

Unfavorable (likelihood of death or
  persistent vegatative state)
Duration weeks to months
Age over 40 years
Absent corneal reflex
Absent pupillary light reflex
Absent motor response
Absent oculocephalic response
Absent somatosensory evoked potentials

Favorable

Duration hours to days
Age under 20 years

Figure 7–11.2 Prognostic Indicators in Coma

It is known only that Mike is unconscious. Patients with prolonged periods of unconsciousness may no longer be comatose but may actually be in a persistent vegetative state (PVS), the most advanced neurologic sequela in coma survivors. PVS (called "permanent" vegetative state after a prolonged period of time, when it is deemed to be irreversible) is a chronic form of eyes-open unconsciousness (see Case 10, "A Religious Objection to the Determination of Brain Death"). Higher cortical function is absent, but, in contrast to whole brain death sufficient brainstem function is retained so that respiration, heartbeat, and function of internal organs continue. Since the cerebral hemispheres govern the perception of sensory input, a patient in PVS, like the patient in coma, cannot experience sensory input, including pain, and does not exhibit any voluntary behavior. In contrast to coma, which is a sleeplike state, PVS is characterized by an arousal response and sleep-wake cycles. Therefore, the eyes may open and random eye movements are seen, but the patient is incapable of voluntarily tracking a visual cue. Wandering eye movements sometimes cause observers to believe the patient is conscious. Conversely, PVS may be diagnosed when less severe derangements exist.[3,4] Inaccurate diagnosis may be partly due to inexperience of the examining physician and partly to the complex mechanisms responsible for arousal.

Short of the vegetative state, a patient who awakens from prolonged coma is almost always left with a severe neurologic deficit, including aphasia, paralysis, or cognitive and behavioral deficits. Intermediate states have been termed *minimally conscious state*. In addition, the prolonged bedridden state also leads to severe contractures of the joints; these deformities could be avoidable with aggressive bedside physical therapy. It is important to recognize that patients with severe deficits have varying degrees of disability, which may range from complete dependency to satisfactory cognitive function with ability to assist in self-care.

Several independent medical centers have claimed "miraculous" recovery from coma, but they have not published data allowing objective evaluation of their results. Rare anecdotal reports have appeared in the literature of patients who regained consciousness after prolonged existence in the vegetative state; in all cases, the patient had severe functional dependence (see Suggested Readings). Incidents of extraordinary return of cognitive function could reflect the complex mechanisms governing arousal and the current inability to distinguish a variety of "unconscious" states from one another. Neurologic distinctions among coma, PVS, and whole brain death are depicted in Figure 7–11.3.

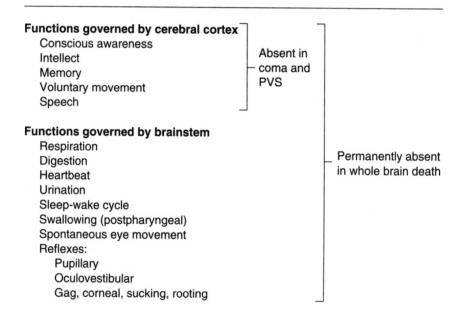

Figure 7–11.3 Neurologic Distinctions among Coma, PVS, and Whole Brain Death

ETHICAL AND LEGAL CONSIDERATIONS

1. How can the best interests of the patient be determined in this case?

In determining the patient's best interests, it is appropriate to balance the benefits of any treatments with the burdens imposed by the treatment or the disease, as discussed in Case 4 ("Management of Life-Threatening Illness"). The prognosis must also be taken into consideration, since in patients with a good prognosis, more burdens might be worth the future benefits gained, but if the prognosis is poor, the balance might tip in the opposite direction. In Mike's case, the prognosis is poor but still somewhat uncertain, making it difficult to weight the scale accurately.

In general, the burdens to a patient from a particular treatment intervention might include pain, suffering, indignities caused by the treatment or the disease, or being subjected to treatment that merely prolongs the process of dying. With patients such as Mike, who is unconscious and incapable of experiencing these burdens, there is dispute as to whether such burdens should weigh heavily in the balance. Many court cases that have considered such situations note that it is appropriate to weigh these factors. Although the patient himself cannot currently experience pain and suffering, most people would and do factor in related concerns, including dignity and quality of life, when making treatment decisions in advance. For example, a reasonable person might not want to be maintained in an irreversible condition or in a state of prolonged unconsciousness from which little or no recovery is expected.

The benefits of continued treatment in Mike's case include prolongation of his life with the possibility, though slight, that he may regain some ability to function. Maintenance of life alone has intrinsic value for some people, regardless of one's functional disabilities. For others, however, the maintenance of biologic life alone is not considered a benefit in the absence of adequate cognitive function or an adequate quality of life. There is concern that quality of life judgments may be unavoidably biased and tend to deprecate the social value of people with fewer capabilities than others. Even given this concern, however, the consideration of the patient's quality of life, as it relates to that specific patient in comparison to his previous quality of life, is generally held to be a legitimate and often essential component of treatment decision making. Numerous commentators have supported the incorporation of the patient's quality of life as part of the mix to be considered when determining benefits and burdens to the patient.[5]

For Mike, a consideration of his quality of life would examine not his value to society now or in the future, but rather his current and projected condition compared to his past lifestyle and the future he would have had, were it not for this accident. Obviously, for someone to move from a functional and healthy existence to a possible vegetative state, the quality of his life has dramatically changed. Because of Mike's poor prognosis, it would be understandable and appropriate if his parents were to consider this drastic change in quality as part of their decision-making process.

2. Would it be appropriate to consider the interests of others (as Mike's father is doing) when examining what serves Mike's best interests?

There is a growing consensus that it is justifiable to consider how treatment decisions affect other involved individuals, such as close family members. This is tied to the consensus that best-interests determinations should be specific to the particular patient. Most people would factor the interests of others into their own decision-making process when determining what kind of treatment they desire for themselves.[5] For many people, the financial and emotional burdens experienced by their family are of as much concern as the burdens they would experience as a patient in such circumstances.

In this case, therefore, a reasonable person might take into account the protracted burdens experienced by Mike's family, particularly in light of Mike's poor prognosis. The family's emotional trauma, the neglect of the younger children, marital discord, and the financial burdens would all be factors that a reasonable person might consider important and influential if he or she were ever in such a situation. Too often, treatment decisions, especially those that entail transfer of the patient to another care setting, fail to consider or acknowledge the impact of such decisions on the involved family members, both in their roles as informed decision makers and as actual givers of physical care to the patient. Lack of consideration of these family interests not only can heighten the burden experienced by the family but can also directly affect the patient's own well-being. The interests of others, such as a close family, do constitute an additional factor in the balance of benefits and burdens in decision making, but it is important to emphasize that they do not replace the central role of the patient's own interests.

It is also important to emphasize that the interests of providers—doctors, nurses, and health care institutions—in contrast to close family, should not influence how the decisions concerning treatment are determined. If a patient's physician objects to the direction of care, perhaps because of a different religious or moral perspective, then the physician should transfer care to someone else. The only interests of the provider that should enter and influence the decision process would be those factors that affect the medical interests of the patient, such as whether or not a particular intervention was medically beneficial.

3. Of what relevance is the patient's age in this decision-making process?

Despite his technical status as child, Mike is very close to the age of legal majority and his involvement in the decision process would be essential if he possessed the capacity to participate. On the cusp of capacity, he would essentially have been treated like an adult in the decision-making process. While Mike's parents are legally and rightfully the decision makers for their son, their determination of his best interests should in general coincide with a best-interests analysis as it would be applied to an adult, particularly because Mike is so close to the age of majority. The concept of the mature or emancipated minor is explored further in Case 30 ("A Teenager Who Wants Cosmetic Surgery") and Case 31 ("An Adolescent with Cancer Who Wants To Discontinue Medical Treatment").

From a medical perspective, Mike's age may be a factor, as discussed above.

4. What procedures should be utilized to resolve the dispute between the parents?

Given the connection and involvement that both parents appear to have with their son, normally they would serve as joint decision makers, bound only by the usual limits placed on parents as decision makers (see Case 29, "A Religious Objection to a Child's Medical Treatment").

If the parents were in agreement, they would be jointly empowered and there would be no basis on which to challenge their decisional authority. However, their disagreement raises a dilemma. By virtue of their equal status as parents, neither has greater decisional authority than the other. The essence of the problem here appears to be highly divergent views as to what should be done, what serves the best interests of their son, and the importance of other family considerations in this protracted trauma.

In order to resolve this dispute between equally empowered decision makers, short of resorting to a court of law, important steps must be taken.

These include providing a supportive and neutral forum in which this dispute can be explored as well as up-to-date and accurate information concerning the boy's condition, prognosis, and treatment options.

The physicians must take pains to ascertain the patient's overall prognosis. If the primary care physician has not already done so, he or she should seek the opinion of a neurologist to perform a meticulous examination, including laboratory tests if indicated, so that the most accurate prognosis possible can be conveyed to the family. A second opinion by a consulting neurologist might also be helpful in resolving the dilemma. It is not possible to predict an individual patient's neurologic prognosis with perfect accuracy, but it would be important for the family to have as realistic a picture as possible before arriving at a decision.

Other issues should be addressed. For example, the physician should discuss the option of a do-not-resuscitate (DNR) order with the family (see Case 12, "Resuscitation Decision in a Patient with Lung Cancer"). In doing so, he should explain that a DNR order does not prevent Mike from receiving other treatments nor would it signal abandonment of Mike by involved clinicians.

If there is still a conflict, the physician should arrange for a family conference to include both parents and any appropriate health professionals involved in the patient's care. Caregivers might include one or more physicians, including a neurologist, nurses, and nurse aides, in order to give an all-around view of the patient's medical condition. Other participants might include a social worker, patient representative, clergy who has been closely involved, or friends to whom Mike might have confided his wishes regarding care. This team/family conference should be held in a supportive and relaxed setting so that those involved would be able to speak frankly and openly. Although all interested parties would be encouraged to attend, the group should not be so large as to be unwieldy or intimidating, particularly to the parents, who are assigned the responsibility of making the decision.

The forum of family or team conference may help to set out the facts clearly and help family members or other surrogates to arrive at a more informed decision. If this type of forum does not resolve the dispute, in many institutions a forum for discussion is made available through the hospital ethics committee (see Case 4). This multidisciplinary group of professionals and other interested individuals is knowledgeable about the decision-making process but is not directly connected with the case. For Mike's family, this type of forum might also provide a nonthreatening and objective perspective to allow a range of issues to be fully and reasonably explored. The committee could respond in a variety of ways and one or more members might well meet with Mike's parents on one or more occasions.

The forum of the ethics committee allows for the proposal of strategies to accommodate the parents' apparent competing perspectives. For example, perhaps the mother's point of view supporting aggressive treatment could be placed into a more time-limited perspective; that is, certain interventions could be continued or attempted, with their benefits or burdens assessed after a specific time interval. Likewise, the broader interests incorporated by the father's position should be explored, perhaps to assure the patient's mother that it is the *patient's* interests, insofar as they can be determined, that are truly central in this decision process. It is even possible in these situations that one of the parents may lack the capacity to make the decision because he or she is too distraught to view the situation realistically.[6] This process of exploration and mediation may take some time, given the complexity and diversity of the interests to be considered, but the time taken is in keeping with the goals of mediation, namely, to undergo a *process* of deliberation involving all parties, rather than to weigh facts quickly and reach a binding decision for the parents.

At all levels of mediation, it is essential that both parents have accurate medical information concerning the patient so that they can make a truly informed decision. It is not uncommon for decisions to be based on misinformation or misunderstanding of available information. A neutral forum with the availability of the patient's physician to provide up-to-date and accurate information might end the current impasse.

It is important that these mechanisms for dispute resolution exist *within* the institution. The dispute in this case does not relate to who has legal authority, which might require a court proceeding. Rather, it is one involving disagreement between two loving parents. Such a disagreement is best resolved through sensitive and knowledgeable mediation in the clinical setting rather than through the more harsh and public forum of a court of law, which should always be the option of last resort. Fortunately, it is exceptionally rare for a dispute between equally empowered family members to require a judicial process for resolution.

REFERENCES

1. C. Bassetti et al., "Early Prognosis in Coma after Cardiac Arrest: A Prospective Clinical, Electrophysiological, and Biochemical Study of 60 Patients," *Journal of Neurology, Neurosurgery, and Psychiatry* 61 (1996): 610–615.
2. P. Safar, "Cerebral Resuscitation after Cardiac Arrest: Research Initiatives and Future Directions," *Annals of Emergency Medicine* 22 (1993): 324–349.
3. K. Andrews et al., "Misdiagnosis of the Vegetative State: Retrospective Study in a Rehabilitation Unit," *British Medical Journal* 313 (1996): 13–16.
4. N.L. Childs et al., "Accuracy of Diagnosis of Persistent Vegetative State. *Neurology* 43 (1993): 1465–1467.
5. President's Commission for the Study of Ethical Problems in Medicine and Biomedical and Behavioral Research. *Deciding To Forgo Life-Sustaining Treatment* (Washington, DC: U.S. Government Printing Office, 1983), 135–136.
6. A. Buchanan and D. Brock, *Deciding for Others* (Cambridge: Cambridge University Press, 1989), 215–266.

SUGGESTED READINGS

Arts, W.F.M. et al. 1985. Unexpected improvement after prolonged posttraumatic vegetative state. *Journal of Neurology, Neurosurgery, and Psychiatry* 48: 1300–1303.

Bernat, J.L. 1992. The boundaries of the persistent vegetative state. *Journal of Clinical Ethics* 3: 176–180.

Choi, S.C. et al. 1988. Enhanced specificity of prognosis in severe head injury. *Journal of Neurosurgery* 69: 381–385.

Choice in dying. Map: State laws addressing minors and end-of-life decision making. 1998. *Right To Die Law Digest*, March.

Council on Scientific Affairs and Council on Ethical and Judicial Affairs. 1990. Persistent vegetative state and the decision to withdraw or withhold life support. *Journal of the American Medical Association* 263: 426–430.

Covinsky, K.E. et al. 1994. The impact of serious illness on patients' families. *Journal of the American Medical Association* 272: 1839–1844.

Dubler, N.N., and Marcus, L.J. 1994. *Mediating bioethical disputes*. New York: United Hospital Fund.

Higashi, K. et al. 1988. Five-year follow-up study of patients with persistent injury related to patient's age. A longitudinal prospective study of adult and pediatric head injury. *Journal of Neurosurgery* 68: 409–416.

Jennett, B. et al. 1981. Disability after severe head injury: Observations on the use of the Glasgow Outcome Scale. *Journal of Neurology, Neurosurgery, and Psychiatry* 44: 285–293.

Kinney, H.C. et al. 1994. Neuropathological findings in the brain of Karen Ann Quinlan. The role of the thalamus in the persistent vegetative state. *New England Journal of Medicine* 330: 1469–1495.

Levin, H.S. et al. 1992. Severe head injury in children: Experience of the Traumatic Coma Data Bank. *Neurosurgery* 31: 435–444.

Levine, C., and Zuckerman, C. 1999. The trouble with families: Toward an ethic of accommodation. *Annals of Internal Medicine* 130: 148–152.

Levy, D.E. et al. 1981. Prognosis in nontraumatic coma. *Annals of Internal Medicine* 94: 293–301.

Levy, D.E. et al. 1987. Differences in cerebral blood flow and glucose utilization in vegetative versus locked-in patients. *Annals of Neurology* 22: 673–682.

The Multi-Society Task Force on PVS. 1994. Medical aspects of the persistent vegetative state. *New England Journal of Medicine* 330: 1499–1508; 1572–1579.

Payne, K. et al. 1996. Physicians' attitudes about the care of patients in the persistent vegetative state: A national survey. *Annals of Internal Medicine* 125: 104–110.

Plum, F., and Posner, J. 1980. *The diagnosis of stupor and coma*. Philadelphia: Davis.

Rogove, H.J. et al. 1995. Old age does not negate good cerebral outcome after cardiopulmonary resuscitation: Analysis from the brain resuscitation clinical trials. The Brain Resuscitation Clinical Trial I and II Study Groups. *Critical Care Medicine* 23: 18–25.

Rosenberg, G.A. et al. 1977. Recovery of cognition after prolonged vegetative state. *Annals of Neurology* 2: 167–168.

Snyder, B.D. et al. 1983. Delayed recovery from postanoxic persistent vegetative state (abstract). *Annals of Neurology* 14: 153.

Steinbock, B. 1989. Recovery from persistent vegetative state? The case of Carrie Coons. *Hastings Center Report* 19: 14–15.

Volicer, L. et al. 1997. Persistent vegetative state in Alzheimer disease. Does it exist? *Archives of Neurology* 197, no. 54: 1382–1384.

Zandbergen, E.G.J. 1998. Systematic review of early prediction of poor outcome in anoxic-ischaemic coma. *Lancet* 352: 1808–1812.

LEGAL CITATIONS

Statutory Examples

Arkansas Rights of the Terminally Ill or Permanently Unconscious Act, Ark. Code Ann. Sec. 20-17-214.
Statute permits parents to execute a written declaration on behalf of an unmarried minor to be effective in the event of terminal illness or permanent unconsciousness.

Louisiana Protection of Terminally Ill Children Act, La. Rev. Stat. Ann. Sec. 1551 to 1563.
Statute permits a parent or guardian to make a declaration ordering the withholding or withdrawal of life-sustaining treatments from a minor child.

CASE 12

Resuscitation Decision in a Patient with Lung Cancer

Phil is a 50-year-old man with non-small-cell lung cancer who is admitted to a large city teaching hospital after collapsing on the street. He was previously hospitalized here for superior vena cava syndrome, which was partially treated with radiation therapy, followed by a course of chemotherapy. The course of chemotherapy was complicated by pneumonia and bacteremia, from which Phil recovered. His medical records, which include his outpatient chart and records of his prior hospitalizations, have been sent to the floor.

Phil obtains sporadic medical care in the outpatient medical clinic, where patients are treated primarily by interns and residents under the supervision of attending physicians. Although his insurance plan covers his care adequately, he frequently misses his regular appointments.

Phil has been divorced from his wife for many years. He has not had contact with his two adult children, who live in another state, for some time. Their names and addresses, however, are listed on the outpatient chart.

In the emergency room, Phil was found to be minimally responsive. CT scan of the brain showed a large metastasis and his physical findings are consistent with pneumonia. Treatment with intravenous fluids and broad spectrum antibiotics was initiated, and Phil was sent to the floor. Now, several hours after admission, Phil's intern approaches the patient to obtain a blood sample, but she discovers that the patient's breathing is agonal and his pulse is not palpable. Earlier the intern had begun to review Phil's medical chart with the resident, and it was concluded that the overall prognosis was very poor. There had not been time to address the subject of a do-not-resuscitate (DNR) order for Phil, however, as the hospital ward had been exceptionally busy, and there were numerous admissions of seriously ill patients. The intern, who graduated from medical school just two months earlier, runs to find her resident to inform him that Phil is having a cardiac arrest. The resident tells the intern to "call a code," and walks slowly to the patient's bedside.

ISSUES TO CONSIDER

- Survival rate after cardiopulmonary resuscitation
- Presumption of consent to emergency interventions
- Do-not-resuscitate orders
- "Slow code" and professional integrity
- Medical futility
- Definitions of *terminal* illness

MEDICAL CONSIDERATIONS

1. What was Phil's prognosis on admission?

Phil presented initially with superior vena cava syndrome due to non-small-cell lung cancer. Superior vena cava syndrome, in which the superior vena cava is compressed by tumor, indicates that the cancer is not surgically resectable. Surgically unresectable non-small-cell cancer of the lung has a poor prognosis and is only moderately responsive to chemotherapy. Recurrent advanced disease, which Phil has, is poorly responsive to additional chemotherapy or other treatment modalities. Although further chemotherapy is nonetheless sometimes offered—for example, motivated patients whose performance status is otherwise satisfactory—it would not be considered in someone so ill at the time of admission.

2. If cardiopulmonary resuscitation is initiated for Phil, what is the likely medical outcome?

Prognosis post-CPR after in-hospital cardiopulmonary arrest is poor in patients with cardiac arrest due to medical illness other than uncomplicated arrhythmia or drug overdose. The reasons for this are obvious, though often ignored when a decision is made to institute CPR in someone with incurable medical illness. Cardiac resuscitation is directed at the conducting system of the heart. Lasting success of CPR depends on adequate functioning of the cardiac pump and other organ systems. When cardiac arrest results from end-stage disease in other organs, CPR may restore heartbeat and secondarily respiration, but it cannot permanently restore cardiopulmonary function in organic isolation. Thus, it would not be expected to do so in a patient such as Phil, whose cardiac arrest was the result of noncardiac illness and his respiratory failure at least in part the result of cardiac arrest. (Respiratory arrest differs from cardiorespiratory arrest in that the prognosis would depend on the cause of the respiratory arrest and the degree of reversible lung disease, in addition to the patient's overall medical condition.)

Cardiopulmonary arrest, if not quickly reversed, may lead to anoxic encephalopathy among those initially resuscitated. Among patients who are in a coma following resuscitation, fewer than one-third achieve good neurological recovery.[1] The neurologic prognosis is worse when the arrest is the result of noncardiac illness, as in the case of Phil.

It is virtually certain that if Phil is resuscitated, he will not survive to be discharged from the hospital, and there would be a good possibility that he would require advanced life support in an intensive care unit for a period before death.

ETHICAL AND LEGAL CONSIDERATIONS

1. How could the issue of DNR have been raised in advance, thus possibly averting this dilemma?

Because of the nature of Phil's illness, the subject of CPR would have been important to raise before this hospitalization, as a resuscitation attempt in a patient such as Phil might drastically change the manner in which he dies, which may have been quite important to him. By addressing the issue of DNR in advance, a physician might have pointed out that while CPR would in no way affect the incurable nature of his illness, it might disrupt an otherwise peaceful demise. The issues of pain, suffering, and quality of life would have been important for the patient to know about in advance, while he had capacity, so he could have considered them and exercised some control.

Given his mental state throughout this brief hospitalization, it obviously would not have been possible to discuss CPR with Phil during this admission. The next alternative would have been to contact those close to him, possibly his adult children. Although they had not been in recent contact, they might have provided enough information to authorize a DNR order and probably could have done so over the telephone.

The estrangement and distance of Phil's children would have posed the practical problem of reaching them in a timely fashion. Although he did not have one consistent primary care physician, Phil's condition and circumstances were known to at least certain providers. It would have been appropriate during one of his outpatient visits, or perhaps during an earlier, less serious hospitalization, for the gravity of his illness to be discussed and his preferences toward end-of-life care documented, including his wish concerning CPR. While such a discussion obviously requires tact and sensitivity, and may even have to occur over several visits, it would be wrong not to raise such issues with a patient whose disease progression is clear. Furthermore, it is important for a patient to consider these questions while he possesses decisional capacity. Particularly in a situation such as Phil's, where informed, authorized surrogate decision makers would not likely be available, it would have been valuable to create sufficient evidence of Phil's own wishes and values as a way to guide treatment decision making, in the event he lost decisional capacity.

It is unfortunate that DNR was not discussed with Phil because it was a lost opportunity to provide the patient with some level of control over his dying. The erratic nature of his health care and the absence of a consistent primary care physician made this difficult. If Phil had authorized a DNR order in advance of this crisis, his decision would have been valid and binding under this current circumstance. The difficulties encountered in implementing DNR orders made in advance of hospitalization and the strategies that can be used are discussed in detail in Case 8 ("Withdrawing Mechanical Ventilation at the Request of a Patient with Decisional Capacity").

Additional obstacles present themselves once a patient has been admitted to a hospital. There is not always time to evaluate the clinical situation and determine a prognosis before onset of an emergency. This problem is often magnified in situations such as that of Phil, who has not had an ongoing set of permanent providers. Moreover, although Phil was not alert enough to participate in a discussion of DNR, in other circumstances physicians are often reluctant to raise this issue early in the hospitalization. This reluctance stems from a fear of unnecessarily frightening a patient whose medical and emotional state might be fragile (see Case 5, "'Don't Tell Mother': Withholding Information from a Patient"). If the patient is not known to the physician in charge, it is difficult to establish the proper rapport to carry out such a serious and sensitive discussion in the first several hours of hospitalization.

These practical issues leave open the possibility that a patient could experience a medical emergency or loss of capacity without the physician having the benefit of the patient's wishes regarding an emergency procedure such as CPR. This unfortunate dilemma now confronts Phil and his doctors. Ideally this scenario could be limited to a small percentage of patients if physicians aggressively pursued advance planning with their patients. Barring this, physicians are guided by the usual standard of care in emergency situations (see below).

2. In view of the need to obtain informed consent before performing a procedure, what would be the justification for performing CPR without Phil's consent?

In contrast to the usual case, in which consent must be given by the patient or an authorized surrogate before the initiation of a treatment intervention, in CPR, consent is requested to *withhold* the treatment. There is a legal presumption that patients consent to attempts of the administration of CPR when it is medically indicated. This is based on an established principle that in a medical emergency a patient unable to give consent is presumed to consent to the medically indicated standard of care unless he has previously stated his objection. Many have interpreted this to mean that if a patient has not authorized a DNR order, a physician is always obliged to perform CPR. The justification given for this interpretation is that the initiation of CPR is the acceptable standard of care and any variation on what is usual should occur with the patient's input, if not consent. However, the standard of care concerning the use of CPR is evolving. Since the early 1960s, there has been a gradual extension of CPR from its use in limited circumstances to its widespread application in serious systemic illness.[2] In the 1980s, a series of published studies began to document the poor prognosis of CPR in medical inpatients, confirming what might have been predicted—the unphysiologic nature of CPR in advanced systemic disease. From this, there is a growing consensus that CPR is *not* indicated in many emergency situations.

The presumption of consent in an emergency covers the use of treatment interventions that are medically indicated. This presumption *does not* mandate the use of every possible emergency intervention in all circumstances. Thus, the presumption that a patient would consent to CPR does not mandate its use in every case of cardiopulmonary arrest, regardless of the patient's underlying condition. Second, in cases in which no DNR order has been issued, CPR might still be withheld if, at the time of the arrest, the physician, using reasonable medical judgment, concludes that such intervention would be medically futile. As discussed below, however, there is not yet unanimity of opinion regarding the precise definition of the concept of medical futility. Therefore, a decision not to initiate attempts at CPR for a patient without a DNR order would have to be carefully considered and justified, based upon a clear understanding of the patient's diagnosis, prognosis, and the clinical judgment about the medical benefits of CPR versus the harms for a person in the patient's condition. Even so, such a decision might be considered controversial by some. A judgment that resuscitation would be futile should not, however, be used as an excuse for not discussing DNR orders in advance with capable patients or authorized surrogates. If a physician believes that CPR would be medically futile, then he or she should explain this to the patient or surrogate, discuss the value of a DNR order under the circumstances, and offer DNR as an available option. In Phil's situation, there might have been time to authorize a DNR order. However, when there is insufficient time to gather information in order to determine an accurate prognosis, one cannot justify the determination of futility regarding CPR or other treatments.

Written institutional policies regarding DNR are mandated by the Joint Commission on Accreditation of Healthcare Organizations and provision of information regarding DNR to patients is required by the federal Patient Self-Determination Act, which came into effect in 1991. Many states also have specific statutes governing DNR orders both within hospitals as well as in the community.

3. Given the absence of consent to a DNR order and the gravity of Phil's medical condition, how might the resident justify his slow response, and are there alternatives?

The resident's actions suggest that he intends to perform a "slow code" or "show code," that is, moving slowly to the bedside or going through the motions of standard code (resuscitation) procedures, without the intent or desire that active attempts at resuscitation actually occur. Such actions are sometimes taken when there is no DNR order in place but the physician expects CPR to be unsuccessful or to produce more harm than good for the patient. Although there are legitimate alternatives, which are discussed below, a number of factors might motivate a physician to perform a sham procedure. A physician might be reluctant to go on record by writing a chart note that CPR would be medically futile, for fear of legal liability. Going through the motions of resuscitating the patient gives the appearance of conforming to what the physician may mistakenly believe is the standard of care. In other situations a motive might be that the patient or the patient's surrogate has requested or expected CPR and physicians feel compelled to appear as though they were responding to such wishes.

Many physicians believe that performing CPR in a situation where resuscitation is thought to be futile compromises their professional integrity. However, professional integrity is maintained when alternatives are used, and most physicians recognize that a slow code itself compromises professional integrity.

Several basic guidelines can be followed in these situations. First, when there is clinical justification to support a conclusion of medical futility, thus making the use of CPR medically inappropriate, the physician should be prepared to explain this to the patient or family ahead of time and to clarify any misunderstandings or false expectations they may have concerning CPR.

Second, in cases in which patients or families remain unconvinced or insist that CPR occur, and the physicians feel compelled to respond in some manner, then they must make an honest attempt at CPR if a code is called. Once a procedure is in progress, however, there do remain the elements of physician discretion and clinical judgment. If, for example, a code is initiated but it quickly becomes clear that the patient is not responding, there is nothing to compel the physician to continue the resuscitation attempt. Physicians may always exercise discretion in this situation and can end the resuscitation attempt at any point that it appears useless or unsuccessful. When patients or families insist on CPR, or when consent is presumed, the obligation on the physician is only to attempt CPR to the best of his or her abilities. There is no obligation to continue the procedure when the failed consequence of the effort becomes clear. In addition, a patient's or family's insistence on a treatment intervention does not in itself obligate the physician to respond accordingly (see Case 21, "'Do Everything': Physician Obligations in the Face of Family Demands").

Third, no action or intervention should ever occur in the clinical setting when the provider cannot justify his or her actions and document them in the chart. If a physician truly believes CPR is medically futile, then he or she should be able to stand by this assertion. If there is some doubt, then he or she should earnestly attempt CPR but conclude efforts if it becomes clear that such efforts are fruitless. If a patient such as Phil were resuscitated but could not be subsequently weaned from life support, it would then be possible to discontinue life support, as discussed in Case 8.

4. When is a treatment considered medically futile?

What constitutes medical futility is the subject of intense debate. This is an important question because of the implication that futile treatment may be withheld or withdrawn without the patient's consent. In addition, insurance companies and other third-party payers may refuse to pay for treatment that is deemed medically futile.

In one view, CPR would be medically futile if it did not do what it was developed to do—restart the patient's heart and allow his brain to be perfused so that he could breathe spontaneously. Thus, under this view, it could not be said that CPR would be medically futile for Phil because there is a possibility that these responses will occur, at least temporarily. Such a definition of futility is extremely narrow, however, since it is applicable only to the purely physiologic consequences of a treatment. For example, using this definition, it would be absolutely certain that CPR would be futile only if a patient were found decapitated or in rigor mortis with extreme dependent lividity.

In contrast, many would consider CPR futile in Phil's case because although it might temporarily restore his cardiac function, it does not affect or alter his *underlying* condition, which is likely to cause his death some time soon. Such a definition does not refer primarily to the immediate physical consequences of the intervention, but rather to the broader meaning of that outcome in the context of the patient's circumstances.

While probably more commonly accepted, this broader view of futility carries with it the potential for varying interpretations, unrecognized value judgments, and perhaps disregard for certain conditions in life. This second view of futility takes into consideration facts beyond the patient's medical condition alone and *judges* these facts from a certain value perspective. For example, a physician might decide not to resuscitate Phil because even if the resuscitation is technically successful, the terminal nature of his condition remains unchanged and the quality of his life might even diminish further if the outcome is reliance on machinery for continued survival. It is perfectly supportable for the patient to decide to avoid CPR in order to avoid risking a worse quality of life, however, it is debatable whether it is appropriate for a physician to make this value judgment *for* the patient, in the guise of futility.

Thus, in Phil's case, it would be ethical and justifiable to withhold CPR if his physicians were convinced that it would not bring about the restoration of his cardiac or respiratory function, given his deteriorated medical condition. If, however, the physicians withheld CPR because they believed that his quality of life is so poor at this point that no justification exists to try to maintain it, then it must be recognized that such a conclusion relies on more than just a medical evaluation. It is preferable to have the patient or his family be a part of this broader evaluation, as different individuals may have different perspectives concerning this issue.

Currently, there is not a consensus in society that would support physician decisions based on value judgments, rather than medical criteria, to the exclusion of the patient or the patient's spokesperson. Physicians who withhold or withdraw treatment based on this broader concept of futility do so without legal authority or perhaps societal support at this time; however, as physicians, regulators, and society as a whole develop more experience and understanding of the concept of medical futility, it may be that there will be ethical agreement on a firmer middle ground. This, in turn, might lead to use of CPR based only on certain medical indications or criteria, rather than confused reasoning concerning the extent of legal or moral obligations under the circumstance. Recent pronouncements concerning the determination of futility favor a procedural approach rather than an outright substantive definition of what constitutes futile treatment in various circumstances.

5. How do treatment decisions in Phil's case differ from those made for a patient with advanced cardiomyopathy? Stroke? Amyotrophic lateral sclerosis?

The same principles should govern the patient with any serious disease—namely, that resuscitation should be performed unless the patient or his surrogate would object or unless there is a consensus that CPR would be medically futile. Yet diseases that carry the same prognosis are associated with somewhat varying physician behaviors regarding DNR orders.[3] This is probably related to the fact that the prognosis in some diseases (e.g., congestive heart failure) is less clear-cut than others (e.g., metastatic cancer). Nonetheless, many diseases can be progressive and irreversible; when they are so severe that they lead to cardiopulmonary arrest, the likelihood of survival does not appear to differ from diseases such as metastatic cancer. Nevertheless, the question sometimes arises whether liver failure, heart failure, or other incurable diseases are terminal in the same sense as advanced cancer. It becomes important to carefully define what is meant by a *terminal* illness when delineating standards to be followed in health care legislation. Some states with living will legislation require that the patient be "terminally ill" in order to activate the living will, a requirement generally not applicable in the use of health care agents. The concept of a terminal illness is open to interpretation, however; some states define a terminal condition as one from which there is no recovery and which can be expected to cause death in 6 months while other states might use a more liberal standard of 12 months. Of course, it is often not possible to predict a patient's survival with precision, and thus such a criterion may unnecessarily exclude certain patients from the option of having treatment withheld or withdrawn in jurisdictions where *terminal* is defined in a time-limited fashion. Another example of this controversial prognostication is that in order for a patient to be eligible for hospice benefits, the physician must certify that it is likely the patient will die in six months (see Case 13, "A Dispute over DNR Status in a Patient Who Wants Palliative Surgery"). For a few examples of the different definitions of "terminal" to be found in state legislation, see the statutory examples at the end of this case.

Another definition of the concept of *terminal* centers on the likelihood that death will occur unless life-sustaining treatment is given. In this definition, one could argue that progressive conditions such as amyotrophic lateral sclerosis or advanced Alzheimer's disease are terminal, when the patient can no longer live without life support (respirator in the case of ALS; artificial nutrition and hydration in the case of Alzheimer's disease). Alternatively, terminal could be defined as the inevitability of death even if life-sustaining treatment is given. Therefore, a patient with ALS might not be considered terminal under the law if continued respirator treatment was given, nor a patient with advanced Alzheimer's disease if artificial nutrition and hydration were provided. Other examples would be conditions with a fixed but profound neurologic deficit like a major stroke or persistent vegetative state. Even if there is resistance to define these conditions as terminal, it might be argued that there should not be separate legal standards for these conditions and for diseases with a more predictable course, such as advanced cancer. This dilemma is related to the fact that definitions of terminal rely on discrete time intervals or probability of survival with or without life-support, and when the law invokes such definitions, it fails to take into account an evaluation of the patient's quality of life. Thus, it is possible that a family member, acting on behalf of a patient through a living will, might request the withdrawal of life support from someone with a disease or condition not regarded as terminal under the law, and thus this request might be turned down.

REFERENCES

1. H.J. Rogove et al., "Old Age Does Not Negate Good Cerebral Outcome after Cardiopulmonary Resuscitation: Analysis from the Brain Resuscitation Clinical Trials. The Brain Resuscitation Clinical Trial I and II Study Groups," *Critical Care Medicine* 23 (1995): 18–25.

2. W.B. Kouwenhoven et al., "Closed-Chest Cardiac Massage," *Journal of the American Medical Association* 173 (1960): 1064–1067.

3. R.M. Wachter et al., "Decisions about Resuscitation: Inequities among Patients with Different Diseases but Similar Prognoses," *Annals of Internal Medicine* 111 (1989): 525–532.

SUGGESTED READINGS

Blackhall, L.J. 1987. Must we always use CPR? *New England Journal of Medicine* 317: 1281–1285.

Choice in Dying. 1998. Statutes authorizing do-not-resuscitate orders. *Right To Die Law Digest*, March.

Council on Ethical and Judicial Affairs, American Medical Association. 1999. Medical futility in end-of-life care. Report of the Council on Ethical and Judicial Affairs. *Journal of the American Medical Association* 281: 938–941.

Curtis, J.R. et al. 1995. Use of the medical futility rationale in Do Not Attempt Resuscitation orders. *Journal of the American Medical Association* 273: 124–128.

DeBuono, B.A. 1997. New York's DNR law does not require futile resuscitation. *Archives of Internal Medicine* 157: 467–468.

de Vos, R. et al. 1999. Quality of survival after cardiopulmonary resuscitation. *Archives of Internal Medicine* 159: 249–254.

Diem, S.J. et al. 1996. Cardiopulmonary resuscitation on television. Miracles and misinformation. *New England Journal of Medicine* 334: 1578–1582.

Ebell, M.H. et al. 1998. Survival after in-hospital cardiopulmonary resuscitation. A meta-analysis. *Journal of General Internal Medicine* 13: 805–816.

FitzGerald, J. et al. (for the SUPPORT investigators). 1996. Functional status among survivors of in-hospital cardiopulmonary arrest. *Archives of Internal Medicine* 156: 72–76.

Futility in clinical practice (series). 1994. *Journal of the American Geriatrics Society* 42: 861–905.

Gray, W.A. et al. 1991. Unsuccessful emergency medical resuscitation: Are continued efforts in the emergency department justified? *New England Journal of Medicine* 325: 1393–1398.

Hakim, R.B. et al. 1996. Factors associated with do-not-resuscitate orders: Patients' preferences, prognoses, and physicians' judgments. SUPPORT Investigators. Study To Understand Prognoses and Preferences for Outcomes and Risks of Treatment. *Annals of Internal Medicine* 125: 284–293.

Hoffman, J.C. et al. 1997. Patient preferences for communication with physicians about end-of-life decisions. *Annals of Internal Medicine* 127: 1–12.

Murphy, D.J. et al. 1994. The influence of the probability of survival on patients' preferences regarding cardiopulmonary resuscitation. *New England Journal of Medicine* 330: 545–549.

Schneiderman, L.J. et al. 1996. Medical futility: Response to critiques. *Annals of Internal Medicine* 125: 669–674.

Consensus Statement of the Society of Critical Care Medicine's Ethics Committee regarding futile and other possibly inadvisable treatments. 1997. *Critical Care Medicine* 25: 887–891.

Thel, M.C., and O'Connor, C.M. 1999. Cardiopulmonary resuscitation: Historical perspective to recent investigations. *American Heart Journal* 137: 39–48.

Tresch, D.D. et al. 1994. Cardiopulmonary resuscitation in elderly patients hospitalized in the 1990s: A favorable outcome. *Journal of the American Geriatrics Society* 42, no. 2: 137–141.

Waisel, D.B., and Truog, R.D. 1995. The cardiopulmonary resuscitation-not-indicated order: Futility revisited. *Annals of Internal Medicine* 122: 304–308.

LEGAL CITATIONS

Case Examples

Reported legal cases addressing various aspects of medical futility:

Gilgunn v. Massachusetts General Hospital, Mass. Super. Ct., No. 92-4820, verdict 21 (1995).

In re Baby "K", Nos. 93-1899, 93-1923, 93-1924, 4th Cir. (Va. Feb. 10, 1994).

In re Conservatorship of Wanglie, No. PX-91-283, Minn. Dist. Ct., Hennepin Cty. (July 1991).

Statutory Examples

New York Pub. Health Law Sec. 2961(9) (McKinney, 1993 Suppl. 1998).
State statute that defines the term *futile* resuscitation as that which is unsuccessful in restoring cardiac or respiratory function or in circumstances when the patient would experience repeated arrests within a short time before death.

Examples of different definitions of "terminal" found in state legislation:

Oklahoma Rights of the Terminally Ill or Persistently Unconscious Act, Okla. Stat. Ann. Title 63, Sec. 3101.1 to 3101.6 (West Supp. 1996).

"Terminal condition" means an incurable and irreversible condition that, even with administration of life-sustaining treatment, will, in the opinion of the attending physician and another physician, result in death within six (6) months."

California Natural Death Act, Cal. Health & Safety Act, Sec. 7185 to 7194.5 (West. Supp. 1996).

"Terminal condition" means an incurable and irreversible condition that, without the administration of life-sustaining treatment, will, within reasonal medical judgment, result in death within a relatively short time.

CASE 13

Dispute over DNR Status in a Patient Who Wants Palliative Surgery

Maria, a previously healthy woman, developed breast cancer at age 37. Now, three years later, her cancer has metastasized to bone and pleura. Further chemotherapy or hormonal therapy is not expected to prolong her life. She recently underwent pleurodesis to prevent recurrent pleural effusion. Her insurance carrier, a managed care corporation, has a contract with a local home hospice program, and she has recently enrolled. Prior to her enrollment in hospice, her bone pain was poorly controlled. Hospice nurses have seen to it that Maria receives sufficient doses of oral morphine, and her pain is fairly well controlled.

Recently, Maria sustained a pathologic fracture of the hip. An orthopedic surgeon in the emergency room explained that she may benefit from reconstructive surgery for the hip, which could restore her ability to walk. He further explained that he has performed this kind of operation on hospice patients in the past. Maria was eager to undergo the surgery, stating, "I want to die with my boots on." On admission, she requested a do-not-resuscitate (DNR) order, as she had done on a previous admission when she was hospitalized for treatment of her pleural effusion. To her surprise, she was informed that the DNR order would be suspended while she was in the operating room, recovery room, and surgical intensive care unit.

Her husband asked the surgical attending physician why this was being done. The surgeon stated that this was the policy of the departments of surgery and anesthesiology, and that it was adopted because their "hands would be tied" and they would be "unable to function" without such a policy. The surgeon said that even if he himself agreed to go along with the patient's request, his department would not agree and it would be impossible to find an anesthesiologist for the surgery. "Besides," he said, "things can go wrong, and if we just stand by it would amount to killing your wife."

Maria is uncertain about proceeding as planned under this restriction. After another day goes by, the surgeon receives a call from the hospital's case manager, who informs him that the days that Maria waits for surgery will be disallowed by Maria's managed care company, and the decision must be made quickly or Maria will have to be discharged.

ISSUES TO CONSIDER

- The specificity of a DNR order
- Suspending DNR orders during invasive procedures
- Physician interests and obligations in the context of patients' rights
- Insurance coverage under managed care and hospice programs

MEDICAL CONSIDERATIONS

1. What medical procedures can a hospice patient receive?

Hospice status does not automatically limit the type of procedure that a patient can receive. In the United States, the term *hospice* generally refers to a reimbursable system of palliative care delivery to dying patients, and though care under hospice is generally delivered at home, it is not uncommon for hospice patients to undergo invasive palliative procedures, since the goal of hospice care (and other modes of palliative care delivery) is to relieve symptoms and to maximize function. Thus, Maria's pleurodesis and proposed hip surgery are not inconsistent with the goals of her hospice program. Furthermore, she could obtain radiation to specific sites of bony metastases if this were indicated for pain relief. Despite this, reimbursement within hospice may place some practical limitations on the course of her treatment, as discussed below.

2. What are the medical implications of agreeing to perform surgery with a DNR order in place?

The physician has alluded to the restrictions posed by DNR orders from the perspective of the surgeon. The events that trigger the need for resuscitative measures in the surgical patient are generally very different from the circumstances of the medical patient who experiences cardiorespiratory arrest. Surgical patients who experience cardiorespiratory arrest tend to be of certain groups—trauma victims undergoing emergency surgery, patients who experience left ventricular failure during cardiac surgery, or patients with serious underlying disease associated with high operative risk. In elective surgery, cardiopulmonary arrest is usually due to problems extrinsic to the disease process.

If the term *resuscitation* is meant to include any procedure or intervention used to maintain life during a cardiac arrest, then theoretically a surgeon operating with a DNR order in place would be prohibited from using any and all resuscitation measures when the arrest occurred, regardless of circumstances. But the spectrum of events that can occur in connection with surgery and anesthesia includes some that can be resolved easily. It is not surprising then that the surgeon would feel that his "hands would be tied" if he could not intervene in easily remediable situations. Events unrelated to the disease process that may trigger an arrest or near-arrest during surgery range from the expected physiologic events resulting from anesthesia to unexpected but known emergencies such as airway problems, to accidents caused by human error.

As one anesthesiologist has pointed out, induction of general anesthesia is intrinsically a procedure that creates hemodynamic instability for which resuscitation is a linked follow-up maneuver.[1] Thus, by its very nature, the use of anesthesia may require at least limited resuscitation, even in the physiologically healthy patient. Patients who typically request DNR orders are among the sickest and would be more likely to develop severe hemodynamic instability. In contrast to this anticipated, finely controlled situation, in which resuscitation plays a role, is a frank, unanticipated cardiorespiratory arrest during surgery. This could be due to inappropriate treatment, for example, an anesthesia overdose or accidental esophageal intubation. In such a case, the physician would likely feel compelled to attempt to reverse a process for which he felt responsible. Not to do so might place him in a morally or legally untenable situation, in which he might feel he was involved in "killing" the patient, as the surgeon on Maria's case feels. Iatrogenic arrest could also occur despite appropriate care, for example, as an unexpected reaction from appropriate use of anesthesia (laryngospasm or severe hypotension). Even without an explicit link of responsibility for the event, the physician might still feel obligated to act. In fact, the majority of intraoperative cardiac arrests appear to be iatrogenic, especially when emergency operations and patients with underlying medical risk factors are excluded.[2,3]

The intensity of monitoring during surgery and the immediate availability of a resuscitation team would presumably enhance the likelihood of a good outcome. Survival to discharge after perioperative arrest ranges from approximately 48 to 92 percent when the arrest is directly linked to anesthesia, although prognosis is highly dependent on the patient's underlying condition. In one study of DNR patients receiving surgery, 54 percent survived to discharge and 30 percent survived at least four months,[4] which is generally much higher than among nonsurgical patients (see Case 12, "Resuscitation Decision in a Patient with Lung Cancer"), suggesting that only those with relatively good surgical risk would receive surgery, despite their decision to have a DNR order.

It would be difficult to predict the precise outcome for Maria if she were to have a cardiopulmonary arrest during surgery, although her age and baseline neurologic and cardiac status are predictive of a favorable outcome. More likely than an intraoperative arrest in this patient might be a prolonged postoperative intubation, since her pulmonary status is somewhat impaired. This possibility, and strategies to deal with it, would be very important to address in advance. This element in Maria's case, which is independent of the DNR dilemma, points out the complexity of such cases and the numerous medical uncertainties to consider other than those directly surrounding the question of DNR.

3. What would be the implications of a DNR order for a neurologically impaired patient who was undergoing percutaneous endoscopic feeding gastrostomy (PEG)? Hemodialysis?

PEG has practically replaced operative gastrostomy, but it is an invasive procedure that requires some form of sedation, usually intravenous benzodiazepines with or without opioids. This form of light anesthesia poses a small but real risk of respiratory suppression or hypotension, especially in the frail patients who are the most common recipients of this procedure. In hemodialysis, accidental death related to electrical or mechanical failure of the procedure or contamination of the dialysate is exceedingly rare. By contrast, hypotension requiring administration of intravenous saline occurs in at least 30 percent of dialyses overall and is extremely common in certain subgroups, for example, patients over the age of 70 years. Severe hypotension can produce shock, loss of consciousness, and cardiac arrest, all of which would normally be followed by resuscitative measures.

Thus, in these invasive procedures, the same dilemma concerning DNR orders might arise. Physicians might be reluctant to participate in these interventions because of the limits placed on their ability to respond if the patient experienced an arrest during the procedure. In these cases it would, of course, be important to be sure that the procedure itself was in keeping with the patient's wishes and overall treatment goals.

ETHICAL AND LEGAL CONSIDERATIONS

1. What are the justifications for performing an invasive procedure on a patient who requests a DNR order?

A patient's decision not to be resuscitated is a specific wish to forgo cardiopulmonary resuscitation and is not synonymous with a decision to give up or refuse other sorts of treatment interventions that might provide some benefit, such as symptom relief or even life prolongation. Thus, "do not resuscitate" does not mean "do not treat." Maria's desire not to be resuscitated has been made after an assessment of the risks and benefits that CPR would hold for her, given her prognosis and goals of care, and these risks and benefits would be similar whether the arrest resulted from her disease or from a perioperative event.

At the same time, she might decide that the risks associated with surgery are worth the potential benefit of being ambulatory, which would improve the quality of her remaining life. She might be willing to take the risk of dying during surgery, for example, because being able to walk again means so much to her. Her decision not to be resuscitated can logically coexist with decisions to consent to other sorts of interventions, even if they are invasive or aggressive.

On a practical note, for many patients, a decision not to be resuscitated *does* indicate a certain perspective concerning their circumstances and what they desire from medical care at that point. The discussion concerning a DNR order is often an appropriate time to consider broader end-of-life treatment options and goals, about which the patient may have equally strong feelings.

2. What are the ethical implications of operating with a DNR order in place?

If Maria and her doctors agreed that the DNR order should remain in place during surgery, presumably this would be done with the mutual understanding that either complications from the surgery itself or the patient's underlying condition might cause a cardiac arrest. Although Maria has experience with DNR orders, she should be made aware of the potentially different circumstances surrounding an arrest in the operating room and how those circumstances might affect her assessment of potential benefits, burdens, and outcomes. In general, any time a DNR patient is about to undergo an invasive procedure or has a drastic change in circumstance, the decision to continue the DNR should be reviewed, rather than automatically suspended. The review ensures that the patient understands the nature of the procedure and its potential complications, including the possibility of a cardiac arrest not directly related to her underlying condition. The choice of whether or not to continue the DNR order should be that of the patient, but the decision should be an informed one.

Assuming there is a mutual understanding, the patient still desires to have a DNR order, and her doctors agree to perform surgery under such conditions, then the surgeons and anesthesiologists would be bound by the terms of the DNR order should the patient arrest during surgery. If she experienced an arrest and no attempt was made to resuscitate her, her doctors would not be "killing" the patient or be responsible for her death, but rather would be acting in accordance with their obligation to respect their patient's right to self-determination. It would be unethical and theoretically challengeable in a court of law if her doctors agreed to the DNR order but subsequently refused to honor it during the procedure, because the patient's consent to surgery would then have been obtained under fraudulent circumstances.

3. If the surgeon insisted that there be no DNR order during the surgery, would this be a violation of Maria's rights?

As discussed in Case 12, there is a general legal presumption that a patient consents to treatment during emergency circumstances and, in the case of cardiac arrest, to CPR, unless a DNR order has been previously authorized. In cases such as Maria's, there is no reason that the issue of the DNR during surgery could not be discussed in advance. If, however, the anesthesiologist accidentally placed the endotracheal tube in her esophagus, he would be acting in good faith if he corrected the situation, which might include CPR. It would be important for the doctors involved to anticipate this type of situation and discuss it with Maria in advance (see below).

If Maria desires to continue her DNR status but her physicians remain unwilling to operate on her with these restrictions, Maria cannot demand that they do so. A patient cannot insist that a physician practice in a manner that the physician would evaluate as compromising his or her professional integrity; doctors do have the right to decide under what conditions they want to operate. These limits of provider obligations are discussed in detail in Case 1 ("A Religious Objection to a Blood Transfusion"). Maria would need to either seek out alternative surgeons or make her decision regarding surgery with the understanding that the DNR order would be suspended. It could be that as part of her assessment of the surgery's risks and benefits, Maria will have to account for the unwillingness of physicians to oblige her choice to maintain her DNR status during surgery. Thus, unwilling to risk resuscitation, she may unfortunately have to forgo the surgery if she cannot work out a compromise or cannot find alternative providers.

If Maria gave her consent to surgery with the understanding that the DNR order would continue, but her doctors had no intention of honoring it, such action would both violate the patient's right to self-determination and constitute a fraud on the patient, particularly if her consent were obtained with explicit reference to the issue of DNR. If, however, no discussion of the matter of DNR occurred, and all parties, in good faith, acted according to their presumptions under the circumstances, then there could be no claims of fraud. It would still be unethical to suspend the DNR order without involving Maria in the decision. Thus, physicians must be alert to this possibility and be cognizant of patients' rights and preferences.

4. Is there a solution to this dilemma?

First, it is important to weigh carefully the advantages and disadvantages of even performing the proposed surgery. Maria is eager to remain ambulatory, and the procedure, which will not cure her disease, may nonetheless achieve her goal of improving the quality of her remaining life. In contrast, Nathan, the patient in Case 3 ("Urgent Surgery in a Stuporous Patient"), was in a situation with much greater operative risk. For Nathan, the proposed surgery might not have been as clear an option, and other methods of palliation, such as heavy sedation, might have been more in keeping with his goals. Because the potential benefits of surgery are quite clear for Maria, and her surgical risk is lower, it is essential to confront the troublesome issue of what to do about the DNR order.

The surgeon should discuss details of the intervention with the patient. He should explain that if there were a problem that could be easily reversed—for example, if the ventilator became unplugged or if anesthesia-related hypotension occurred—then these would rapidly be attended to, and, because of her underlying good cardiac and brain function, the outcome would likely be positive and would not increase the risk of prolonged illness in the intensive care unit. Likewise, if Maria choked on a piece of food while in the hospital her doctors would want to take swift action to remedy the situation, under the presumption that resuscitating her in these circumstances was not what she meant by DNR and that honoring her DNR order was not relevant to the situation at hand. If there were misunderstanding or disagreement over these issues, they could best be addressed at this point. It is possible that the patient's and her husband's misgivings can be relieved once the facts of the situation are made clear.

Any policy that calls for the blanket rescinding of DNR orders may be too rigid, as it does not take into consideration a patient's desire not to end up in a worse condition. DNR decisions can be negotiated on a case-by-case basis. This would take into account the physician's interest in being allowed to effectively treat the patient, while also respecting the patient's wish for protection should something go terribly wrong. A negotiated compromise could best be reached if the surgeon or anesthesiologist took the time to inform the patient carefully of all the risks, to assure her that any remediable events would be quickly corrected. It should also be explained, however, that if an unexpected event occurred that was not directly related to the surgery and that could not be corrected, her wish not to be resuscitated would be honored. Informing the patient in such detail has the added benefit of enhancing the patient's ability to make an informed decision.

5. What if the patient experienced intraoperative cardiac arrest related to sudden and massive bleeding from a surgically damaged artery? From an artery invaded by tumor?

In the first situation, the cause of the arrest could be considered iatrogenic, whereas in the latter, one could argue that the bleeding was disease induced. Regardless of the origin of the mishap, the risk to the patient is the same and could be as serious as permanent brain damage or death following a prolonged stay in the ICU. As this is undoubtedly a major concern of most DNR patients, it should be explained to Maria that life support could be discontinued if she found herself in an irreversible condition that she would not tolerate. In fact, before the surgery Maria could stipulate a time and treatment schedule that she would be willing to undergo if an untoward event occurred during surgery and life-prolonging measures were instituted. In that way, she could try to realize the benefits of surgery but could also set limits if her condition deteriorated. She should be advised as well that, if she has not yet done so, she should execute an advance directive (either a health care power of attorney, living will, or both) so that if such decisions needed to be made, they could be made swiftly on her behalf and in keeping with her wishes.

6. What limitations does Maria's hospice status place on her ability to obtain the surgery?

Depending on the source of reimbursement for Maria's hospice care and whether this surgery is viewed as a strictly palliative procedure or something more, Maria may need to temporarily discontinue her hospice enrollment in order to obtain the surgery. Medicare is the primary source of reimbursement for hospice care in this country, primarily serving patients over 65 years of age. Currently, 42 states also cover hospice care through Medicaid, and most managed care providers also provide a hospice benefit, though the extent of coverage may vary from one plan to another. As most hospices are Medicare certified, in order to be eligible for Medicare reimbursement, even non-Medicare hospice patients are affected by the rules and regulations of the Medicare hospice reimbursement program.

Hospice care is primarily home-based care, aimed primarily at pain and symptom control interventions. It is a palliative approach to care, designed neither to hasten death nor to prolong the dying process. Occasionally, hospice patients do require admission to an acute care setting, either for respite care for involved caregivers or for aggressive, intensive pain or symptom management. Whether or not Maria's surgical repair of her hip would be considered a palliative procedure that is eligible for reimbursement under hospice is questionable. If necessary, however, Maria could discontinue enrollment from hospice care to be eligible for coverage of an acute care surgical procedure and then subsequently reenroll in hospice upon discharge from the hospital, assuming she continues to meet the hospice eligibility requirements.

When the Medicare hospice benefit was created in 1982, fairly strict eligibility criteria limited access to hospice for patients at the very end of life. Under more recent revisions of the hospice Medicare benefit with the enactment of the Balanced Budget Act of 1997, eligibility requirements have become more flexible. While physicians still need to certify that the patient has a prognosis of six months or less, there is no maximum number of months a patient can remain in hospice, as long as the physician continues to recertify the prognosis for each benefit period. Therefore, currently, the Medicare hospice benefit has an initial 90-day benefit period, followed by a subsequent 90-day period, and then finally an unlimited number of subsequent 60-day benefit periods as long as the patient continues to meet the program eligibility criteria. Patients in hospice always have the right to discontinue enrollment from hospice and return to more aggressive, cure-oriented care whenever they wish, and can always reenter hospice at a subsequent time as long as their doctor is able to certify their eligibility.

If Maria's insurance coverage is provided through a managed care organization, then the extent of her hospice coverage and her ability to switch back and forth between hospice and more cure-oriented care would be dictated by the terms of the managed care contract. One area of potential concern, however, might be coverage of the inpatient days while Maria and her physicians determine the feasibility of a DNR order during the surgical procedure. It is possible that the days spent discussing this issue, and the subsequent delay of the surgical procedure, might lead to a determination on the part of the managed care organization not to pay for much of this hospitalization. Cost containment pressures exerted by the managed care company to minimize days of hospitalization might therefore affect the nature of the discussion and the outcome of this dilemma.

REFERENCES

1. R.D. Truog, "'Do-Not-Resuscitate' Orders during Anesthesia and Surgery," *Anesthesiology* 74 (1991): 606–608.
2. R.L. Keenan and C.P. Boyan, "Cardiac Arrest Due to Anesthesia. A Study of Incidence and Causes," *Journal of the American Medical Association* 253 (1985): 2373–2377.
3. G.L. Olsson and B. Hallen, "Cardiac Arrest during Anaesthesia. A Computer-Aided Study in 250,543 Anaesthetics," *Acta Anaesthesiologica Scandinavica* 32 (1982): 653–664.
4. N.S. Wenger et al. "Patients with DNR Orders in the Operating Room: Surgery Resuscitation and Outcomes SUPPORT Investigators. Study to Understand Prognoses and Preferences for Outcomes and Risks of Treatment," *Journal of Clinical Ethics* 8, no. 3 (1997): 250–257.

SUGGESTED READINGS

American College of Surgeons 1994. Statement on advance directives by patients: "Do not resuscitate" in the operating room. *Bulletin of the American College of Surgeons* 79 no. 9:29 (see Appendix A).

Casarett, D.J. et al. 1999. Would physicians override a do-not-resuscitate order when a cardiac arrest is iatrogenic? *Journal of General and Internal Medicine* 14: 35–38.

Christakis, N.A., and Excarce, J.J. 1996. Survival of Medicare patients after enrollment in hospice programs. *New England Journal of Medicine* 335: 172–178.

Clemency, M.V., and Thompson, N.J. 1993. "Do not resuscitate" (DNR) orders and the anesthesiologist: A survey. *Anesthesia and Analgesia* 76: 394–401.

Clemency, M.V., and Thompson, N.J. 1997. Do not resuscitate orders in the perioperative period: Patient perspectives. *Anesthesia and Analgesia* 84: 859–864.

Cohen, C.B., and Cohen, J. 1991. Do-not-resuscitate orders in the operating room. *New England Journal of Medicine* 325: 1879–1882.

Committee on Care at the End of Life, Institute of Medicine. 1997. The health care system and the dying patient. In *Approaching death. Improving care at the end of life,* eds. M.J. Field and C.K. Cassel, 87–121. Washington, DC: National Academy Press.

Council on Ethical and Judicial Affairs, American Medical Association. 1991. Guidelines for the appropriate use of do-not-resuscitate orders. *Journal of the American Medical Association* 265: 1868–1871.

Hospice Association of America. 1997. *Hospice Facts and Statistics* (see Appendix A).

LaPuma, J. et al. 1988. Life-sustaining treatment. A prospective study of patients with DNR orders in a teaching hospital. *Archives of Internal Medicine* 148: 2193–2198.

Lumley, J., and Zideman, D.A. 1989. Perioperative CPR. *Clinical Critical Care Medicine* 16: 123–134.

Seale, C. 1991. A comparison of hospice and conventional care. *Social Science and Medicine* 32: 147–152.

Sontag, M.A. 1991. Hospice values, access to services and the Medicare hospice benefit. *American Journal of Hospice and Palliative Care* 9: 17–21.

Walker, R.B. 1991. DNR in the OR. Resuscitation as an operative risk. *Journal of the American Medical Association* 266: 2407–2412.

Youngner, S. J. et al. 1991. DNR in the operating room. Not really a paradox. *Journal of the American Medical Association* 266: 2433–2434.

CASE 14

Suicide Risk in a Managed Care Patient

John is a 63-year-old man who has been seeing a psychiatrist, Dr. Offenbach, for two years because of an accumulation of life stresses. John's managed care insurance plan permits 20 psychiatry outpatient visits per year. John began to see Dr. Offenbach when he lost his job as a midlevel executive for a large corporation and was unable to find comparable employment or succeed in a lawsuit he filed against his employer for age discrimination. During this time, his wife developed cancer and deteriorated rapidly.

On Monday morning, weeping uncontrollably, John called Dr. Offenbach at home. His wife had died the previous Wednesday and was buried on Saturday. "Life isn't worth living," he said over and over again. John refused to come to the psychiatry emergency room but agreed to meet Dr. Offenbach in her office. When he arrived unshaven and disheveled, John was inconsolable, and when asked what he was going to do, he replied, shaking his head, "I'm not sure, I'm not sure. Things just keep getting worse and worse." Although John has denied a suicidal plan in the past, Dr. Offenbach is aware that her patient is an avid hunter and owns a rifle and would like to admit him to the hospital for close observation. Before it will agree to pay the hospital bill, however, John's managed care company must approve the admission and Dr. Offenbach will therefore need to carefully justify this admission in order to obtain this "precertification."

Several months ago, another managed care company refused to certify an admission for Dr. Offenbach's patient, Karen, a woman with borderline personality disorder, who had recently broken up with her boyfriend. Karen had a history of impulsive behavior and had threatened suicide on several occasions. A psychiatry resident in the emergency room had told the company's case manager the patient was "suicidal," to which the case manager replied, "How is she suicidal?" The resident wavered, saying, "she's not sure what she's going to do, but I'm sure she's going to do something." Precertification was refused, and the patient was referred for outpatient follow-up with Dr. Offenbach. Karen went home and called Dr. Offenbach at her office, stating she had "just taken 50 Pamelor [nortriptyline]." Karen's mother took her to a local emergency room, where appropriate measures were taken. Although it appeared as though Karen had exaggerated the number of pills taken, she was admitted to a medical ward and was discharged in good physical condition.

Dr. Offenbach had discussed that "close call," with several of her colleagues, who had had similar experiences and were increasingly disgruntled about managed care (see Case 13, "A Dispute over DNR Status in a Patient Who Wants Palliative Surgery"). Now she wants to take no chances, and tells the company's case manager that John has a clear plan, has stated that he owns a gun, and intends to shoot himself. The admission is approved. John is admitted and is treated with antidepressants, sedation, and psychotherapy.

Continued hospitalization requires preapproval every two days; without this approval, the hospital will not be paid. The managed care company uses published criteria,[1] which require discharge to home or outpatient day program by Day 4 if the patient is "capable of activities of daily living," and is "neither suicidal or self-mutilative." By Day 3, John is calmer and has taken a shower. "I'm still not sure what I'm going to do," he says. Dr. Offenbach feels the patient should be observed for a while longer while psychotherapy and medications continue and instructs the hospital's case manager to tell the company the patient is sticking to his suicide plan. The doctor is concerned about the patient's risk and documents her concerns on the chart and adds, "patient still suicidal."

ISSUES TO CONSIDER

- Establishing risk of outpatient management
- Fraudulent documentation
- Physician versus insurance company liability

MEDICAL CONSIDERATIONS

1. How is suicide risk determined?
It is not possible to know in an individual case whether or not a person is going to commit suicide, but certain factors have been consistently associ-

ated with suicide or suicide attempts serious enough to require a medical hospitalization. These risk factors include advanced age, living alone, male sex, Caucasian or native American, recent conflict with or loss of a loved one, recent personal or financial loss or other major life stressors, a history of psychiatric disease, alcohol, drug, or multiple substance abuse, and poor physical health. Specific psychiatric illnesses often associated with suicide or attempted suicide include major depression, depression with psychotic symptoms, bipolar disorder, and borderline personality disorder. John has at least six aspects of this risk profile.

2. What are the limitations of the managed care company's criteria for admission and continued hospitalization in a patient at possible risk for suicide?

The criteria generally required by managed care companies include a specific suicidal plan or ruminations about suicide, access to the means of committing suicide, prior history of suicide attempt, or hallucinations instructing the patient to commit suicide. These criteria are very often absent,[2] however, or are not disclosed to a health care provider. Therefore, Dr. Offenbach's concern about John, who satisfied none of the criteria, were probably well grounded, and the managed care company's criteria appear to be overly rigorous if the goal is to prevent suicide.

People who attempt suicide (as opposed to those who complete suicide) tend more often to be women and have psychiatric illnesses associated with impulsivity, such as personality disorders or bipolar disorder, and attempt suicide by drug overdose or other less certain means than gunshot. Attempts are more often impulsive than carefully thought out and deliberated, so their risk profile would be less likely to fulfill the managed care requirements than a person at risk for suicide completion. Suicide attempts can be severe enough to cause death or serious morbidity, however, and a history of suicide attempt is in itself a risk factor for suicide. Although suicidal patients often discuss details of their intentions with their provider, someone with serious suicide intent might well keep his intentions and plan to himself. The majority of people who have committed suicide have seen a doctor within the month prior to the suicide, suggesting that physicians often fail to identify suicidal patients. It is thus possible—if not likely—that strict managed care criteria might pose a further obstacle to suicide prevention.

Although "Day 4" probably represents the fourth *phase* of the course of the patient's illness, physicians, case managers, and others interpret these specific intervals in various ways. Moreover, even if there appears to be a decrease in suicide risk, stabilization of a patient often takes longer. Additional time may be required to see if medication regimens will be successful and the dose tolerated. Even though the symptoms may appear to have stabilized, discharging the patient might not be safe. John, for example, will return to an empty home and will be far from resolving the concerns that led to his crisis. Social issues can also be a problem if patients return to a home situation where family members are poorly equipped, poorly motivated, or reluctant to follow through on a patient's care needs. Similar issues arise in medical illness, as comorbidity and, in particular, functional impairments are not often considered in reimbursement for continued hospitalization. In patients undergoing surgery, preoperative days are often disallowed, because reimbursement is modeled on the assumption that the patient is medically prepared to undergo surgery within the first 24 hours. Unfortunately, many patients do not neatly fit the profile on which such reimbursement is modeled (see also Case 13).

Practice guidelines commonly used by managed care organizations[1] have been the subject of intense debate, and are constantly evolving. In response to bad publicity, consumer backlash, irate physicians, and economic urgencies of health care institutions, efforts are underway to assist health care professionals to interpret existing guidelines, and to revise the guidelines so they conform more closely to the realities of patient care needs and the health care system in general.

3. What are the consequences of a "disallowed" acute care day, and what can the physician do about it?

Under managed care contracts, if the company determines that reimbursed services were not rendered, the hospital is not reimbursed for the disallowed days. On the other hand, the physician generally will be reimbursed for his or her visits—at the in-hospital rate. Although nonreimbursement can often be anticipated, the managed care company can review the admission retrospectively and retroactively disallow payment to the hospital. Usually the physician is asked to intervene by speaking directly to the company case manager, and if unsuccessful, to the company's physician, in order to prospectively certify the days. In some instances, the physician can clarify the medical need; for example, if a patient undergoing surgery had unstable cardiac disease, the physician might explain that longer inpatient monitoring would be needed. Comorbidity or frailty is more likely to be taken into account under non–

managed care Medicare, but managed care companies often adhere firmly to strict criteria, regardless of the argument given. Physicians often refuse to take the time to make these calls, which are time consuming and often unsuccessful, and not infrequently the company makes it difficult to reach the physician. Few company case managers are on site for consultation, and efforts need to be made by telephone. The company representatives may reside in a distant state, and the company physician might actually be a consultant who resides elsewhere (even in a third state), and arrangements need to be made before the consultation can occur. Not only is this time consuming, but it raises the question of how fully company representatives appreciate the local circumstances leading to the request for hospitalization. The time required to accomplish these administrative tasks acts as a disincentive for the physician to pursue recertification or even admission itself. Ultimately, the patient might be placed at risk.

If third-party payers retroactively disallow days, the hospital can dispute this and will often ask the physician to write a strong letter supporting the medical need for the hospital stay. Since the physician's reimbursement will not be disallowed, he or she lacks a direct a financial incentive in the dispute and may refuse to take the time to write a letter often deemed purposeless.

ETHICAL AND LEGAL CONSIDERATIONS

1. Given the limitations and potential conflicts of interest inherent in a managed care setting, are there particular ethical obligations physicians owe to patients?

The primary goal of managed care is to control health care expenditures. By integrating the control of treatment costs squarely into the treatment decision process, and by shifting the financial risks of expensive and ever-escalating health expenditures onto physicians and hospitals, managed care systems have introduced new sources of tension, conflict, and potential for abuse into the health care decision-making arena. In the previous fee-for-service reimbursement system, incentives were aligned to encourage excess treatment and the utilization of expensive options—a system that encouraged and financially rewarded physicians for doing more. Overtreatment does not always further the best interests of patients, however, though few patients perceived, or complained about, this potential for harm. But fee-for-service was unsustainable in the long run, with its minimal control over increasing health expenditures. To address such cost concerns, managed care was embraced by corporate employers and public systems of health insurance. Yet managed care comes with its own set challenges. With its strong financial incentives on physicians and institutions to limit, restrict, or even deny access to treatment, both physicians and patients are now confronted with uncertainty about their interests and obligations.

The mainstream approach to clinical ethics has identified respect for patient autonomy, with its strong emphasis on informed consent, as a preeminent obligation of clinicians, followed closely by the need to promote patient well-being, prevent harm, and to act fairly and justly by treating like patients alike. These ethical obligations help cement a fiduciary relationship between patient and physician, so that patients are comfortable seeking out care, revealing their secrets and collaboratively working with physicians to arrive at individually appropriate decisions. While this ethical framework has always been more of an ideal than a reality, it has nonetheless provided a set of aspirations that have served to anchor the physician-patient relationship in trust and reliance. The question then becomes, with so many of the sources of authority and control now well beyond the decision-making reach of individual patients and their physicians, can these same obligations be carried out with integrity and meaning? Furthermore, are there additional obligations that arise as a result of this managed care framework?

Studies surveying physicians generally, and psychiatrists in particular, report negative perceptions of managed care. Included among the reported concerns are limits placed on hospital admissions, lengths of stay, and access to specialists, and pressures to limit one-on-one time with patients. Concern has been generated that activities intended to control cost may also be compromising the quality and standard of care and may negatively affect established and developing physician-patient relationships. Financial incentives create potential conflicts of interest for physicians to place personal financial interests above patient interests. Included among these incentives are income withholds, capitated payments, and rewards for frugally practicing physicians. Furthermore, the imposition of practice guidelines, intended to standardize and streamline treatment decisions, may not always adequately address the particular aspects of an individual case. At times, a patient's special circumstance may place the treatment scenario outside of an easily categorized framework. This is especially true in psychiatric care, where patients may respond quite differently to diverse treatment options and where the fragile bond between physician and patient, critical to therapeutic success, may not easily withstand the buffeting brought on by managed care dictates. These limits and incentives also underscore the necessity of strong patient advocacy, a heightened concern when vulnerable populations such as the elderly or mentally ill are increasingly enrolled in managed care systems. Mental health care, now accounting for 10 percent of all health care expenditures, is a particular target for cost controls in managed care systems.

Given this array of competing interests and potential conflicts, do physicians incur any special obligations to patients? An ethical framework of professional responsibility and integrity may be difficult to uphold, yet more necessary than ever for physicians and other clinicians, given the managed care environment. Most critical and yet most fragile is the need to sustain patient trust in their providers, so that the alliance necessary to provide appropriate and responsive treatment is maintained. Especially for patients such as John, whose instability and fragility make them poor advocates for themselves, physicians may need to take on heightened levels of advocacy, even while recognizing the real world limitations of these efforts.

At a minimum, physicians practicing in a managed care context need to be acutely aware of the sources of pressure and incentive that may influence the course of care. While such incentives and pressures may inevitably inform responses to patient medical needs, they should not outright determine the goals of care and course of treatment independent of the particular medical needs and individual values of the patient. Financial incentives and practice guidelines may inevitably influence treatment protocols, but they must do so within the context of the individual needs and values of the particular patient. When conflicts do emerge, physicians should be guided by two particular principles: advocacy and honesty. To the extent that physicians become aware of conflicts of interest that may work to the detriment of their patients, they must use their positions, in individual cases as well as within the larger system, to advocate on behalf of patient needs. Particularly in circumstances where patients may lack the ability to appreciate conflicts or to advocate on their own behalf, there is a heightened need for physicians to accept such a role. So, for a patient in John's condition, fragile and vulnerable due to life's circumstances and his deepening illness, Dr. Offenbach's instincts to advocate on her patient's behalf are laudable and supportable.

Even while such efforts may be supportable, it may be difficult to justify deception or fraud in the name of advocacy. Dr. Offenbach's instinct to color and exaggerate John's circumstances in the medical record in order to ensure continued reimbursement for his hospitalization are understandable, but it sets a dangerous precedent. Medical records are legal documents that record and communicate patients' circumstances, to the institution, to insurers, as well as to other involved care providers. Not only do misstatements in the record put a physician at theoretical legal risk (perhaps imperiling her continued relationship with the hospital and the insurance plan, as well as risking formal legal sanctions), but they also pose potential harm to the patient, whose situation might then be misinterpreted by other involved clinicians. Dr. Offenbach's concerns about John are well placed, as his situation may not neatly fit within the practice guidelines recommendations, and a more hasty discharge to an unsupported environment may imperil him further. It is not clear, however, that misstating his situation in the medical record is the ethically appropriate or justifiable response.

Candor within the system and advocacy on behalf of this vulnerable patient, both within the hospital (which may shoulder unreimbursed expenses if subsequent insurance denial surfaces) and with the insurer, is a more ethically supportable response, though it does risk the possible discharge of the patient against the advice of the physician. While this advocacy may also jeopardize the physician's standing within the hospital and with the insurer, it is clearly the right path to take, given Dr. Offenbach's genuine concerns about the welfare of her patient.

2. If John were discharged in his current condition, due to the decisions of the managed care company, and he then went on to take his own life, could the managed care company be held accountable in some way?

The question of whether or not managed care organizations can be held accountable for harmful outcomes to patients within their systems is perhaps one of the most contentious debates currently ongoing in the legal and policy arenas addressing managed care. At the center of this dilemma is a core question regarding the primary function of managed care organizations: Do they merely manage health insurance benefits, making determinations about the availability and extent of coverage, or are their activities so integral to the current practice of medicine that their coverage decisions directly influence treatment decisions, thus opening the door for liability if harm befalls the patient?

This debate over the role and function of managed care organizations is exacerbated further by federal legislation that currently shields many managed care organizations from state level litigation. In 1974 Congress passed the Employment Retirement Income Security Act (ERISA), which was originally intended to address and standardize the management of pension plans across the country. Over the years, as the parameters and breadth of ERISA have been tested in courts of law, judges have determined that ERISA also applies to the management of health insurance benefits, so that health plans that fall under ERISA are exempt from state law and shielded from state-level litigation. Any company that operates a self-insured or self-funded health plan is covered by ERISA. As 90 percent of Fortune 500 companies currently have self-insured or self-funded health plans, their employees are therefore unable to sue these plans in state courts. This amounts to more than 120 million individuals whose health plans are covered by ERISA.

The reality of these ERISA exemptions can have far-reaching implications. Through a series of judicial cases, it has been established that under ERISA, litigation involving health plans is not permissible in state courts and that such health plans can be sued only in federal court. Furthermore, the damages that can be sought in federal court do not include compensatory or punitive damages in situations where patients have experienced harmful outcomes or even death as a result of treatment decisions. The only damages that can be sought under ERISA in federal court, as a result of poor outcomes for patients, is the value of a benefit that was found to have been wrongfully denied the patient. For example, if a patient's plan refused to pay for a mammogram, and the patient later died of metastic breast cancer that was not detected until its late stages, the only potential liability the plan might incur would be the cost of the mammogram. While health plans and corporate employers argue that as benefit managers, these plans should only be accountable for the value of a benefit wrongfully denied a patient, consumers and other patient advocates argue that for all intents and purposes, denial of a benefit in the context of managed care usually translates to denial of the actual treatment, thereby potentially causing tragic harm to a patient as a result. In the 1997 case of *Andrews-Clarke v. Travelers Insurance Company,* the family of a suicide victim who was wrongfully denied coverage for inpatient hospitalization, attempted to hold the insurance company accountable for the tragic death of their loved one. The judge, while openly acknowledging the legitimacy of the family's claim, was forced to conclude that under ERISA, which protected this health plan, the family's attempt to hold the plan liable could not go forward.

Plans that are not covered under ERISA, however, do not have the same protections, and there have been several cases at the state level, including cases involving the suicide of a patient denied ongoing inpatient treatment, which have suggested that in certain situations, such plans may be held liable for not only compensatory but also punitive damages for denial of treatment coverage that can directly be linked to harm that results to a patient. Several multimillion-dollar verdicts and settlements against health plans have been reported on the state level. Patients who individually purchase managed care plans, or those who are employed by state or local governments, are able to bring suit against health plans for tort or contract violations on the state level. Patients enrolled in Medicaid or Medicare managed care plans also have the option to bring suit against their managed care plans in state court. Federal employees, however, are under similar restrictions to those imposed on ERISA plans.

Several states, however, have begun to challenge the seemingly impenetrable ERISA barrier, and litigation has begun to surface, which suggests the picture may be evolving. In 1997, Texas became the first state to enact state legislation permitting its citizens to bring suit against health insurance plans for malpractice if their health has been adversely affected by a treatment decision made by the plan. The Texas law defines a health care treatment decision to include "a decision which affects the quality of the diagnosis, care, or treatment provided to the plan's insured or enrollees." In essence, what Texas has attempted to do is to hold health plans accountable for the medical decisions resulting from their prospective or concurrent utilization review determinations. While the Texas law has been challenged in court as being in violation of the ERISA preemption, such challenges have so far been unsuccessful. The Texas law does require patients and their families to first pursue remedies under internal or external appeals processes prior to initiating state litigation. Recently, the first lawsuit under this new legislation has been filed, by the family of a patient who committed suicide hours after being discharged from a psychiatric hospital over the objections of his treating physician. The family alleges that the plan's denial of continued inpatient hospitalization to treat the patient's depression directly contributed to the patient's death. While the outcome of this litigation is uncertain at this time, it does suggest that health plans may be subject to malpractice if it can be demonstrated that their actions in fact were tantamount to treatment decisions that directly harmed the patient. While no other state has yet to pass legislation quite like the Texas statute, some have begun to eliminate state prohibitions on the corporate practice of medicine, statutes to which health plans had previously pointed as shielding them from liability for actual medical decisions.

Finally, it is also clear that ERISA preemptions do not insulate treating physicians from malpractice liability in these circumstances. Physicians would not be relieved of their professional obligations to the patient by asserting that the managed care plan would not pay for needed treatment.

3. Has any activity occurred on the state or federal level to address the concerns raised by patients and providers about the actions of managed care organizations?

Much activity and debate has taken place at both the federal and state level examining and regulating the current managed care environment. On the federal level, while limited legislation has been enacted to address such discrete treatment decisions as insurance coverage for postmastectomy breast reconstruction, attempts to examine the broader implications of managed care and patient rights in the managed care environment have so far been unsuccessful. Tremendous lobbying efforts have been underway on the federal level to emphasize the heavy costs to be borne by more tightly regulating managed care organizations. Such organizations and their corporate backers underscore that the more regulated the industry actions, the more costly it will be to provide coverage, thus throwing us back into serious concerns previously raised in the fee-for-service context. As more and more frail and vulnerable patients who were traditionally covered by such government programs as Medicare and Medicaid are enrolled in managed care, however, it is likely that the federal government will have no choice but to address some of the more serious concerns about patients' rights in the managed care context. Already, federal law now prohibits managed care organizations providing care to the Medicare enrollees from imposing "gag orders" (i.e., communications restrictions) on physician providers.

On the state level, the legislatures have passed an extraordinary number of bills addressing a range of managed care benefit management and patient enrollment practices. As of March 1999, 39 states had passed some type of patient protection act or comprehensive consumer bill of rights for managed care enrollees. States that have not yet passed such legislation have bills that are now pending. The scope of coverage of these bills, however, and the thoroughness of their protections, vary significantly from one state to another. Broadly speaking, the areas under legislative protection include the following:

- Emergency room access. More than 30 states now have *prudent layperson* standards to ease managed care restrictions and coverage denials when patients seek out care in a hospital emergency room. Essentially these statutes require managed care coverage of emergency room services if a prudent layperson would believe immediate treatment was necessary.
- Bans on financial incentives. At least 22 states have passed legislation prohibiting managed care organizations from financially rewarding physicians due to the selection of less costly treatments or drugs.
- Independent external reviews. At least 21 states now mandate an independent, external review process to which patients can appeal their managed care organizations' denial of coverage.
- Gag orders. Almost every state now has legislation that prohibits managed care organizations from restricting communication between physicians and their patients about treatment options, even if such options are not covered by the managed care plan.

In addition, states have addressed concerns about the quality of care available through managed care organizations by requiring plans to issue "report cards" concerning consumer satisfaction and health outcomes, by mandating that medical directors be licensed, and by requiring plans to promptly pay providers for services rendered within specified periods of time.

This significant array of legislative activity, often motivated by consumer complaints, reflects a serious concern that in the effort to contain costs and rationally allocate our ultimately limited pool of resources, we must not lose sight of fundamental patients' rights in the process.

REFERENCES

1. *Healthcare Management Guidelines*. Vol. 1. Inpatient and Surgical Care (Milliman and Robertson Inc., 1998 [see Appendix A]).
2. R.C.W. Hall et al., "Suicide Risk Assessment: A Review of Risk Factors for Suicide in 100 Patients Who Made Severe Suicide Attempts," *Psychosomatics* 40 (1999): 18–27.

SUGGESTED READINGS

Baldwin, D.C. et al. 1998. Unethical and unprofessional conduct observed by residents during their first year of training. *Academic Medicine* 73: 1195–2000.

Dwyer, J., and Shih, A. 1998. The ethics of tailoring the patient's chart. *Psychiatric Services* 49: 1309–1312.

Feldman, D.S. et al. 1998. Effects of managed care on physician patient relationships, quality of care, and the ethical practice of medicine: A physician survey. *Archives of Internal Medicine* 158: 1626–1632.

Ginzburg, E. 1999. The uncertain future of managed care. *New England Journal of Medicine* 340: 144–146.

Hall, M.A., and Berenson, R.A. 1998. Ethical practice in managed care: A dose of realism. *Annals of Internal Medicine* 128, no. 5: 395–402.

Hirschfeld, R.M.A., and Russell, J.M. 1997. Assessment and treatment of suicidal patients. *New England Journal of Medicine* 337: 910–915.

King, J.Y. 1997. Practice guidelines and medical malpractice litigation. *Medicine and Law* 16: 29–39.

Meehan, P.J. et al. 1991. Suicides among older United States residents: Epidemiologic characteristics and trends. *American Journal of Public Health* 81: 1198–1200.

Miller, T.E. 1997. Managed care regulation: In the laboratory of the states. *Journal of the American Medical Association* 278: 1102–1109.

Nather, D. 1998. Legal appeal rights playing a critical role in managed care debate. *Bureau of National Affairs Health Care Policy Report* 6, no. 16: 675–678.

Orentlicher, D. 1998. Practice guidelines: A limited role in resolving rationing decisions. *Journal of the American Geriatrics Society* 46: 369–372.

Reed, R.L., and Hepburn, K.W. 1999. Managed care for older people: A primer for the geriatrician. *Journal of the American Geriatrics Society* 47: 241–249.

Rodwin, M.A. 1998. Conflicts of interest and accountability in managed care: The aging of medical ethics. *Journal of the American Geriatrics Society* 46: 338–341.

Schlesinger, H. et al. 1996. Managed care constraints on psychiatrists' hospital practices: Bargaining power and professional autonomy. *American Journal of Psychiatry* 153, no. 2: 256–260.

Slovenko, R. 1999. Malpractice in psychotherapy. *Psychiatric Clinics of North America* 22: 1–15.

Stone, A.A. 1999. Managed care, liability and ERISA. *Psychiatric Clinics of North America* 22: 17–29.

Vickizer, T.M. et al. 1999. Controlling inpatient psychiatric utilization through managed care. *American Journal of Psychiatry* 153, no. 3: 339–345.

Yoskowitz, E. 1998. Clinical responsibility and legal liability in managed care. *Journal of the American Geriatrics Society* 46: 37–77.

LEGAL CITATIONS

Case Examples

Wilson v. Blue Cross of Southern California, 222 Cal. App. 3d 660, 271 Cal. Rptr. 876 (2d Dist. 1990).
Patient treated and hospitalized for major depression and substance addiction was discharged after a 10-day stay, even though the treating physician recommended a three- to four-week hospitalization. Twenty days after the patient's discharge, he committed suicide. The patient's family brought suit against his insurance plan. The Court held that the harms caused by a utilization review decision not to authorize continued hospitalization for mental illness provided a basis for liability sufficient to permit the plaintiffs to go to trial. This case is important for suggesting potential liability for utilization review decisions.

Muse v. Charter Hospital of Winston-Salem, 45 S.E.2d 589 (N.C. App. 1995).
The parents of a 16-year-old suicide victim brought suit against the hospital and the hospital's parent corporation, after their son was prematurely discharged from his inpatient psychiatric care. The parents were awarded $7 million in compensatory and punitive damages after proving the hospital had a policy to discharge patients when insurance coverage ended, regardless of the treating physician's medical judgment.

Andrews-Clarke v. Travelers Ins. Co., 984 F. Supp. 49 (1997).
A patient with a depressive disorder and substance abuse was covered by a health plan provided by his employer, AT&T. Inpatient care was limited by the plan on several occasions, despite clear risk of harm the patient posed to himself. Ultimately, the patient was forced to enter a public facility, where he received no meaningful treatment and where he was sexually assaulted by another patient. The patient eventually committed suicide and his family brought suit against the insurance plan. The Court reluctantly concluded that this corporate insurance plan was protected under ERISA and therefore, even though the court found that the plan acted improperly in refusing to authorize treatment, ERISA prohibited the imposition of compensatory or punitive damages on the plan.

Statutory Example

Texas Senate Bill 386. An act relating to review of and liability for certain health care treatment decisions (effective Sept. 1, 1997).

Groundbreaking Texas statute addressing managed care plan liability for treatment decisions. The statute states, "A health insurance carrier, health maintenance organization, or other managed care entity for a health care plan has the duty to exercise ordinary care when making health care treatment decisions and is liable for damages for harm to an insured or enrollee proximately caused by its failure to exercise such ordinary care."

CASE 15

Assisted Suicide in a Man with Amyotrophic Lateral Sclerosis

Frank is a 64-year-old insurance executive with amyotrophic lateral sclerosis (ALS). He first developed this condition three years ago and was forced to retire. Currently he is very weak and confined to a wheelchair. As recently as six months ago, he shopped with his wife, using a motorized wheelchair, but he does less now because he lacks stamina.

Frank has read a lot about ALS and is very fearful of what lies ahead. He has heard about one patient who "couldn't move a muscle," but was wide awake, maintained on mechanical ventilation and tube feeding. Last year Frank was hospitalized for pneumonia and respiratory failure and required mechanical ventilation for several days. He recovered but was left weakened and has been wheelchair dependent ever since. He has purchased a copy of *Final Exit* and has told his wife he thinks "Dr. Kevorkian is a great man." She agrees.

He has told his doctor that he intends to "end it before things get really bad. I married my wife for better or for worse—not to change my diapers." He requested a prescription for sufficient medication to accomplish this when the time comes. The doctor refused, but told him "there are alternatives." On the next visit, Frank was accompanied by his wife. He told the doctor that he has "developed a nervous condition and insomnia," and the doctor wrote a prescription for bupropion (BuSpar), because he felt it was less likely than others to depress respiration. Frank reported that the medication was ineffective and asked for something stronger, and the doctor wrote him a succession of prescriptions, including triazolam (Xanax), temazepam (Restoril), and lorazepam (Ativan). Claiming that these do not work, Frank requested barbiturates. The doctor, concerned about the patient's intentions, asked if he plans to use the pills for anything but sleep, and the patient said no. After the third prescription refill, the patient raised the issue of suicide again and asked the doctor for more information. The doctor replied that he will do everything in his power to make the patient comfortable through the end of his illness, but that it would be illegal for him to do anything beyond that. He assisted Frank in appointing his wife as a health care agent and in executing a living will and executed a nonhospital DNR order.

The physician then agreed to write Frank a prescription for secobarbital (Seconal) but admonished, "You have to be very careful of these pills. They can be very dangerous in your condition. You take 20 or 30 and you're dead. You drink booze with these pills and you're history, no doubt about it. If you only take a few you can end up in worse shape. So, be careful."

One week later, Frank's wife calls the doctor to tell him she has found her husband dead in bed. She apologizes for calling him but says she "was afraid to dial 911." The doctor comes to Frank's home, examines him, and pronounces him dead. He asks about the Seconal, and Frank's wife says "it was used up, and all the bottles are gone." Though aware of state regulations concerning suspected suicides, the physician does not report the case to the medical examiner. On the death certificate, he writes that the cause of death is "amyotrophic lateral sclerosis." As he leaves the house he sees two wine glasses on the kitchen counter next to an empty bottle of Chardonnay.

ISSUES TO CONSIDER

- Physician-assisted suicide
- Active euthanasia
- Dying at home
- Palliative care

MEDICAL CONSIDERATIONS

1. What medical options could the doctor have offered that might have prompted Frank to reconsider his plan?

Hospice physicians and pain experts assert that attention to palliative care issues greatly reduces requests for euthanasia or assisted suicide among dying patients.[1,2] Prospective studies would be needed to document this observation. One recent survey of palliative care units in England revealed that suicides and suicide attempts did occur in that setting,[3] suggesting that better counseling and preparation may be needed in some centers.

Others say that merely having a cache of medications sufficient to commit suicide provides enough relief of anxiety so that the patient's desire to commit suicide disappears.

It would be very important to know if Frank was receiving adequate control of symptoms. In ALS, troubling symptoms include weakness, loss of physical function, breathlessness, difficulty speaking and communicating, choking, and inability to swallow. These symptoms appear and worsen as the disease progresses. Cognition is usually not impaired, and the patient is well aware of his physical deterioration. In addition, Frank read a lot about the condition and knows that patients who survive until the end are unable to "move a muscle," but can experience pain, and require mechanical ventilation and artificial nutrition and hydration. He was aware of this "locked-in syndrome," in which certain neurological illnesses leave the patient able to hear and see, but unable to move and unable or barely able to communicate. The observations of a patient with locked-in syndrome were elicited with great difficulty and patience, and recently published in a poignant book.[4] Although severe pain is an infrequent accompaniment of ALS, awareness of the specter of suffocation, complete dependency, and the indignity of the loss of bowel and bladder control are frightening and emotionally devastating. Studies in Holland and Oregon revealed that factors other than pain are involved in reasons for assisted suicide, including loss of dignity and concerns over loss of autonomy or control over bodily functions.[5,6]

The physician should have discussed methods of palliative care with Frank. Palliative medicine has been defined as "the active total care of patients whose disease is not responsive to curative treatment. Control of pain, of other symptoms, and of psychological, social and spiritual problems, is paramount. The goal of palliative care is achievement of the best quality of life for patients and their families."[7] Although the traditional model of palliative care is based on management of the patient with advanced cancer, palliative care is appropriate in the management of any disease that is "active, progressive, and at an advanced stage such that death is inevitable within the foreseeable future."[8] In addition, aspects of palliative care can be instituted at the same time that curative treatment is undertaken (see Case 13, "A Dispute over DNR Status in a Patient Who Wants Palliative Surgery"). For example, a palliative care plan would not have obviated the possibility of Frank's involvement in new treatment modalities, if any were available, although currently new treatments, such as riluzole, slow the progression of the disease by only a few months.[9] Frank clearly did not want to end his days on a respirator, but a palliative care plan would not have excluded a trial of a respirator in the event of potentially reversible decompensation or even long-term respirator treatment if he had changed his mind. It is not uncommon for patients with terminal illness to change their minds about assisted suicide or even artificial life support. In general, throughout the course of illness, the proportion of care that is palliative might increase and curative care decrease, but no plan of care is immutable, whether palliative or curative, or a combination, and the patient can elect to amend the entire plan or aspects of it at any time.

Unlike cancer pain, which generally responds well to opioid analgesics,[10] symptoms of ALS might be less overt, subjective, and less often communicated. Functional impairments should be addressed with a multidisciplinary approach that involves occupational, physical, or speech therapy, incorporating assistive devices (most covered by Medicare), and modification of the home where possible. Dyspnea should be addressed as discussed in Case 8 ("Withdrawing Mechanical Ventilation at the Request of a Patient with Decisional Capacity"), and pain, when it occurs, should be treated with analgesics or nonpharmacologic modalities such as massage therapy. When patients have difficulty swallowing, the choice and consistency of food should be tailored to the patient's needs before artificial nutrition and hydration are offered as the only solution (see Case 9, "Withholding Tube Feeding in a Woman with Advanced Dementia").

Psychological symptoms are particularly important, as these may be the most prominent symptoms in ALS. Fear, anxiety, hopelessness, and depression are common in terminal illness. Clinical depression is often unrecognized and symptoms are often undertreated. Patients with terminal illnesses are frequently depressed, and, although most evidence indicates that only a small minority of terminally ill people actually commit suicide,[11,12] depression alone produces severe psychic pain that should be addressed and treated aggressively. Although Frank might have denied that he was depressed, the physician should have inquired about specific symptoms that he reported, such as insomnia, as well as other symptoms of depression, such as changes in appetite or loss of interest in activities that he is still able to perform. Supportive psychotherapy and antidepressant medications are important modalities in the management of depression.

In Frank's case, it would have been important to explore his ideas about what was ahead. The majority of patients with ALS can achieve a peaceful, pain-free death if palliative care is delivered painstakingly. Frank should have been given this information in detail in order to alleviate his anxieties. Such patients should be reassured that all measures can be taken to avoid the kind of prolonged dying that Frank feared. Frank's doctor assisted him in executing advance directives and should have discussed the possible scenarios that might occur, so he could avoid them. Frank and his wife and any home attendants or family helpers could have been counseled about the use of nonhospital DNR orders and how to avoid emergency resuscitation. Frank could have considered enrollment in a hospice program (see Case 13), where personnel are available for repeated counseling about emergency decisions. Certified hospice programs offer bereavement counseling to family members after the patient's death, which might be particularly important if it was a suicide.

A physician caring for a patient like Frank needs to anticipate questions that he or his family might *not* be asking. He should reassure them that they will not be abandoned. He should offer medications such as morphine along with specific instructions on how to use such medications for dyspnea, explaining that control of symptoms, even by using "risky" doses, is not illegal and will not lead to criminal prosecution (see Case 8). Patients and families are often concerned over the illegality of medicinal use of controlled substances, confusing adequate pain control with illegal acts, such as assisted suicide (see Table 7–15.1). Conversely, writings accessed by the lay public, like *Final Exit*, may provide incorrect information and following such guidelines could lead to prolonged suffering.[13]

Health professionals and family involved in Frank's care should recognize that suffering is an individual phenomenon. What might be tolerable to one person might be intolerable to another. One patient might be able to withstand great pain or loss of function, and even feel that his stoicism is heroic, while another patient might find the indignity of dependence unbearable and would not want to live if he could not be a "whole person."[14] Specific approaches to palliative care are discussed further in Case 2 ("Determining If a Patient Has Decisional Capacity"), Case 8, and Case 13.

2. What can be done for patients whose chronic pain cannot be controlled?

Failure to recognize pain and undertreatment of pain are major barriers to pain management. Although this has been best documented in cancer patients, patients with acquired immunodeficiency syndrome (AIDS) commonly have pain and are frequently undertreated. Among the latter

Table 7–15.1 "Euthanasia": terminology

Term	Description	Example
Active voluntary euthanasia	direct action to take a person's life at the person's request (also called "mercy killing")	lethal injection
Nonvoluntary euthanasia*	euthanasia when a person has lost capacity	person who desired assisted dying† but lapsed into a coma
Assisted suicide	providing the means for the patient to take his or her own life	prescription for lethal dose of medication
Double effect	unintentional hastening of death during symptom control when death is near	cautious escalation of opioid or sedative dose in patient with hypotension or respiratory depression
Forgoing life support (also called "passive euthanasia" or "allowing to die")	withholding or withdrawing life-sustaining treatments in a patient who would otherwise die of the disease	DNR order; withholding or withdrawing mechanical ventilation or artificial nutrition and hydration

* to be distinguished from *involuntary euthanasia,* performed regardless or without knowledge of the person's wishes (e.g., one who never had capacity, or never expressed his or her wishes).
† "assisted dying" refers to active euthanasia or assisted suicide

group, physicians may be fearful of prescribing opioids to patients with a history of substance abuse, which is often associated with this disease, although there is evidence that former opioid abusers are likely to maintain good control when using opioids for medicinal purposes.[15] Patients with progressive neurological impairments are at risk for undertreatment if they are unable to communicate pain directly or do so only with grimaces or agitation. Such patients often experience pain more from intrusive treatments and devices than from intrinsic aspects of the disease itself.

Access to palliative care and to opioids may be insufficient. Although education about pain management and palliative medicine is increasing in the United States, and although legislative changes are occurring (see Ethical and Legal Considerations, below), regulatory and legal barriers still exist in certain settings and locations. For example, the availability of hospice in nursing homes has increased, but pharmacy support is generally limited in such settings, and opioids may be often difficult to obtain rapidly, especially at night.

Pain control is usually achievable in patients with cancer and other terminal illnesses. Opioids are the mainstay in cancer pain, but for chronic pain of any etiology, palliative care experts recommend following the "analgesic ladder" proposed by the World Health Organization. A nonopioid, such as acetaminophen, is used first, and if this is ineffective, a weak opioid such as codeine (with or without acetaminophen), and then a strong opioid, such as morphine is instituted. Nonpharmacologic treatments, such as guided imagery and massage therapy may be highly effective. Adjuvant medications, such as corticosteroids, can enhance the analgesic effect of opioids in certain situations, and neurotropic medications, such as anticonvulsants, tricyclic antidepressants, or gabapentin (Neurontin) are often more effective in neuropathic pain. Opioids carry a risk of depressing respiration, as do the sedatives that Frank's doctor prescribed; morphine is generally not needed in the control of pain in ALS, but it sometimes is needed for control of terminal dyspnea, as discussed in Case 8.

Most side effects of opioids are treatable, and tolerance usually develops to nausea and sedation, which occur frequently when opioids are initiated. Most cancer patients achieve sufficient pain control without undue clouding of the sensorium, and some patients achieve relief when psychostimulants such as methylphenidate (Ritalin) or dextroamphetamine (Dexedrine) are added. Epidural administration of opioids, nerve blocks, and other modalities may be useful in difficult-to-treat situations. Although some symptoms may not be amenable to standard treatments, intractable pain, nausea, vomiting, or dyspnea, and even psychic pain can be treated with sedation, using complete anesthesia if necessary (see Case 3, "Urgent Surgery in a Stuporous Patient"). Treatment modalities are reviewed in the references[8,16] and suggested readings.

3. Was Frank's apparent suicide a rational act?

The question of whether suicide can ever be considered rational is the subject of medical as well as philosophic debate (see below). At least 95 percent of known suicides are among people with psychiatric disease.[12] Even among those with serious medical illness, there is evidence that it is still the presence of psychiatric disease that leads to the suicide. Studies from which these numbers are taken, however, do not always define psychiatric illness with precision, and may not distinguish clinical depression from the expected grief that accompanies terminal illness. These figures must also be interpreted in light of the probable underreporting of suicide, because the medically ill who commit suicide might well avoid notice.

Surveys of patients with ALS, cancer, and AIDS indicate that patients would favor assisted suicide if given the option (see Suggested Readings) and these groups are among those who most commonly inquire about assisted suicide.[17] Despite these results, available evidence suggests that only a small proportion actually commit suicide. Specific medical conditions have been associated with an increased risk of suicide, including Huntington's disease, end-stage renal failure requiring dialysis, multiple sclerosis, spinal cord injury, advanced pulmonary disease, cancer, and AIDS, but those reports generally fail to consider associated risk factors, such as a premorbid history of depression or other psychiatric illness, or a family history of suicide or attempted suicide. Likewise, there is evidence that the risk of suicide among people with Huntington's disease may be related in part to neurologic abnormalities of the disease state per se, which may lead to affective disorders that predispose to suicidal behaviors.[18] Delirium, a psychiatric syndrome caused by medical disease, may itself lead to suicidal behaviors. Despite interest among ALS patients in assisted suicide, research has shown they may not be at higher than average risk for committing suicide[11]; however, this could be due to impaired ability to commit suicide in the late stages of the disease.

Suicide risk appears to be highest among elderly men, especially those with chronic disease. Compared to younger suicide victims, suicide among the elderly tends to be more often premeditated and carefully planned, suggesting more rationality. To test the hypothesis that such behavior is rational, however, would require accurate data to construct a normal psychological profile of patients who are either elderly, chronically ill, or terminally ill, and compare it retrospectively with a profile of those completing a suicide.

Among hospitalized medically ill patients, suicides are generally impulsive acts that occur in the setting of delirium, dysphoria, extreme anxiety, or a combination of these.[19] In the case of cancer, most suicides seem to occur in patients with advanced disease, but in a subgroup of patients, the risk of suicide is highest at the time of diagnosis and may decline over time. In some individuals, a recent diagnosis of cancer or AIDS can be a catalyst to suicide, even in the absence of advanced disease. This type of behavior has been associated with personality and affective disorders, in which the patient might exaggerate the significance of physical signs and symptoms. The inability to cope with the new reality leads individuals predisposed to suicidal behavior to resort to catastrophic behaviors, whether or not they have become seriously ill, lending more credence to the idea that suicide among these patients is a result of mental illness and not a rational response to medical disease.[20]

The risk or desire for suicide often wanes as a patient comes to grips with the realities of disease and learns to cope, although a waning risk could also be related to disease progression, as a patient with advanced disease may have grown too weak or dependent to complete a suicide without help. In other cases, the patient might have given up, and the tendency to the aggressive act of suicide has merely given way to passive behaviors.

A waning of suicide risk with disease progression might be more apparent than real. It has long been suspected and it is logical to assume that suicide is underreported. Deaths might be incorrectly attributed, intentionally or unintentionally, to natural causes. Or, when death is expected, the act of suicide might be viewed as less onerous and reporting is avoided to protect family or physician from emotional stress or liability. The assumption that suicide is underreported would of course be difficult to verify. In any case, this remains an obstacle to the study of suicidal behaviors in the medically ill.

Most physicians would agree that clinical depression must be identified and treated in suicidal patients who are medically ill. In the context of clinical depression or other psychiatric illness (with or without medical illness), however, it is difficult to determine a point at which suffering impairs reason, making an act of suicide "irrational."[21]

4. What arguments might Frank have given to end his life at this point, rather than waiting until the disease progressed further?

At the time of his death, Frank appeared cognitively intact and capable of making his own decisions. It was possible that his illness would make him physically too weak to take his own life, and although patients may enlist a family member or friend to assist, others might not wish to involve them out of concern that they would place them at risk for any legal repercussions, or impose an unacceptable emotional burden on them. Although loss of mental capacity is not a common accompaniment of ALS, CO_2 narcosis, stroke, or other intercurrent event might occur, so that providing Frank with the means to take his life or even more actively assisting him at that time would constitute nonvoluntary euthanasia. Finally, although the doctor can offer adequate effective palliative care, this may not be an acceptable alternative to the patient.

5. Was this a case of physician-assisted suicide?

Suicide is defined as the intentional taking of one's own life. *Assisted suicide* denotes that someone intentionally supplied the means to a patient to take his own life; in physician-assisted suicide this might be a prescription for a lethal dose of medication. In contrast, *active euthanasia* denotes that an individual such as a physician not only provides the means of causing death but is actually the agent to bring about the death, for example, by injecting a lethal substance (see Table 7–15.1). In the current case, there is evidence that the patient, Frank, committed suicide by utilizing the medication supplied by his physician. If the physician intended that Frank utilize the prescription for this purpose, this would be a case of physician-assisted suicide. If there were evidence that Frank's wife had collaborated in his plan, it is theoretically possible that she could be implicated (see Ethical and Legal Considerations, below).

It is not certain, of course, that this death was suicide. Suicidal ideation is common among patients with incurable medical illness. Professionals employed in the care of the dying have asserted that it is rare for patients who have obtained lethal amounts of medications to actually use them for suicide and that merely having the medication may provide them with the emotional security to reduce suicidal impulses.

Thus, unless there is an autopsy or Frank's wife provides specific information about the circumstances surrounding his death, it cannot be known with certainty that Frank committed suicide using the drugs supplied by his physician. Likewise, one could argue that he developed respiratory failure from a pharmacologic dose of barbiturate, which is not inconceivable in a patient with neuromuscular disease and a prior history of respiratory failure. In the setting of terminal illness, natural death is expected and those involved, including the physician, may feel the issue of whether or not a suicide occurred is academic and that an autopsy to determine the cause of death is not needed and may cause unnecessary emotional pain for family members.

If, as is suspected, the patient took an overdose of barbiturates combined with alcohol, it could be argued that the physician assisted in this suicide by knowingly writing the prescription and instructing the patient, in the guise of informing him precisely of the drug's dangers. Barbiturates are no more effective than other hypnotic agents in inducing sleep, but are well known to have a narrow therapeutic index (ratio of the dose producing therapeutic effect to that producing toxicity) and are commonly used for suicide. It is not clear that Frank's physician intended to assist his patient with suicide; his actions and words could be more innocently interpreted. Perhaps he was trying to help this anxious, terminally ill patient to get some rest with a time-honored medication that theoretically could help when others had failed, and he described the medication's risk to protect the patient rather than to instruct him in how to end his life. The physician's motive and intent are ambiguous in this case, as were the actions leading to the patient's death. Given the legal risk and moral uncertainty faced by physicians in such situations, such ambiguity is probably not coincidental.

ETHICAL AND LEGAL CONSIDERATIONS

1. Is it illegal for a physician to assist a patient in a suicide?

In earlier times, suicide was considered a crime, and those who were unsuccessful in their attempts were subject to punishment, which could include forfeiture of their assets and estate. In modern times, neither suicide nor attempted suicide is punishable by law, however, the question remains as to whether an individual who *assists* another in committing suicide is liable. For physicians in particular there is the concern that such action might lead to criminal prosecution or professional disciplinary hearings, including the potential loss of licensure.

In all jurisdictions, a physician or other individual who commits active euthanasia, whether at the request of the patient (voluntary euthanasia) or without the patient's permission (involuntary euthanasia) would theoretically be subject to criminal prosecution for homicide. Actively taking a patient's life, even with his or her permission and for beneficent motives, would still constitute some form of criminal homicide. The case of assisted suicide differs in a small but important way, as the physician does not actually cause the death, but rather provides the means. The majority of states have legislation that forbids one individual from assisting another in a suicide.[22] In Michigan, one of the few states that previously did not have such legislation, the issue of physician assistance in suicide became quite explosive when a retired pathologist, Jack Kevorkian, assisted in the suicides of several individuals who were unable to obtain the assistance of a physician in their own states where laws banned this practice. Dr. Kevorkian's "suicide machines" and the publicity surrounding his actions led the state of Michigan to pass legislation outlawing assisted suicide.

As of this writing, Dr. Kevorkian was convicted of second-degree murder in Michigan following the televised broadcast of his activities to bring about the death of an ALS patient who was unable to take his own life.[23] In this circumstance, Dr. Kevorkian went beyond the realm of physician-assisted suicide into the arena of euthanasia, when he directly injected the patient with a lethal dosage of medication with the intent of bringing about the death of the patient. Under Michigan law, consent to injection of a lethal dose of medication is not a defense for a charge of murder. Dr. Kevorkian has stated that he will appeal this verdict.

The state of Oregon is currently the only state that has passed legislation permitting physicians to legally assist patients in their decisions to end their lives. The Oregon Death with Dignity Act sets forth limited, proscribed circumstances, as well as a specific protocol, in which a physician may provide a competent, terminally ill patient with the pharmacologic means to end his or her life.[24] This legislation was fought in the courts for several years, even after it was originally approved by Oregon voters in 1994. In 1997, the matter was once again brought to Oregon voters, who resoundingly defeated a measure to repeal the Act. Since the law's actual implementation in 1998, a total of 15 deaths from physician assistance have been reported in Oregon.[5]

In 1997, the United States Supreme Court ruled on the matter of physician-assisted suicide in two cases, *Washington v. Glucksberg* and *Vacco v. Quill*. In each case, terminally ill patients and their physicians challenged the constitutionality of state statutes that outlawed physician assistance for terminally ill patients who wish to end their lives. In these decisions, the Court declared that it was neither a violation of the Due Process clause of the Constitution nor a violation of the Equal Protection clause for a state to criminalize physician-assisted suicide. The Court held that there was no fundamental liberty interest in determining the manner or timing of one's death. Moreover, it affirmed the important distinction previously made by courts and commentators concerning the distinction between the right to refuse unwanted life-prolonging treatments and the desire for physician-assisted suicide. In a previous case (*Cruzan*), the Court did uphold the fundamental constitutional right of patients to refuse or have withdrawn undesired medical treatments, even if they prolong life. In these most recent cases, however, several concurring opinions began to articulate a right to palliative care for dying patients as a reason that there need be no constitutional right to assisted suicide. These cases also suggest that the Court might be willing to reconsider this issue and that states, through the legislative process, may experiment on this issue, as Oregon has already done.

Physician assistance in a patient's suicide thus carries with it the risk of criminal prosecution, depending on the physician's intent and actual participation, or loss of professional licensure, even if no statute exists to explicitly outlaw such conduct. This risk is theoretical, however, as no physician has yet been successfully prosecuted for such a crime in the United States. In the few cases that have led to litigation, juries, out of sympathy and despite the evidence, have generally been unwilling to convict. In a well-known case, Dr. Timothy Quill of Rochester, New York, described his actions in the *New England Journal of Medicine*.[25] Dr. Quill was investigated but, despite public acknowledgment of his own actions, he was neither indicted by the criminal justice system nor subjected to professional disciplinary hearings.

Currently, the legal risk for physicians remains more theoretical than actual. Although that risk surely remains a powerful disincentive for many, physician reluctance likely also stems from deeper ambivalence over the propriety and morality of a physician using his or her professional expertise to intentionally bring about a patient's death.

It is theoretically possible that Frank's wife could be criminally implicated in Frank's death. Whether or not she could face criminal charges for assisting in his suicide or even more serious charges such as manslaughter would depend upon the cause of Frank's death, her knowledge of and assistance with any suicide plans he had, and her intent as such. There have been a few reported cases of prosecutors bringing criminal charges against a relative whose actions contributed to, or helped bring about, a patient's death, though guilty verdicts or prison terms are usually exceedingly rare, given the jury sympathy for the merciful motives of the relatives. Frank's wife would be unlikely to face criminal charges, since his death certificate lists ALS as the cause of death and the death was not reported as suspicious. For one relative's encounter with the legal system following his participation in his wife's suicide, and the complexities raised by such an act, the reader is directed to the references.[26]

It is important to emphasize that the law clearly distinguishes between activities intended to bring about a patient's death (assisted suicide or active euthanasia) and adhering to the patient's or surrogate's decision to withhold or withdraw life-sustaining treatments (allowing to die). The withholding or withdrawal of treatment from a patient is *not* considered either a suicide on the part of the patient or assistance with suicide on the part of the physician. Adherence to such wishes has, in fact, been repeatedly upheld as lying within the patient's right to determine the nature and course of treatment, and as part of the physician's obligation to respect patient autonomy (see Case 1, "A Religious Objection to a Blood Transfusion," and Case 8). The law also clearly distinguishes assisted suicide and active euthanasia from the theoretical acceleration of death that can result from administration of high doses of symptom-relieving medication—the double effect (see Case 9, "Withholding Tube Feeding in a Woman with Advanced Dementia").

2. Is it unethical for a physician to assist a patient who wishes to commit suicide?

The question of whether physician-assisted suicide can ever be considered ethical is a controversial and unsettled issue. Historically, there has been a taboo against this practice. The Hippocratic oath, which states that a physician shall not "give poison" is generally cited as the source of this traditional prohibition. Some commentators assert categorically that a physician must not intentionally cause the death of a patient and that doing so violates the fundamental role of physician as healer. Others believe that such a position ignores the equally deep historical role of the physician as the reliever of suffering, that the ancient prohibitions never foresaw that medical advances would postpone dying and often make the end of the life less merciful rather than more. In this argument, the role of the present day medical profession in such efforts needs to be reevaluated.

In modern medicine it is probably easier than it was in the past to control a dying patient's pain and symptoms. Anguish is highly individual, however, and the physician can only ameliorate suffering, not eliminate it completely. Moreover, not all patients would find measures such as sedation or total anesthesia acceptable, even if they were the only means to relieve physical symptoms. Others want to choose the precise way or time that they would like to die. For these reasons, some would argue that the principle of autonomy demands that physicians honor requests for assisted suicide or active euthanasia. It has been argued, however, that easing traditional prohibitions could lead down a slippery slope to euthanasia of the helpless, the elderly, and next the incompetent. The logical end point of this slippery slope would be involuntary euthanasia, which would be clearly unacceptable. Thus, the entire justification for physician assistance—namely, the relief of unrelenting suffering—would be lost, and the likelihood of abuse overwhelming.

The slippery slope could be avoided, some argue, by adopting strict guidelines and criteria to ensure against potential abuse. The Oregon Death with Dignity Act, for example, has a strict protocol, which includes the requirement of a written request from a patient with capacity, a formal waiting period, residency requirements for patients, and complete and full documentation and disclosure of the process. Other criteria might include the following:

- The patient has an incurable condition associated with severe unrelenting suffering.
- Alternative measures of comfort care are addressed for the patient.
- The patient clearly and repeatedly requests the assistance and it is evident that the patient's judgment is not distorted.
- There is a meaningful doctor-patient relationship in which this request is fulfilled.
- Another physician is consulted to confirm that these previous steps have been taken.

These proposed criteria governing assisted suicide are similar to those in Holland governing both assisted suicide and active euthanasia. Those criteria, proposed by the Royal Dutch Medical Association and unofficially by the Dutch government, have in effect curtailed prosecutions for physicians involved in assisted suicide and active euthanasia, which technically have been criminal offenses punishable by up to 12 years in prison. Recently, the law in the Netherlands has been amended. Since the end of 1993, when the new law took effect, active euthanasia and physician-assisted suicide still have been technically criminal offenses, but doctors who strictly follow the guidelines can be prosecuted only under exceptional circumstances (involuntary euthanasia remains strictly illegal). Holland was thus the first country in the world to regulate euthanasia and the only country with public acknowledgment that these practices may take place without risk if a specific protocol is followed.

Recent data from the Netherlands shows that a small fraction of deaths (less than 3 percent) in the Netherlands are attributable to euthanasia, although one worrisome finding was that a small percentage of these deaths seem to have resulted from nonvoluntary euthanasia, that is, without the explicit, concurrent request of the patient. While many interpret these data as demonstrative that physician-assisted suicide and euthanasia, under proscribed and limited circumstances, are possible without abuse, others believe the unique Dutch experience is not relevant to our more heterogeneous American society, with our unequal access to health insurance and other discriminating influences on patient care delivery.

Although guidelines governing assisted suicide might be acceptable to many, they would still address neither the contention that assisting in someone's death is morally wrong nor the concern that the criteria might broaden and lead to a slippery slope ending in involuntary euthanasia. For patients too physically impaired to take their own lives, active euthanasia would be the next logical and supportable step and this step would create new pressures on patients. Although patients are always able to desist from committing suicide, there might be subtle pressures on the patient to go ahead with a decision for active euthanasia despite a change of heart, when the physician is ready, willing, and able. Although official guidelines would subject a covert process to better scrutiny, guidelines are not safeguards. According to the Dutch study, an estimated 0.7 percent of all deaths were believed to have occurred from active euthanasia without a patient's explicit or persistent request. This figure represents 27 percent of total deaths from assisted suicide and active euthanasia.[10]

One might criticize Frank's physician for his lack of in-depth involvement with his patient before writing the prescription for barbiturates. It is not at all clear that Frank's symptoms, fears, or possible depression were addressed or that the physician adequately explored Frank's reasons for choosing this solution at this time. While the physician's lack of exploration might have been intentional, to avoid the appearance of being a part of the patient's actions, an exploration might have led to other sorts of solutions, allowing the patient to find additional meaning in his life, rather than opting for the solution of suicide.

REFERENCES

1. K.M. Foley, "The Relationship of Pain and Symptom Management to Patient Requests for Physician-Assisted Suicide," *Journal of Pain Symptom and Management* 6 (1991): 289–297.
2. H. Hendin et al., "Physician-Assisted Suicide and Euthanasia in the Netherlands: Lessons from the Dutch," *Journal of the American Medical Association* 277 (1997): 1720–1722.
3. P. Grzybowska and I. Finlay, "The Incidence of Suicide in Palliative Care Patients," *Palliative Medicine* 11 (1997): 313–316.
4. J-D. Bauby, *The Diving Bell and the Butterfly* (New York: Alfred A. Knopf, 1997).
5. A.E. Chin et al., "Legalized Physician-Assisted Suicide in Oregon—The First Year's Experience," *New England Journal of Medicine* 340 (1999): 577–583.
6. P.J. van der Maas et al., "Euthanasia, Physician-Assisted Suicide, and Other Medical Practices Involving the End of Life in the Netherlands," *New England Journal of Medicine* 335 (1996): 1699–1705.
7. World Health Organization, *Symptom Relief in Terminal Illness* (Geneva: World Health Organization, 1998).
8. D. Doyle et al., eds., *Oxford Textbook of Palliative Care* (Oxford: Oxford Medical Publications, 1998).
9. M. Riviere et al., "An Analysis of Extended Survival in Patients with Amyotrophic Lateral Sclerosis Treated with Riluzole," *Archives of Neurology* 55 (1998): 526–528.
10. V. Ventafridda et al., "A Validation Study of the WHO Method for Cancer Pain Relief," *Cancer* 59 (1987): 850–856.
11. E.C. Harris and B.M. Barraclough, "Suicide as an Outcome for Medical Disorders," *Medicine* 73 (1994): 281–296.
12. T.B. Mackenzie and M.K Popkin, "Medical Illness and Suicide," in *Suicide Over the Life Cycle*, eds. S.J. Blumenthal and D.J. Kupfer (Washington, DC: American Psychiatric Press, 1990), 205–232.
13. B.I. Crouch, "Toxicological Issues with Drugs Used To End Life," in *Drug Use in Assisted Suicide and Euthanasia*, eds. M.P. Battin and A.G. Lipman (New York: Haworth Press, Inc., 1996), 211–222.

14. E.J. Cassel, "The Nature of Suffering and the Goals of Medicine," *New England Journal of Medicine* 306 (1982): 639–645.

15. W. Breitbart et al., "A Comparison of Pain Report and Adequacy of Analgesic Therapy in Ambulatory AIDS Patients with and without a History of Substance Abuse," *Pain* 72 (1997): 235–243.

16. H. Brody et al., "Withdrawing Intensive Life-Sustaining Treatment—Recommendations for Compassionate Clinical Management," *New England Journal of Medicine* 336 (1997): 652–657.

17. J.C. Ahronheim and S.B. Davol, "Pursuit of Assisted Dying: A Pilot Study of Inquiries Made to a National Consumer-Based Organization," *Journal of Pain and Symptom Management* 1999 (in press).

18. R.L. Albin et al. "Abnormalities of Striatal Projection Neurons and N-methyl-D-aspartate Receptors in Presymptomatic Huntington's Disease," *New England Journal of Medicine* 322 (1990): 1293–1298.

19. J.A. Salmon et al., "Mortality Conference: Suicide of an 'Appropriately' Depressed Medical Inpatient," *General Hospital Psychiatry* 4 (1982): 307–313.

20. P.M. Marzuk et al., "HIV Seroprevalence among Suicide Victims in New York City, 1991–1993," *American Journal of Psychiatry* 154 (1997): 1720–1725.

21. Y. Conwell and E.D Caine, "Rational Suicide and the Right To Die—Reality and Myth," *New England Journal of Medicine* 325 (1991): 1100–1103.

22. Choice in Dying, "Map: Assisted Suicide Laws in the United States," *Right To Die Law Digest,* December 1998.

23. P. Belluck, "Dr. Kevorkian Is a Murderer, the Jury Decides," *New York Times,* 27 March 1999, 1(A).

24. Task Force To Improve the Care of Terminally-Ill Oregonians, "The Oregon Death with Dignity Act: A Guidebook for Health Care Providers," (Portland, OR: Center for Ethics in Health Care, Oregon Health Sciences University, 1998).

25. T.E. Quill, "Death and Dignity: A Case of Individualized Decision Making," *New England Journal of Medicine* 24, (1991): 691–694.

26. G.E. DeLury, *But What if She Wants To Die?* (New York: Birch Lane Press, 1997).

SUGGESTED READINGS

Bernabei, R. et al., for the SAGE Study Group. 1998. Management of pain in elderly patients with cancer. *Journal of the American Medical Association* 279: 1877–1882.

Breitbart, W. et al. 1996. Interest in physician-assisted suicide among ambulatory HIV-infected patients. *American Journal of Psychiatry* 153: 238–242.

Breitbart, W. et al. 1996. The undertreatment of pain in ambulatory AIDS patients. *Pain* 65: 243–249.

Burt, R.A. 1997. The Supreme Court speaks. Not assisted suicide but for a constitutional right to palliative care. *New England Journal of Medicine* 337: 1234–1236.

Cleeland, C.S. et al. 1994. Pain and its treatment in outpatients with metastatic cancer. *New England Journal of Medicine* 330: 592–596.

Coyle, N. et al. 1990. Character of terminal illness in the advanced cancer patient: Pain and other symptoms during the last four weeks of life. *Journal of Pain and Symptom Management* 5: 83–93.

Drickamer, M.A. et al. 1997. Practical issues in physician-assisted suicide. *Annals of Internal Medicine* 126: 146–151.

Emanuel, E.J. et al. 1996. Euthanasia and physician-assisted suicide: Attitudes and experiences of oncology patients, oncologists, and the public. *Lancet* 347: 1805–1810.

Field, M.J., and Cassel, C.K., eds. 1997. *Approaching death. Improving care at the end of life*. Washington, DC: Committee on Care at the End of Life, Institute of Medicine, National Academy Press.

Foley, K., and Hendin, H. 1999. The Oregon Report. Don't ask, don't tell. *Hastings Center Report* 29 no. 3: 37–42.

Ganzini, L. et al. 1998. Attitudes of patients with amyotrophic lateral sclerosis and their caregivers toward assisted suicide. *New England Journal of Medicine* 339: 967–973.

Ganzini, L., and Lee, M.A. 1997. Psychiatry and assisted suicide in the United States. *New England Journal of Medicine* 336: 1824–1826.

Groenewoud, J.H. et al. 1997. Physician-assisted death in psychiatric practice in the Netherlands. *New England Journal of Medicine* 336: 1795–1801.

Hendin, H. 1997. *Seduced by death. Doctors, patients, and the Dutch cure*. New York: WW Norton & Company.

Hirschfeld, R.M.A., and Russell, J.M. 1997. Assessment and treatment of suicidal patients. *New England Journal of Medicine* 337: 910–915.

Humphry, D. 1997. *Final exit: The practicalities of self-deliverance and assisted suicide for the dying*. 2nd ed. New York: Dell.

McCarrick, P.M. 1992. Active euthanasia and assisted suicide (scope note 18). *Kennedy Institute of Ethics Journal* 1: 79–99.

Meehan, P.J. 1991. Suicides among older United States residents: Epidemiologic characteristics and trends. *American Journal of Public Health* 81: 1198–1200.

Meier, D.E. 1998. A national survey of physician-assisted suicide and euthanasia in the United States. *New England Journal of Medicine* 338: 1193–1201.

Moyer, L.A. 1989. Validity of death certificates for injury-related causes of death. *American Journal of Epidemiology* 30: 1024–1032.

Portenoy, R.K. 1996. Adjuvant analgesic agents. *Hematology/Oncology Clinics of North America* 10: 103–119.

Quill, T., and Cassel, C.K. 1995. Nonabandonment: A central obligation for physicians. *Annals of Internal Medicine* 122: 368–374.

Quill, T.E. et al. 1998. The debate over physician-assisted suicide: Empiric data and convergent views. *Annals of Internal Medicine* 128: 552–558.

Robberson, T. 1997. A new way of death in Colombia—One of the easiest places in the world to die is rocked as its highest court allows euthanasia. *The Toronto Star* 13 August, 19(A).

Rowland, L.P. 1998. Assisted suicide and alternatives in amyotrophic lateral sclerosis. *New England Journal of Medicine* 339: 987–988.

Sachs, G.A. et al. 1995. Good care of dying patients: The alternative to physician-assisted suicide and euthanasia. *Journal of the American Geriatrics Society* 43: 553–562.

Stuart, B. et al. 1996. *Medical guidelines for determining prognosis in selected non-cancer diseases*. 2nd ed. Washington, DC: National Hospice Organization.

Sulmasy, D.P. et al. 1998. Physician resource use and willingness to participate in assisted suicide. *Archives of Internal Medicine* 158: 974–978.

Symptom relief in terminal illness. 1998. Geneva: World Health Organization.

U.S. Department of Health and Human Services. 1994. *Management of cancer pain. Clinical Practice Guideline*. AHCPR Publication No. 94-0592. March.

Van der Maas, P.J. et al. 1991. Euthanasia and other medical decisions concerning the end of life. *Lancet* 338: 669–674.

Ventafridda, V. et al. 1987. A validation study of the WHO method for cancer pain relief. *Cancer* 59: 850–856.

LEGAL CITATIONS

Case Examples

Vacco v. Quill, 117 S. Ct. 2293 (1997).
Washington v. Glucksberg, 117 S. Ct. 2258 (1997).
Decisions by the United State Supreme Court that held that there is no constitutional right to physician-assisted suicide under either the Due Process Clause or the Equal Protection Clause of the Constitution.

Statutory Example

The Oregon Death with Dignity Act, Oregon Rev. Stat. Sec. 127.800–127.897
First state statute to legalize physician-assisted suicide under certain statutorily defined circumstances.

CASE 16

A Married Man Contracts Syphilis

Steve is a 38-year-old married man who frequently travels in the course of his business. Recently, he developed a vesicle on his penis. After an examination by his physician, Steve is diagnosed as having primary syphilis. His physician informs him that this diagnosis will have to be reported to the State Department of Health, in accordance with state law governing sexually transmitted disease (STD). When asked what this will mean, the physician explains that the health department might then trace all of Steve's sexual contacts to inform them of possible exposure and the need for treatment.

Steve is clearly uncomfortable with this reporting requirement. He states that he must have contracted the disease on a business trip in Miami, where he had a "brief affair." He tells his doctor that he has not had any sexual contact with his wife since that out-of-town interlude and he would appreciate it if his doctor would not mention this to anyone, especially his wife. The doctor has trouble making that sort of commitment, and wonders what his obligations are in this case.

ISSUES TO CONSIDER

- Patient confidentiality
- Obligations to third parties
- The duty to protect
- Public health concerns in the context of individual rights

MEDICAL CONSIDERATIONS

1. How important is it that Steve's wife be notified about her husband's sexually transmissible disease?

If Steve has truly not had sexual contact with his wife since his affair, and if he had no previous extramarital contacts, then there would be no risk that Steve had exposed his wife to an STD. However, as disclosure to his wife would be embarrassing and probably troublesome for Steve, it is uncertain if his assertions about his contacts can be accepted at face value. Even if he has not had sexual relations with his wife since the affair, this does not guarantee that he will avoid subsequent sexual contact with his wife or anyone else before the resolution of his condition or in the future.

The incubation period of primary syphilis is approximately 21 days, but it can be shorter and it can be as long as 3 months. It would be important to know if the clinical evidence supports the dates that Steve ascribes to the sexual contact. In addition to confirmatory antibody testing, does the nontreponemal serologic test (VDRL or RPR) suggest recent (high reagin titers) rather than remote infection (low titers)? Was *Treponema pallidum* demonstrated by direct examination of the vesicle fluid using methods such as dark-field microscopy? Is there clinical evidence that the vesicle represents a different STD, such as herpes simplex virus? If so, the vesicle could reflect postprimary infection acquired at a much earlier date. All of this clinical information would be important to ascertain the time of infection in a patient who may have had other contacts but whose history might not be reliable.

Another possibility to consider is whether the wife herself had contracted the disease from her own extramarital activity and transmitted it to Steve. This would be an odd coincidence given Steve's story, but it would be important to go over the sequence of events carefully so that this could be ruled out. Suggesting that the source of infection comes from elsewhere might also encourage Steve to be more forthcoming.

Assuming that the facts cannot be verified, it would be important for Steve's wife to be notified of her possible health risk so she could undergo prompt testing. Early syphilis in non–HIV-infected patients is treated with a one-time dose of intramuscular penicillin, or two weeks of oral antibiotics for those allergic to penicillin. Management of disease of more than one year's duration (late latent syphilis) or of uncertain duration may require a spinal tap followed by two weeks of intravenous antibiotics. Though rare in immunocompetent individuals, neurosyphilis can occur early as well as late in the disease. If Steve's wife were to become pregnant, the developing fetus would be at risk. Although prenatal testing for syphilis is routine, *T. pallidum* can cross the placenta any time during pregnancy, and fetal infection could cause potentially irreversible damage even before a woman seeks prenatal care. In fact, the highest organism load occurs in early rather than late infection, so that the fetus whose mother has recently acquired infection may be at highest risk.

2. Should Steve be tested for human immunodeficiency virus (HIV), given the diagnosis of primary syphilis?

In the United States, a syphilis epidemic paralleled the HIV epidemic in the 1980s, and a significant decline in the incidence of syphilis since 1990 has paralleled public health initiatives that came in the wake of the HIV epidemic. Behaviors that are associated with acquisition of either disease are similar, namely, multiple sexual partners, crack cocaine use, and sex for money. Although crack cocaine use and sex for money have declined, prostitutes in endemic HIV areas in the United States, such as parts of the South, have an elevated rate of HIV infection as well as syphilis, and it would be important to have more details about the person with whom Steve had an affair. It is not certain that the presence of either infection increases the likelihood of acquiring the other since HIV is associated with different STDs in some other parts of the world, and the association may be related to epidemiologic factors rather than pathophysiologic ones. HIV may modify the patient's serologic response to syphilis, however, and may alter the course of the latter disease, perhaps necessitating a different treatment approach than would be adopted in a non–HIV-infected individual. Thus, many experts argue that any patient diagnosed with syphilis should be tested for HIV.

In contrast to all other diagnostic blood tests, there may be disincentives to HIV testing. In some jurisdictions, HIV blood testing cannot be done without written informed consent (see below, and Case 25, "Prenatal Counseling of a Pregnant Woman at Risk for HIV Infection"). It is not unusual for a physician to avoid disclosing to a patient all specific tests to be performed on a blood specimen, in order not to cause the patient undue concern. In the case of HIV infection, however, the decision to perform a blood test, ordinarily a routine medical judgment, becomes a more complex issue given the current political climate surrounding AIDS and HIV infection. There might be situations in which HIV positivity is possible but unlikely, for example, in a patient without HIV risk factors who now has unexplained weight loss or who develops infection with an unusual organism. A requirement to obtain written informed consent might be a disincentive for the physician to perform HIV testing unless the indication was very strong.

There is strong medical justification for HIV testing in this patient. Informing Steve of the association between syphilis and HIV would be helpful regardless of whether or not he agreed to HIV testing, since it would impress on him the need for testing now, and for more caution in the future.

ETHICAL AND LEGAL CONSIDERATIONS

1. What obligations to maintain confidentiality does a physician have in this circumstance?

Confidentiality has long been considered a basic element of doctor-patient relations. One justification is that without the assurance of confidentiality, the patient might withhold information that would be needed for an accurate diagnosis and appropriate treatment, or he might be discouraged from seeking out necessary care. For most people, the desire to maintain confidentiality comes in precisely the kind of situation that Steve fears and that might concern other patients. Will my wife discover I've had an affair? Will my mother find out that I'm homosexual? Will my boss learn of my cancer? Revelation to those close to the patient, where the consequences may be most devastating, could inhibit a patient from seeking medical attention and disclosing information if confidentiality is not assured.

These arguments supporting confidentiality could be applied to Steve's situation, given the embarrassment and potential marital difficulties that could ensue. Like many patients, Steve may assume that his disease will be cured readily with an antibiotic, and after obtaining a prescription, he might not return to his physician again. If he were to acquire an STD in the future, he might seek treatment elsewhere, perhaps under an assumed name. If the assurance of confidentiality is what will keep Steve in treatment and lead to his education concerning STDs and the ways to avoid future problems, then the most judicious course might be to work with Steve so that he will, on his own, quickly disclose his condition to his wife or any other contacts. This strategy could be justified only if disclosure came immediately and were verified, so that his wife could be treated in the earliest possible stages of the disease if she had it.

The increased incidence of syphilis, gonorrhea, and other sexually transmitted diseases in the early part of the twentieth century led states to develop contact tracing and partner notification mechanisms. Thus, in most states, physicians have a legal obligation to report patients with such transmissible conditions to state departments of health, which in turn will attempt to notify sexual contacts of the patient that they have been exposed to a sexually transmitted disease. Whether such contact tracing programs have successfully limited the spread of sexually transmitted diseases is questionable. This is of particular concern, given the breach of patient confidentiality that inevitably results from partner notification and given the increasing state interest in utilizing such techniques for HIV-positive patients as well. In fact, in situations in which mandatory reporting is not required, state licensing laws and in some instances case law, state health codes, or other state and federal regulations require the physician to keep information strictly confidential.

Arguments in favor of maintaining confidentiality have been made forcefully in the case of HIV-infected patients who are the objects of discrimination in housing, insurance, and employment, but whose HIV status in and of itself does not pose a risk to third parties. These problems have led to laws specifically designed to protect the civil liberties of patients affected by a dangerous communicable disease. For example, in most states, patients must be given a special informed consent form before a blood test for HIV can be administered. Given the advances in HIV treatment, however, and the prolonging and enhancement of quality of life that has accompanied the advent of protease inhibitors, there is a strong public health interest in identifying persons with HIV infection as soon as possible after an infection has occurred. This public health concern poses a formidable counterconcern to the very legitimate interest in the rights of patients in confidentiality and privacy.

2. What exceptions exist to the physician's obligation to maintain confidentiality?

In the modern era of medical services delivery, other members of the health care team directly caring for the patient need to be aware of the patient's medical condition, and third-party payers require specific information before they will agree to pay for services rendered. Steve, like most patients, is likely to accept these types of disclosures, if he is even aware of them. In some situations, however, a breach of confidentiality might be difficult for the individual patient to accept, but in society's judgment, it is important for the well-being of others or the public. Steve faces this situation; although disclosure to his insurance company might not even be needed (if he pays out of pocket), disclosure to a public health agency and ultimately to his wife might be mandated by law.

If the need to protect a third party or the public health outweighs the benefits to a particular patient of maintaining confidentiality, a physician may be legally mandated to breach confidentiality and make certain select disclosures. An important example is a communicable disease, in particular one spread by intimate contact, when halting unchecked spread of the disease is both important and possible. Other traditional examples of sanctioned breaches of confidentiality include reporting of gunshot wounds and suspected child abuse.

It is noteworthy that the physician's obligation under partner notification regulations is usually to disclose to a public agency, *not* to the intimate contact of the patient. Whether or not the agency then acts on this information by conducting a contact tracing is beyond the authority of the physician. If a physician's breach of confidentiality is legally mandated and limited only to this particular situation, the patient might still be able to feel a sense of privacy in his relationship, allowing for continued honest dialogue between doctor and patient and commitment to treatment.

3. Does the physician have any moral or legal obligation to Steve's wife, who might be harmed but who has not received information concerning her husband's behavior and disease acquisition?

If Steve's wife were infected with syphilis but unaware of it, there would be obvious health consequences, as outlined above. In this type of situation, the physician may believe that his obligation as a citizen to protect a third party overrides his responsibility as a physician to his patient. If he acted on this belief, he would be bucking a long legal and ethical tradition protecting patient confidentiality. A few states have attempted to address this conflict specifically in the case of AIDS. For example, while underscoring the need to maintain patient confidentiality, several states permit, but do not require, physicians to directly contact identifiable third parties who are at risk of infection due to the activities of the HIV-infected patient. Indiana, for example, permits physicians to make such disclosures with immunity from civil or criminal liability if done in good faith.

If efforts fail to convince Steve to disclose, the physician may feel that his moral obligation to alert Steve's wife outweighs any theoretical risk of liability imposed by breach of confidentiality. Cases do exist in some jurisdictions in which a physician was found to be legally liable for failure to disclose information to a third party who might be harmed by a patient. The classic cases in this category have involved a psychotherapist and a patient, who, during the course of therapy, reveals plans to harm a third person. In the most prominent of these cases, *Tarasoff v. Regents of the University of California*, it was found that the psychotherapist had a legal obligation to breach confidentiality in order to protect a specifically identified third party. The case involved a patient who disclosed to his therapist his intention to kill a woman who had jilted him and who then actually carried out his plan. Since *Tarasoff*, other parties have won lawsuits based on what is now considered a limited legal duty to warn and protect third parties, within the context of a therapist-patient relationship.

There have also been court cases that have found sexual partners liable for failure to disclose a diagnosis of STD before engaging in sexual contact with the injured party. In New York, criminal prosecution was also brought against an HIV-infected patient on felony charges of reckless endangerment by continuing to have unprotected sex with identifiable teenagers despite his knowledge of his positive HIV status. Could liability extend to a patient's physician? At least one case has been reported where liability of health care providers was found for failure to warn the fiancee of a hemophiliac patient, likely to have become HIV infected by tainted blood provided by these providers.

Despite these precedents, a physician who elected to disclose this type of information might also be taking a personal risk since the patient could still attempt to hold the physician liable for unauthorized disclosure of confidential information. Medical organizations have taken a variety of stands on this issue focusing on HIV infection, ranging from the ethical permissibility to disclose to the obligation to disclose.

As previously mentioned, another example of an exception to the obligation of confidentiality is in the case of known or suspected child abuse. It is legally recognized in all jurisdictions that known or suspected cases of child abuse must be reported to the authorities, despite the harm that such disclosure may cause to the relationship that the physician has with the child's parents. Analysis of benefits and burdens has come down in favor of child protection regardless of the cost in other ways. The obligations of the physician in such circumstances are clear, though there may be disagreement concerning precisely what behavior can be defined as child abuse. Other exceptions to the obligation of confidentiality are discussed in Case 19 ("An Elderly Driver").

SUGGESTED READINGS

Alexander, L.A. 1984. Liability in tort for the sexual transmission of disease: Genital herpes and the law. *Cornell Law Review* 70: 101–140.

American Psychiatric Association. 1988. AIDS Policy. Confidentiality and disclosure. *American Journal of Psychiatry* 145: 541.

Andrus, J.K. et al. 1990. Partner notification: Can it control epidemic syphilis? *Annals of Internal Medicine* 112: 539–543.

Anfeng, S.A., and Applebaum, P.S. 1996. Twenty years after Tarasoff: reviewing the duty to protect. *Harvard Review of Psychiatry* 4: 67–76.

Bindman, A.B. et al. 1998. Multistate evaluation of anonymous HIV testing and access to medical care. *Journal of the American Medical Association* 280: 1416–1420.

Bok, S. 1983. The limits of confidentiality. *Hastings Center Report* 13: 24–31.

Council on Ethical and Judicial Affairs. 1992. Principle IV of medical ethics (confidentiality); Opinion 5.05 (confidentiality). In *Code of Medical Ethics: Annotated Current Opinions*. Chicago: American Medical Association.

Cowan, F.M. et al. 1996. The role and effectiveness of partner notification in STD control: A review. *Genitourinary Medicine* 72: 247–252.

Elifson, K.W. et al. 1999. HIV seroprevalence and risk factors among clients of female and male prostitutes. *Journal of Acquired Immune Deficiency Syndrome and Human Retrovirology* 20: 195–200.

Garnett, G.P. et al. 1997. The natural history of syphilis: Implications for the transmission dynamics and control of infection. *Sexually Transmitted Disease* 24: 185–200.

Gostin, L. et al. 1998. HIV infection and AIDS in the public health and health care systems. *Journal of the American Medical Association* 279: 1108–1113.

HIV prevention through early detection and treatment of other sexually transmitted diseases—United States recommendations of the Advisory Committee for HIV and STD Prevention. 1998. *Morbidity and Mortality Weekly Report* 47(RR12): 1–24 (see Appendix A).

Hook, E.W., and Marra, C.M. 1992. Acquired syphilis in adults. *New England Journal of Medicine* 326: 1060–1069.

Martin, J.A. 1995. California court expands physicians' duty to warn HIV patients. *The Journal of Law, Medicine, and Ethics* 23: 209–210.

Peterman, T.A. et al. 1997. Partner notification for syphilis: A randomized controlled trial of three approaches. *Sexually Transmitted Disease* 24: 511–518.

Plummer, F.A. et al. 1991. Cofactors in male-female sexual transmission of human immunodeficiency virus type 1. *Journal of Infectious Disease* 163: 233–239.

Primary and secondary syphilis—United States, 1997. 1998. *Morbidity and Mortality Weekly Report* 47: 493–497 (see Appendix A).

Richardson, L. 1998. Man faces felony charge of exposing girl to HIV. *New York Times,* 20 August.

Rolfs, R.T. et al. 1990. Risk factors for syphilis: Cocaine use and prostitution. *American Journal of Public Health* 80: 853–857.

Siegler, M. 1982. Confidentiality in medicine—A decrepit concept. *New England Journal of Medicine* 307: 1518–1521.

West, K.A., and Stark, R.A. 1997. Partner notification for HIV prevention: A critical reexamination. *AIDS Education and Prevention* 9 (3 Suppl.): 68–78.

LEGAL CITATIONS

Case Examples

Doe v. Borough of Barrington, 729 F. Supp. 376 (D. N.J. 1990).
Borough of Barrington found liable for unauthorized police disclosure of citizen's HIV status to neighbors.

Duke v. Housen, 589 P. 2d 334 (Wyo.), *cert. denied,* 444 U.S. 863 (1979).
The court held that one who negligently exposes another to a contagious disease, which the other party contracts, can be held liable for damages.

Garcia v. Santa Rose Health Corporation, 925 S.W.2d 372 (Tex. 1996).
Texas court extended the *Tarasoff* duty to warn to health care professionals who were found liable for not protecting or warning the fiancee of a hemophiliac patient who had received HIV-infected blood from these health care providers.

N.O.L v. District of Columbia, 674 A.2d 498 (D.C. 1996).
Physician found liable for breach of confidentiality for disclosing patient information to sex partners.

Tarasoff v. Regents of University of California, 17 Cal. 3d 425, 551 P.2d 334, 131 Cal. Rptr. 14 (1976).

Whalen v. Roe, 429 U.S. 589 (1977).
United States Supreme Court case upholding the right of the State of New York to require mandatory reporting of certain prescription drugs for the purpose of controlling substance abuse by doctors or patients; also upheld the mandatory reporting of gunshot or stab wounds.

Statutory Examples

U.S. Code Fed. Reg. Sec. 58.1-58.6 (1997).
Federal regulations permitting the nonconsensual testing for HIV of military personnel.

Indiana Code Ann. Sec. 16-41-7-1 (1994).
A person infected with HIV has a duty to warn or cause to be warned by third-party people with whom he or she is engaged in activities that carry a high risk of HIV transmission.

Section 16-41-7-3(b)(2): A physician may notify persons at risk directly if she has reason to believe that they have been exposed to HIV, that they will not be informed by any other person, and she has made reasonable efforts to inform the patient of her intent to notify the persons at risk.

Section 16-41-7-3(d): A physician who provides notification in good faith is immune from civil or criminal liability.

Michigan Stat. Ann. Sec. 14.15 (5 131)(7) (1991).

A person who notifies a partner of an HIV-infected individual shall not include information that identifies the infected individual unless the identifying information is determined by the person making the disclosure to be reasonably necessary to prevent a foreseeable risk of transmission of HIV.

Texas Health & Safety Code Sec. 81-051 (g)(1) (1997).

A partner notification program shall notify the partner of a person with HIV infection with or without the consent of the person infected with HIV.

CASE 17

A House-Bound Woman with Tuberculosis

Margaret is a 90-year-old housebound woman. She walks only with assistance and is cared for by home attendants 24 hours a day. One of her attendants, Violet, is a recent immigrant from Asia who has been employed privately at the behest of Margaret's niece.

Margaret has developed a lingering febrile illness and cough. Tuberculosis (TB) has been diagnosed and antimicrobial treatment has been instituted. Violet herself has had a cough for a few weeks, which began about the same time as Margaret's diagnosis. Violet attributes her cough to her chronic asthmatic condition, however, the visiting nurse assigned to Margaret's case believes that Violet should have a skin test for tuberculosis and a chest X-ray, and she makes a formal recommendation to the visiting nurse service. Violet refuses, stating that she has no health insurance and cannot afford to take time off from her job.

Margaret and Violet live in a large metropolitan area. Margaret's only visitor has been her niece, who has been well and has no known exposure to TB. The other home attendants are well. Nursing personnel from the patient's home care program are aware that Violet comes from a developing country where drug-resistant TB is common.

ISSUES TO CONSIDER

- Public health concerns in an era of drug-resistant infections
- Social consequences of certain diagnoses
- Directly observed therapy for transmissible infections

MEDICAL CONSIDERATIONS

1. Why is a workup for the home attendant being recommended?

Although it is likely that Violet's symptoms are due to a condition other than tuberculosis, the fact that she comes from a country where resistant

TB is prevalent, and the recent diagnosis of her patient make it essential both for her own well-being and that of others that active TB be ruled out. Clinical TB develops in a significant proportion of geriatric patients as a result of reactivation of prior infection, but primary (newly acquired) tuberculosis may also occur. Overall, approximately 50 percent of new cases of TB in some U.S. urban areas are due to recent infection. It is not possible on clinical or radiographic grounds to ascertain whether Margaret's infection was primary or recrudescent. Thus, it is uncertain whether the home attendant is at risk of being (or already has been) infected by the patient or the patient was infected by the home attendant. In addition, as a health care worker Violet is likely to work closely with other patients in the future. If there is evidence that she has active TB, it is irrelevant where or when she became infected because she could transmit the disease to others regardless of the source or timing of her infection. The risk of developing active tuberculosis is enhanced in those very patients—the chronically ill—with whom she will come into contact.

If Violet's skin test is negative and she is not anergic, it is almost certain that she is not infected with *Mycobacterium tuberculosis*. If her skin test is positive but chest radiograph and relevant smears or cultures are negative, and her symptoms are attributed to a nontuberculous condition, Violet has approximately a 10 percent lifetime risk of developing clinical tuberculosis on the basis of skin test positivity alone. This risk could be reduced or eliminated by prophylactic treatment with isoniazid (INH). If there were evidence that she had been exposed to a resistant strain, additional antimicrobial agents might be recommended. In either case, knowledge about her tuberculin status would provide information that could be of importance to other contacts, including her friends and family.

2. What are the public health implications of undiagnosed and untreated tuberculosis?

After a resurgence of tuberculosis in the United States in the late 1980s, strict public health measures have led to a decline in the disease. Recent evidence shows, however, that from one-third to one-half of new cases are due to recent transmission, and clusters of cases exist in medically underserved, or difficult-to-serve, low-income populations, with an incidence similar to that of third-world countries. These and other high-risk populations, such as immigrants from countries where tuberculosis is endemic, are likely to serve as a reservoir for new cases. Despite fluctuations in the incidence in the United States, tuberculosis remains a worldwide problem. The greatest incidence is in Africa and Southeast Asia, with high incidence seen in Haiti, Brazil, India, and certain other countries.[1] Immigrants from these countries—whether patient or health care worker—comprise an important risk group. Violet might well have been infected in her country of origin, or she could be at risk of acquiring TB from her patient.

A call for stringent public health measures emerged with the appearance of multidrug-resistant tuberculosis (MDR TB), which is associated with a higher mortality rate than nonresistant TB. Although the rate of MDR TB has subsequently declined nationally, the observed national decline in TB and MDR TB may be misleading, because it reflects a disproportionate decline in New York City, where the resurgent epidemic was first noted and where strict public health measures were first instituted. During that same time, MDR TB spread geographically to include 42 states and the District of Columbia. MDR TB also continues to occur disproportionately in certain groups, namely, people who are foreign born, HIV positive, or who have had a prior history of TB. This risk may continue to rise, as appropriate four-drug regimens have only been used in a minority of cases.

Rates of MDR TB are particularly high in the former Soviet Union, Asia, the Dominican Republic, and Argentina.[2] It is not possible to know the future of the tuberculosis epidemic in North America and Europe. Declines in incidence in the United States seem to parallel the institution of public health measures.[3,4] Eradication of TB in a given patient depends on strict compliance with a regimen consisting of two or more antimicrobial agents for 2 to 24 months, depending on whether a patient is HIV infected, and on the degree of drug resistance. In general, symptoms resolve within two weeks of initiation of treatment, and the incentive to continue the prolonged treatment regimen may wane. Patients initially infected with sensitive strains of TB may acquire infection with resistant strains if an improper regimen has been prescribed or if the patient fails to adhere to an appropriate regimen, because each antimicrobial agent selects out spontaneously occurring mutants that are inherently resistant to that drug. Nonadherence to a multidrug regimen encourages the proliferation of these mutants, which may eventually lead to clinical disease as well as transmission of infection to others in the community.

It would be very important for someone like Violet, along with any of Margaret's other contacts, to be promptly and carefully evaluated. Rapid identification of infected individuals, with subsequent treatment if indicated, may slow the spread of the epidemic. Delayed treatment would increase the burden of microorganisms in an infected patient, leading to more rapid spread of infection; under the right conditions (patients or contacts who were immunosuppressed or failed to adhere to the recommended regimen), this would also increase the likelihood that resistant strains would develop.

3. What other emerging resistant organism should create concern? What strategies should be implemented to reduce this threat?

Drug-resistant strains of HIV have emerged and may be responsible for some instances of treatment failure. Although spontaneous emergence of resistant strains occurs, these have variable significance. In contrast, nonadherence by patients to a recommended regimen is directly correlated with failure to respond to antiretroviral treatment. Adherence of less than 95 percent is associated with a high rate of failure to suppress viral load. This has implications for the public health as well as the individual patient. Given the complex medication regimens a patient with AIDS may require, 95 percent adherence is extremely difficult to achieve. Nonadherence in HIV treatment is multifactorial, and may be due to side effects, practical difficulties taking a complex medical regimen, feeling discouraged or depressed, fears about drug effects, misunderstanding of the instructions, or other factors. Because of complex pharmacokinetics, some medications need to be taken at precise times during the day, at spaced intervals before or after meals, in order to maximize bioavailability and ensure adequate antiviral levels. Even so, pharmacokinetics are highly variable in individual patients, and peak and trough levels of drug in serum cannot necessarily be predicted. Abundant research has shown that adherence to any medication regimen consisting of two or more doses per day, is poor, and declines steadily with increasing complexity of the regimen, in depression, and in chronic illness, when medications must be taken indefinitely. Although government entitlements and drug manufacturers' compassionate use programs are available for some patient groups, drug cost is an important obstacle to adherence in any patient who has low or even moderate income and no insurance coverage. Although a number of methods have been proposed to enhance adherence, directly observed therapy is likely to prove the most successful method.[5]

A number of once highly sensitive bacteria are increasingly associated with antimicrobial resistance. Of great importance is *Streptococcus pneumoniae*, the most common cause of community acquired pneumonia. Resistance has been attributed to incorrect prescribing and incorrect use of antibiotics, on a background of spontaneous mutations. Vancomycin-resistant enterococci are an important cause of nosocomial infections as well as asymptomatic colonization, and *Staphylococcus aureus* with intermediate resistance to vancomycin, has recently been reported.[6] In these cases, improper prescribing and suboptimal infection control are contributory, but drug resistance is an inherent characteristic of many microorganisms. Other bacteria for which resistance may become a threat in the near future include *Helicobacter pylori*, an important factor in the pathogenesis of peptic ulcer, and *Clostridium difficile*, which is responsible for antibiotic associated colitis. Antimicrobial resistance is discussed in the Suggested Readings selections.

ETHICAL AND LEGAL CONSIDERATIONS

1. Under the principle of patient autonomy, does Violet have a right to refuse to be tested for tuberculosis?

In the usual provider-patient context, patients with decisional capacity do have the right to refuse any treatment intervention, even at peril to their own health, so long as their actions do not bring about harm to others (see Case 1, "A Religious Objection to a Blood Transfusion"). In this case, however, Violet is not only a patient, she is also a provider of health care to others. Regardless of whether Violet is an employee of a home care agency or has individually contracted with Margaret, she has obligated herself to promote the health and well-being of the patient in her charge. While this commitment was perhaps not made explicitly, implicit in her relationship with Margaret is the obligation to do no harm in the course of providing care. Violet's autonomy does not provide justification to override this obligation. In fact, screening for the presence of tuberculosis is a common procedure for all health care workers with patient contact, both at the time of initial employment and periodically throughout the course of employment. This testing is justified on public health grounds, out of concern that employees may acquire TB through the course of their clinical work or spread the disease themselves through patient contact in clinical settings. If Violet had been employed through a licensed home care agency, it is likely she would have been given a TB test in a preemployment health screen.

2. What might be Violet's reasons for refusing to cooperate and how might they be addressed?

Violet's concerns over lack of time or money to pay for the testing and perhaps for follow-up care are very legitimate. Home attendants, even those employed by agencies, are often not covered by health insurance and may not be paid much more than a minimum wage salary. If Violet acquired TB in the course of her work, however, and was able to prove this, her medical expenses might be covered by workers' compensation, if her employer had obtained such coverage. Violet's employer, whether an agency or family member, has ultimate responsibility for Margaret, and it should be the employer's responsibility to arrange time off for Violet.

Violet's stated reasons for declining testing might also be excuses masking other serious concerns. Perhaps she believes that a positive skin test for TB would harm her lifestyle or freedom of association. Perhaps she has not been made fully aware of the consequences to herself, or that she could have been infected by Margaret and not the other way around. Perhaps her refusal stems from fear of losing her job or concern about her immigration status. If she were a permanent resident alien (holder of a "green card"), a diagnosis of communicable disease would not hamper her immigration status, so long as she agreed to undergo the needed workup and treatment. Her precise immigration status is not known, however, and her fears about contact with the formal health care system might mean that exposure of her presence and employment in this country could lead to deportation proceedings against her. Health professionals should be sensitive to such concerns when counseling a patient about the need for testing. If legitimate concerns were recognized and addressed, it is likely that Violet might be more willing to cooperate and be tested.

3. Given the public health implications of untreated tuberculosis, can Violet be forced to undergo a workup?

The question of government empowerment in the context of communicable disease raises serious concerns about individual civil liberties versus legitimate concerns about safeguarding the broader public health of a community.

Diseases such as tuberculosis and HIV have brought this potential conflict of interest to the public's attention in recent years. The health care system has tried to limit the spread of these communicable diseases while balancing concerns regarding the individual rights of infected patients, a great number of whom already belong to stigmatized, marginalized, or vulnerable populations in our society. The potential for coercive action based upon gross categorizations or stereotypes rather than verifiable data and concrete clinical information looms large.

At the beginning of the AIDS epidemic there was public outcry for quarantine and other forms of coercive government action with respect to HIV-infected patients. It soon became apparent that such restrictive measures were not warranted or justifiable, however, as HIV is not spread by casual contact. Coercive measures were seen as unnecessarily burdensome, given the goals to be addressed. Quarantining HIV-infected individuals makes little sense, as it is not their mere presence in the community that spreads the virus but rather their engagement in specific activities. By contrast, with TB, casual, nonpurposeful contact may unknowingly spread the disease. Moreover, adherence to a specific TB treatment regimen can eliminate infectiousness and ultimately render a patient disease free, while untreated TB can fulminate, spread easily, become unresponsive to available treatment, and ultimately be fatal. Given the nature of TB and its transmission, the question then arises as to whether coercive measures to compel testing and treatment are ever justifiable despite the infringements and restrictions on individual rights that will come about as a result.

Forcing Violet to undergo a workup or treatment against her will would amount to curtailing her individual liberties. If the government were to sanction such action, the questions to be addressed would be: Are there compelling justifications for such coercive measures and can they be achieved by less restrictive methods? A constitutionally based, "least restrictive" due process standard has been developed by the Supreme Court over a series of cases involving restrictions on the fourteenth Amendment liberty interest. It is employed as a way to guide decision making in the most equitable way. Society grants that, at times, the government must take actions in the name of public good that may infringe on the rights and liberties of specific individuals; in that process, however, it must also be recognized that individual rights are to be respected and upheld as far as possible. Even if sufficient justification exists to curtail liberties, the government action must be undertaken in a manner that is least likely to infringe on these rights, that is, the least restrictive alternative must be put in place.

The majority of states do grant public health officials the legal authority to order a medical examination to diagnose active TB. Because this involves significant bodily invasion, the authority is usually predicated on the requirement that officials have good cause to order such an examination, which cannot be done at the mere whim of a physician and that a fair process be in place to examine the request to compel testing. Many states require the issuance of a court order before such an examination can be imposed. Compulsory treatment is also an option for public health officials in about half the states following a positive test.

4. Under what circumstances can a patient infected with TB be detained and forcibly treated?

Whether or not a person is a health care worker, if he or she has active TB and refuses to adhere to a treatment regimen, then there might be sufficient justification for more restrictive measures, such as detention, at least on a short-term basis, until the patient is noninfectious. Involuntary detention of a patient for infectious TB would only be justified after a fair process that reviewed the need for curtailment of individual liberties in the specific case. A patient is considered "probably" no longer infectious after he or she has received appropriate antimicrobial agents for two to three weeks, there has been a reduction of cough and/or resolution of fever, and smears have shown a progressively decreasing quantity of bacilli.[7] There might be concern, however, that a person who was initially uncooperative might not adhere to a long-term voluntary treatment regimen in the community. Nonadherence would result in incomplete eradication of the organism, posing a risk not only to the patient but to society as well, as noted earlier. The dilemma is how to address that concern without overly restricting individual rights.

At the moment, there is no reason to believe that Violet would fail to voluntarily follow long-term treatment recommendations if she were diagnosed with tuberculosis. Several studies have demonstrated that even TB patients with severely compromised social circumstances that challenge their ability to adhere to a treatment regimen usually are able to be treated on a voluntary basis if the right support systems and incentives are in place. Of course, there are well-documented cases of individuals who have steadfastly refused to undergo the needed treatment for tuberculosis or are unable to voluntarily follow a treatment regimen in the community. The extent of government intrusion in these situations would depend on the nature of the circumstance and the laws of the particular jurisdiction. The most restrictive approach might be to detain a patient in a health care environment until he or she could be declared disease free. Although short-course therapy (as little as 2 months) might be effective for some patients, up to 24 months of treatment might be necessary for others, depending on the degree of antimicrobial resistance, the patient's adherence to treatment, time to conversion to sputum negativity, and time to clinical response. The need for this type of drastic action has been considered and used in certain jurisdictions for a limited number of individuals who have refused or been unable to consider their actions in the context of the greater public good. Given the fact that these people are not criminals, however, locking them up for a period of time would obviously be a last resort. Furthermore, detention would only be justified in a secure health care setting rather than a criminal context, such as a jail or prison.

A less drastic and perhaps equally effective alternative has been direct observation therapy. In this type of program, patients remain in the hospital until their immediate threat of harm to third parties has passed. They then return to the community to continue their treatment, which may last many months. In order to ensure that they will complete their treatment regimen, patients are seen daily, at home or in another community setting, where health workers actually observe the patient taking the medication. This lesser infringement on individual liberty may achieve the same effect as detention, but at much less cost to the freedom of the individual patient. The direct observation approach is already in place in many areas. In most circumstances, voluntary participation in directly observed therapy programs is successful, though there have been circumstances where involuntary participation in such programs has been mandated through a court order.

Directly observed therapy is considered highly desirable for all HIV-infected patients with tuberculosis. Treatment of such individuals can involve a highly complex regimen of both antituberculosis and antiretroviral agents with the potential for drug interactions and frequent lapses in adherence. Nonadherence in such patients not only leads to the risk of developing resistant strains of *M. tuberculosis* and HIV, but also to failure of treatment.

5. What about HIV-infected patients who are unable or unwilling to adhere to a treatment regimen? Should their access to treatment then be limited or denied, given the potential for the development of multidrug-resistant HIV?

With the advent of protease inhibitors, treatment for HIV and AIDS has taken an enormous leap forward. Using the appropriate combination of protease inhibitors, HIV viral loads can be squelched to undetectable levels in HIV-positive patients, and many patients can return to a state of near-normal health. Such advances, however, have been achieved at enormous cost—both fiscal and physical. From a fiscal perspective, the costs of the combination therapies of protease inhibitors can be staggering. Access to and adherence with treatment regimens may be beyond the monetary means of many HIV-infected patients, particularly those without adequate insurance coverage or those in developing countries. From a physical perspective, adherence to daily treatment regimens often requires enormous discipline and organization. Different medications require different daily schedules, have different criteria for food intake and result in a variety of side effects. Thus, adherence requires enormous will to succeed and support for many patients. This may be an especially challenging requirement for patients outside of formal support structures, whose erratic lifestyles, limited financial supports and lack of secure housing may limit their ability to strictly adhere to treatment regimens. This is a growing concern as evidence begins to mount that even a few skipped doses of protease inhibitors may lead to treatment failure.

The question then arises as to whether it is ever ethically justifiable to withhold treatment from HIV-positive patients for fear that their inability to adhere to a treatment plan will lead to resistant strains of HIV, a danger to both themselves and to the broader public health. Given the characteristics of HIV infection and treatment with protease inhibitors, the means currently used to compel treatment in TB-infected patients would be unrealistic and unmanageable. Complicated treatment regimens mean that both voluntary and involuntary directly observed therapy is practically not possible for HIV-infected patients. Since protease treatments must be taken permanently to sustain reduction in viral load, involuntary detention would amount to a life sentence for HIV-infected patients. Therefore, public health measures employed to combat TB are not available for HIV infection.

Given these factors, some commentators have begun to argue that in limited, defined circumstances, it may be ethically justifiable to withhold protease inhibitors from some HIV-infected patients. Such decisions would have to result from a fair procedural protocol and could certainly not be based upon any gross categorizations or generalizations based on the patient's lifestyle, racial or ethnic identity, or even on prior behavior and treatment adherence. Moreover, the reasons for past or suspected nonadherence would have to be carefully examined and addressed prior to such a decision. For example, it is now suspected that depression and alcohol abuse are strongly correlated with lack of ability to adhere to treatment.

A decision to withhold access to treatment would have to screen for and address such conditions prior to reaching a justification for denial of access to treatment. Furthermore, such decisions would need to be periodically reevaluated in light of changing conditions. Nonetheless, it is possible that due to the looming threat of resistant strains of HIV, the interests of the public health might require that protease inhibitors be withheld from a limited and well-defined select group of patients.

Finally, it is important to note that incorrect prescribing and dosing could also result in resistant strains of HIV. Therefore, physicians have a professional responsibility to accurately prescribe medication and monitor patient health in accord with the most current HIV treatment guidelines available.

REFERENCES

1. M.C. Raviglione et al., "Global Epidemiology of Tuberculosis. Morbidity and Mortality of a Worldwide Epidemic," *Journal of the American Medical Association* 273 (1995): 220–226.

2. A. Pablos-Mendez et al., "Global Surveillance for Antituberculosis-Drug Resistance, 1994–1997," *New England Journal of Medicine* 338 (1998): 1641–1649.

3. M.R. Gasner et al., "The Use of Legal Action in New York City To Ensure Treatment of Tuberculosis," *New England Journal of Medicine* 340 (1999): 359–366.

4. L.O. Gostin, "Controlling the Resurgent Tuberculosis Epidemic. A 50-State Survey of TB Statutes and Proposals for Reform," *Journal of the American Medical Association* 269 (1993): 255–261.

5. J. Stephenson, "AIDS Researchers Target Poor Adherence," *Journal of the American Medical Association* 281 (1999): 1069.

6. T.L. Smith et al, "Emergence of Vancomycin Resistance in *Staphylococcus aureus*. Glycopeptide-Intermediate *Staphylococcus aureus* Working Group," *New England Journal of Medicine* 340 (1999): 493–501.

7. S.W. Dooley et al, "Guidelines for Preventing the Transmission of Tuberculosis in Health-Care Settings, with Special Focus on HIV-related Issues," *Morbidity and Mortality Weekly Report* 39(RR-17) (1990): 1–29.

SUGGESTED READINGS

Advisory Committee for Elimination of Tuberculosis. 1990. The use of preventive therapy for tuberculous infection in the United States. *Morbidity and Mortality Weekly Report* 39(RR-8): 9–12.

Annas, G. 1993. Control of tuberculosis—The law and the public's health. *New England Journal of Medicine*. 328: 585–588.

Askew, G.L. et al. 1997. Mycobacterium tuberculosis transmission from a pediatrician to patients. *Pediatrics* 100: 19–23.

Bass, J.B. et al. 1994.Treatment of tuberculosis and tuberculosis infection in adults and children. *American Journal of Respiratory and Critical Care Medicine* 149: 1359–1374.

Bayer, R., and Stryker, J. 1997. Ethical challenges caused by clinical progress in AIDS. *American Journal of Public Health* 87: 1599–1602.

Bishai, W.R. et al. 1998. Molecular and geographic patterns of tuberculosis transmission after 15 years of directly observed therapy. *Journal of the American Medical Association* 280: 1679–1684.

Brindle, R.J. et al. 1993. Quantitative bacillary response to treatment in HIV-associated pulmonary tuberculosis. *American Review of Respiratory Disease* 147: 958–961.

Campbell, G.D., and Silberman, R. 1998. Drug-resistant *Streptococcus pneumoniae*. *Clinical Infectious Disease* 26: 1188–1195.

Campion, E.W. 1999. Liberty and the control of tuberculosis. *New England Journal of Medicine* 340: 385–386.

Chaulk, C.P., and Kazandjian, V.A. (for the Public Health Tuberculosis Guidelines Panel). 1998. Directly observed therapy for treatment completion of pulmonary tuberculosis. Consensus statement of the Public Health Tuberculosis Guidelines Panel. *Journal of the American Medical Association* 279: 943–948.

Chaulk, C.P. et al. 1995. Eleven years of community-based directly observed therapy for tuberculosis. *Journal of the American Medical Association* 274: 945–951.

Ciesielski, C. et al. 1992. Transmission of human immunodeficiency virus in a dental practice. *Annals of Internal Medicine* 116: 798–805.

Climo, M.W. et al. 1998. Hospital-wide restriction of clindamycin: Effect on the incidence of Clostridium difficile-associated diarrhea and cost. *Annals of Internal Medicine* 128(12 Pt. 1): 989–995.

Cohen, M.L. 1992. Epidemiology of drug resistance: implications for a post-antimicrobial era. *Science* 257: 1050–1055.

Dubler, N.N. et al. 1992. *The tuberculosis revival: Individual rights and societal obligations in a time of AIDS*. New York: United Hospital Fund.

El-Sadr, W.M. et al. 1998. Evaluation of an intensive intermittent-induction regimen and duration of short-course treatment for human immunodeficiency virus-related pulmonary tuberculosis. *Clinical Infectious Disease* 26: 1148–1158.

Graham, D.Y. 1998. Antibiotic resistance in *Helicobacter pylori*: Implications for therapy. *Gastroenterology* 115: 1272–1279.

Havlir, D.V., and Barnes, P.F. 1999. Tuberculosis in patients with human immunodeficiency virus infection. *New England Journal of Medicine* 340: 367–373.

Hirsch, M.S. et al. 1998. Antiretroviral drug resistance testing in adults with HIV infection. *Journal of the American Medical Association* 279: 1984–1991.

Iseman, M.D., and Starke, J. 1995. Immigrants and tuberculosis control. *New England Journal of Medicine* 332: 1094–1095.

Kunin, C.M. 1993. Resistance to antimicrobial drugs—A worldwide calamity. *Annals of Internal Medicine* 118: 557–561.

Lerner, B.H. 1999. Catching patients: Tuberculosis and detention in the 1990s. *Chest* 115: 236–241.

Lerner, B.H. et al. 1998. Rethinking nonadherence: Historical perspectives on triple-drug therapy for HIV disease. *Annals of Internal Medicine* 129: 573–578.

Moore, M. et al. 1997. Trends in drug-resistant tuberculosis in the United States, 1993–1996. *Journal of the American Medical Association* 278: 833–837.

New York State AIDS Advisory Council. 1998. *Report of the Ethical Issues in Access to HIV Treatment Workgroup*, September.

Oscherwitz, T. et al. 1997. Detection of persistently nonadherent patients with tuberculosis. *Journal of the American Medical Association* 278: 843–846.

Prevention and treatment of tuberculosis among patients infected with human immunodeficiency virus: Principles of therapy and revised recommendations. 1998. *Morbidity and Mortality Weekly Report* 47(RR-20): 1–51.

Singleton, L. et al. 1997. Long-term hospitalization for tuberculosis control: Experience with a medical-psychosocial inpatient unit. *Journal of the American Medical Association* 278: 838–842.

Wainberg, M.A., and Friedland, G. 1998. Public health implications of antiretroviral therapy and HIV drug resistance. *Journal of the American Medical Association* 279: 1977–1983.

Weis, S. et al. 1994. The effect of directly observed therapy on the rates of drug resistance and relapse in tuberculosis. *New England Journal of Medicine* 330: 1179–1184.

Working Group on Tuberculosis among Foreign-Born persons. 1998. Recommendations for prevention and control of tuberculosis among foreign-born persons. *Morbidity and Mortality Weekly Report* 47(RR-16): 1–26.

LEGAL CITATIONS

Case Example

Nassau City School Board v. Arline, 480 U.S. 273, 107 S. Ct. 1123, 94 L. Ed.2d 307 (1987). United States Supreme Court case that held that the dismissal of a school employee because of employee's contagious illness violates the federal Rehabilitation Act of 1973.

Statutory Examples

California Education Code at Sec. 49406 (Deering 1993).
State statute mandating tuberculosis testing before employment in the school system.

New York City Health Code Sec. 11.47(d) (1994).

New York City Department of Health regulation that permits the Commissioner of health to compel examination, treatment, direct observation or detention in certain limited circumstances of suspected or actual tuberculosis infection.

CASE 18

Surgical Delay in a Patient Infected with HIV

Richard is a 39-year-old man in whom renal failure has developed. He has been admitted to a large public teaching hospital, where he attends the human immunodeficiency virus (HIV) clinic for symptoms of acquired immunodeficiency syndrome (AIDS). In addition to HIV, he is known to be infected with hepatitis B and C, although he has no overt signs of liver disease.

Richard lives in a men's shelter. He has been receiving hemodialysis twice a week with femoral access, a painful undertaking. A graft procedure has been scheduled to facilitate vascular access in his arm. This will be performed by vascular surgery residents, but the attending physician's presence and expertise will be required. The surgeon did not appear at the scheduled time for surgery and it was rescheduled for the next day. Once again, the attending physician did not appear. He later states that he had emergency procedures, that he has a "huge case load," and the more emergent cases must take precedence. He suggests that the patient's clinical course be observed for a few days and that if his condition stabilizes, the operation can be performed.

ISSUES TO CONSIDER

- Obligations to patients with serious communicable disease
- Medical risks to health care workers
- Exceptions to the obligation to provide care
- Obligations of health care workers with communicable disease

MEDICAL CONSIDERATIONS

1. What is the medical benefit of hemodialysis for a patient such as Richard?

Hemodialysis is required in symptomatic patients with severe renal failure in order to maintain life; dialysis will also reverse many bad symptoms of kidney failure. Dialysis may be needed only temporarily in some instances; HIV-infected patients may develop reversible forms of renal disease, such as acute interstitial nephritis due to trimethoprim-sulfamethoxazole, which is commonly used to prevent and treat *Pneumocystis carinii* pneumonia. Acute tubular necrosis can occur as the result of sepsis or drug toxicity. Hepatitis B and C viruses can also cause serious renal disease.

HIV-associated nephropathy (HIVAN) is the most common cause of end-stage renal disease (ESRD) in HIV-infected patients, and it occurs almost entirely in patients of African descent. HIVAN is often the presenting AIDS illness, and progresses to ESRD within a few months. Recent evidence that HIVAN is actually a late manifestation of disease associated with low CD4+ counts suggests that ESRD could be prevented with highly active antiretroviral therapy (HAART) in HIV-infected individuals.[1] As of this writing, however, there is no evidence that severe renal insufficiency in HIVAN is reversible, although other treatment modalities, including corticosteroids and ACE inhibitors, may have some beneficial effect in less severe renal impairment.

In patients treated in dialysis centers, hemodialysis exposes the patient to serious communicable disease, particularly hepatitis. Richard is already infected, and his presence poses more of a risk to other patients although the risk of hepatitis among chronic hemodialysis patients may be due to improper implementation of universal precautions). An alternative to hemodialysis is ambulatory peritoneal dialysis. Chronic peritoneal dialysis (CAPD) requires a great deal of self-care and is not an option for the very sick unless there is an appropriate caregiver. In Richard's case, he has no appropriate domicile and would have to be treated in a dialysis center, and vascular access would provide some degree of physical comfort over the pain and difficulty with which dialysis is instituted through the femoral vessels.

2. What is a surgeon's risk of contracting HIV during invasive procedures?

The risk of becoming infected with HIV from contact with an infected patient is approximately 0.3 percent after percutaneous exposures by needle stick or other sharp object, such as a scalpel. There is a lower but documented risk due to exposure through mucous membranes. The risk might be higher in deep needle injuries or exposure to larger volumes of blood, and when an infected patient has a very high viral load. Theoretically, surgeons have a higher overall risk of infection because of the invasiveness of their daily work, and this risk would be higher in a large public hospital with a high degree of seroprevalence. Surgeons have not proved to be a higher risk group, however, and there are a few possible but no documented cases of HIV transmission to a surgeon through occupational exposure. Occupationally acquired transmission has been documented in other physicians, nurses, and other health care workers.

3. In order to lower the risk to surgeons and other medical personnel, is it useful to test patients for HIV before invasive procedures?

Starting with the presumption that a positive test result could not be used to deny an otherwise qualified candidate necessary surgery, the question becomes whether or not knowledge of the test result would help to reduce transmission of HIV to members of the operating team. Since seroconversion may not occur for several months following exposure, standard antibody testing may be falsely negative early on. HIV screening without confirmatory testing is also associated with a small false-positive rate. A false-negative test could lead to reduced vigilance in operative behaviors, while false-positive test results might lead to subtle or overt discrimination. In one study the surgical team's knowledge or perception of their patients' HIV status did not reduce the number of intraoperative accidents, such as needle sticks and glove lacerations, that might have led to HIV transmission.[2] In 5 percent of cases, the team assumed falsely that the patient was not HIV infected or was at low risk of HIV infection when he or she actually indulged in high-risk behavior.

It would be unrealistic to demand mandatory testing for patients who require emergency surgery, since there would not be time to determine the patient's HIV status. Although hepatitis B virus (HBV) is currently associated with less mortality than AIDS, it is more easily transmitted during invasive procedures than HIV. The risks associated with occupational exposure to hepatitis C are about one-tenth that of HBV, and prevalence of infection in health care workers is no greater than the population at large.

Thus, presurgical HIV testing for infection control purposes has no proven medical benefit, ignores the reality that other transmissible agents unrelated to HIV exist (and might develop in the future), is quite impractical in a number of situations, and could even be counterproductive. The use of universal precautions is an important and workable alternative. One should also maintain awareness of situations in which the risk of exposure is increased, such as surgery that is prolonged or involves substantial blood loss, or open skin wounds in doctor or patient. Use of protective gear in these situations and adherence to precautions known to afford protection would appear to be reasonable alternatives to HIV testing.

If testing were to be performed for such purposes, common law and, in some states, statutory law would require specific informed consent from the patient, which would have to include the reasons for testing (see also Case 16, "A Married Man Contracts Syphilis," and Case 25). Unless the patient perceived that testing would be in his interest rather than that of the providers, he might be unwilling to consent. Such a refusal could not then be used as the basis to deny the patient otherwise necessary surgery.

4. What is the risk that the surgeon could transmit HIV to a patient during an invasive procedure?

The risk of doctor-to-patient transmission during invasive procedures is exceedingly rare. To date, only two documented cases of providers transmitting HIV have been reported in the world literature, one a dentist who infected six patients, and one, an orthopedic surgeon who probably infected one patient. The precise risk is unknown.[3,4]

The Centers for Disease Control (CDC) recommends that health care workers who perform invasive procedures should know their HIV status and if infected they should avoid performing invasive procedures unless they have received counsel from an expert review panel. The CDC also acknowledges that the probably low risk of transmission to patients by cautious health care workers "does not support the diversion of resources that would be required to implement mandatory testing programs."[5] Provider-to-patient transmission of HBV has occurred more often. For this reason, guidelines for health care workers infected with HBV are more stringent than HIV-infected workers.

5. What are the public health implications of treating HIV-infected individuals in hospital or community dialysis centers?

There are no documented instances of HIV patient-to-patient transmission in dialysis centers in the United States, probably owing to strict infection control practices coupled with lower transmissibility of HIV compared with HBV. Thus, there is no rationale for screening patients for HIV before accepting them for treatment in a general hemodialysis unit. Knowledge of a patient's HIV status could, likewise, lead to a false sense of security and unintentional relaxation of universal precautions, as in the case of the surgical setting. There might be a rationale, however, for recommending that individual patients be tested to delineate treatment plans—for example, an African American presenting with unexplained renal failure who might be at risk for HIVAN.

ETHICAL AND LEGAL CONSIDERATIONS

1. Does the surgeon have the duty to operate in this case?

Physician conduct, professional guidelines, and codes of ethics have varied over the centuries regarding professional obligations in the context of exposure to risk.[6] During the bubonic plague in the Middle Ages, records indicate that many doctors fled, while others stayed behind at great personal risk out of a sense of professional obligation. In the post-Yellow-fever era, the newly promulgated American Medical Association (AMA) code of ethics described an obligation to treat in the face of an epidemic regardless of the danger to the individual physician. Paradoxically, this requirement to treat was deleted from the code in 1957, in the heyday of the antibiotic era.

The "Pax Antibiotica" of the last several decades falsely assured the medical community that lethal infectious diseases were largely a thing of the past.[7] The emergence of new infectious agents and the spread of AIDS necessitated a reconsideration of such concerns, as well as a reexamination of concepts of professional obligation and personal risk in carrying out one's activities as a health care provider.

While in more recent times, organizations such as the AMA have affirmed the freedom of the individual physician to choose his or her patient population, a 1987 statement issued by that organization warned against abandonment of the HIV-infected population, with the statement, "A physician may not ethically refuse to treat a patient whose condition is within the physician's current realm of competence solely because the patient is seropositive for HIV. Persons who are seropositive should not be subjected to discrimination based on fear or prejudice." This statement was reaffirmed by the AMA in 1996 (see Suggested Readings).

From a legal perspective, refusal to treat a patient because of fear of becoming infected would probably constitute violation of federal laws prohibiting discrimination against the disabled. In a recent Supreme Court decision, *Bragdon v. Abbott*, the Court held that a dentist who refused to provide dental services to an asymptomatic HIV-infected patient violated the Americans with Disabilities Act (ADA), which prohibits discrimination against disabled individuals who have a substantial impairment of a major life activity. HIV infection was considered a disability, and in the case of the patient in *Bragdon*, her HIV infection was found to substantially impair her reproductive activities, considered a major life activity by the Court. The ADA only permits discrimination against such individuals if they pose a direct threat or significant risk to others. In *Bragdon*, the Court found that health care professionals who fear infection deserve no special deference. Their discriminatory actions must be supported by objective, scientific evidence of a significant risk, which includes examination of the mode and probability of transmission. The accused discriminator bears the burden of proving the risk of harm is significant. For services and settings not covered by the ADA, many states have also passed legislation or had judicial determinations that protect HIV-infected patients otherwise eligible for services from unwarranted discrimination.

Physicians who refuse to care for patients with AIDS could also face disciplinary hearings, as professional licensing laws often consider refusal to provide services based on race, creed, color, or national origin to constitute professional misconduct. Physicians who refuse to treat patients with AIDS because of dislike of the person's background or lifestyle, or because of fear of becoming infected themselves, rather than out of evaluation of the patient's medical needs, could therefore face loss of license to practice.

These narrow legal considerations of the obligation to treat do not sufficiently examine whether there is a moral obligation to treat patients with AIDS or other communicable diseases. In essence, does the nature of being a physician include the obligation to treat patients who pose risk to the physician? Furthermore, if it does include such an obligation, does that obligation have any limits?

To begin to answer these questions, the goals of medicine must be considered. There is little disagreement that the main goal of medicine is to relieve the suffering of the sick and to heal the patient if possible. Physicians, in fact, have been given significant societal support in their pursuit of such goals. Although the government does not subsidize medical education directly in most cases, public- and government-funded hospitals are commonly used as training sites for physicians and a large portion of medical research is supported by public funds. Moreover, physicians have been granted a near monopoly over medical practice through state licensing laws. Society has placed great power and trust in the hands of physicians, with the expectation that they will use their skills for such purposes and will be accountable in times of need. In essence, the assumption is that in return for the societal investment, there is an obligation to provide necessary treatment. For physicians to withhold their special skills at their own discretion from those in need would seem unjustifiable and deceitful in the face of public reliance on, and faith in, the medical community.

Moreover, the argument can be made that part of the essential nature of being a physician is the obligation to do all for the patient, including accepting some personal risk if necessary. The profession of medicine differs from many professions that perform services. Given the vulnerability of the sick, the special powers of the physician, and the special place of health in the ability to live life, devotion to patient well-being even at some personal risk is a fundamental obligation of the physician. When entering the profession, a physician assumes such risks, just as a firefighter assumes the risks of burns or smoke inhalation. In essence, a physician cannot enter the medical profession yet choose to opt out of some of the risks associated with it. This view of the physician is often attributed to a virtue-based perspective of the practice of medicine, in which the virtues embodied by the good physician include faithfulness, devotion to those in need, and courage in the face of risk. Martyrdom is not expected, but reasonable risk within the context of available precautions are.

Others argue, however, that because the scourge of AIDS was not a known risk when many physicians entered the profession, there is no obligation to take on such risk. While such an argument may seem a tidy solution to the dilemma, it has several basic problems. First, medicine has never been a risk-free profession even though the nature of the risks may change over time. If a physician chooses not to face a particular risk, then his or her privilege to practice medicine in general must be called into question.

Moreover, a system that would allow some but not other physicians to opt out creates fundamental inequities within the profession, posing undue burdens on those physicians who agreed to provide unpopular or riskier care. It would also pose problems for patients in need, stigmatizing those who already face great obstacles in the ability to receive medical care. It could be argued that better care would be available with a voluntary system, as those providing care would be truly devoted to their work and expert in it. Such a system nonetheless would constitute an abandonment of the essential professional identity of physicians, however, damaging the integrity of the profession. In the case of Richard, the attending surgeon is creating a de facto inequitable system because the surgical residents probably have less freedom to avoid performing the surgery and would perhaps be putting themselves at greater risk than their superior.

If there is a moral obligation to provide care to patients with dangerous communicable diseases, are there any exceptions to such an obligation? Legally, certain providers could never be exempted, namely those providing emergency care and those who practice in public (nonvoluntary) hospitals. In such circumstances, under federal and state law, hospital personnel cannot discriminate but must provide care regardless of the disease, because the public expectation of available care has been created (see Case 20, "A Difficult Patient and the Limits of Provider Obligations").

There is no obligation to provide treatment that is not medically indicated, provides no benefit to the patient, or is futile for the intended purposes, whether the disease is AIDS or any other. If this were applicable to the present case, the question would be whether Richard could benefit from the dialysis and the graft, not whether the physician would undergo risk by treating him. The concept of medical futility is more fully explored in Case 12 ("Resuscitation Decision in a Patient with Lung Cancer"). A physician would also be excused from treating a person with AIDS if the nature of the patient's illness was clearly beyond the bounds of the physician's expertise. Once again, such an exemption is not based upon the risks posed by AIDS but rather is a customarily acknowledged exemption to the obligation to provide medically indicated care. This exemption, however, should not be the motivation for otherwise qualified physicians to purposely decline the opportunity to acquire skills to treat persons with AIDS. In such cases, as well, appropriate referral would be obligatory.

Is there ever an exemption to the obligation to treat in other situations? It is conceivable that if the benefit to the patient would be so small, and the risk to the provider so large, at a certain point the balance would tip in favor of not treating. When universal precautions are applied, the risks of contracting HIV while performing an invasive procedure are substantially reduced; however, the transmission of AIDS-associated infectious diseases, such as tuberculosis, is harder to prevent. If a physician or other health care worker were immunosuppressed, he or she could justifiably choose to transfer care to someone else. A decision not to intervene would have to be made on an individual basis after careful evaluation of the reasons for the decision, the alternatives for the patient, and the honesty and integrity of the decision process.

Another possible exemption might exist, namely for pregnant physicians, given the possible risk to the fetus and a physician's competing obligation to the fetus and the patient. Although the physician's risk of contracting HIV itself is extremely small, there is a theoretical possibility of fetal risk if the mother were exposed to cytomegalovirus (CMV), toxoplasmosis, or perhaps other pathogens while treating a patient with AIDS. Toxoplasmosis and CMV can be transmitted to a fetus and can cause serious disease in the neonate. There is no evidence that the risk of contracting CMV is greater among health care workers than the general population, but current diagnostic methods may not be able to assess the actual risk. For mothers not immune to toxoplasmosis, simple precautions such as hand washing and use of gloves should suffice. Nonetheless, there is insufficient information on which to base recommendations. Accommodations are generally made for health care workers who lack immunity to specific diseases, and it is customary to advise pregnant patients to avoid contact with certain pathogens despite the lack of data to support specific precautions. In such a case, it could be argued that the physician should be given the alternative of temporarily transferring care of the patient until the risk has passed.

Finally, the justification put forth by the surgeon in this particular case must be considered. This surgeon's purported justification is the classic triage argument: Resources are limited and must be apportioned according to which patients would stand to benefit most. Once again, such an exemption would have little to do with the diagnosis of AIDS, but rather with the allocation of limited resources, the determination that in fact resources are limited, the benefits to patients of those resources, and the likely prognosis with or without the intervention. In this particular case, the surgeon would need to demonstrate that he was a "scarce resource" to justify a triage argument. Even in situations of genuine scarcity, such as intensive care units or organ transplant, there is still debate as to whether such rationing schemes are justifiable or whether more objective criteria should be used, such as a place on the queue. With this exemption, as with the others, the physician's justification would of necessity rest on his honesty and integrity when making the determination that nonintervention is justified, rather than on his concern about personal risk of infection from the patient.

2. Should there be any limits on the clinical activities of HIV-infected health care workers? Do patients have a right to know if their physician or other care providers are HIV positive?

Health care providers clearly have a professional obligation not to harm their patients or to place their patients at risk, unless the patient has provided informed consent. The question is whether the mere status of a clinician's HIV positivity poses a risk to patients or whether the assessment of risk must be individualized to the particular circumstances of the clinician-patient contact. A few cases of HIV transmission from infected clinicians to patients have been noted in the literature. Current AMA policies state that HIV-positive physicians should not engage in clinical activities that create an identified risk of transmission and that such physicians should consult colleagues regarding professional activities that do not pose risks of HIV transmission to patients. This is consistent with current guidelines from the Center for Disease Control.

Under the ADA, hospitals that chose to remove infected clinicians from clinical duties would have to justify such removal based upon the significant risk and direct threat the clinician posed to patients or other clinicians. There have been cases that have upheld such removal, as in the case of a surgical technician. Moreover, patients exposed to possible HIV infection because of situations involving intraoperative accidents, for example, would certainly need to be notified about the possible exposure and resulting need for prophylaxis.

Whether or not a patient in nonsurgical contact with an infected physician would need to be informed of that physician's HIV status would depend on the nature of the clinician-patient contact and the actual risk of exposure. Merely because a clinician is HIV positive, however, does not mean there is an automatic legal or ethical obligation to disclose this to a patient prior to or following a clinical encounter. The need for disclosure would depend upon the nature of the risk posed.

REFERENCES

1. J.A. Winston et al., "HIV-Associated Nephropathy Is a Late, Not Early, Manifestation of HIV-1 Infection," *Kidney International* 55 (1999): 1036–1040.
2. J.L. Gerberding et al., "Risk of Exposure of Surgical Personnel to Patients' Blood during Surgery at San Francisco General Hospital," *New England Journal of Medicine* 322 (1990): 1788–1793.

3. J. Gerberding, "Provider-to-Patient HIV Transmission: How To Keep It Exceedingly Rare," *Annals of Internal Medicine* 130 (1999): 64–65.
4. F. Lot et al., "Probable Transmission of HIV from an Orthopedic Surgeon to a Patient in France," *Annals of Internal Medicine* 130 (1999): 1–6.
5. Centers for Disease Control, "Recommendations for Preventing Transmission of Human Immunodeficiency Virus, Hepatitis B Virus to Patients during Exposure-Prone Invasive Procedures," *Journal of the American Medical Association* 266 (1991): 711–776.
6. A. Zuger and S.H. Miles, "Physicians, AIDS, and Occupational Risk. Historic Traditions and Ethical Obligations," *Journal of the American Medical Association* 258 (1987): 1924–1928.
7. Arras, J.D., "The Fragile Web of Responsibility: AIDS and the Duty To Treat," *Hastings Center Report* 18 (1988): 1020.

SUGGESTED READINGS

American Medical Association. 1996–97. Section 9:131. Physicians' ethical obligations to treat HIV infected patients. *Code of Medical Ethics.* Chicago.

Bell, D.M. et al. 1992. Risk of hepatitis B and immunodeficiency virus transmission to a patient from an infected surgeon during a percutaneous injury during an invasive procedure: Estimates based on a model. *Infectious Agents and Diseases* 1: 263–269.

Cardo, D.M. et al. 1997. A case-controlled study of HIV seroconversion in health care workers after percutaneous exposure. Centers for Disease Control and Prevention Needlestick Surveillance Group. *New England Journal of Medicine* 337: 1985–1990.

Daniels, N. 1991. Duty to treat or right to refuse. *Hastings Center Report.* 21 (2): 36–46.

Golper, T.A. et al. 1997. Peritoneal dialysis. In *Diseases of the Kidney,* eds. R.W. Schrier and C.W. Gottschalk, 2771–2805. 6th ed. Boston: Little, Brown and Company.

Gostin, L.O. et al. 1999. Disability discrimination in America: HIV/AIDS and other health conditions. *Journal of the American Medical Association* 281: 745–752.

HIV transmission in a dialysis center—Columbia, 1991–1993. 1995. *Morbidity and Mortality Weekly Report* 44: 404–405, 411–412.

Miles, A.M., and Friedman, E.A. Center and home chronic hemodialysis: Outcome and complications. In *Diseases of the Kidney,* eds. R.W. Schrier and C.W. Gottschalk, 2807–2838. 6th ed. Boston: Little, Brown and Company.

Murphy, T.F. 1994. Health care workers with HIV and a patient's right to know. *Journal of Medicine and Philosophy* 19: 553-569.

Parmet, W.E. 1998. The Supreme Court confronts HIV: Reflections on *Bragdon v. Abbott. The Journal of Law, Medicine and Ethics* 26: 225–240.

Public Health Laboratory Service Communicable Disease Surveillance. 1997. Transmission of hepatitis B to patients from four infected surgeons without hepatitis B antigen.

The Incident Investigation Teams and others. *New England Journal of Medicine* 336: 178–84.

Public Health Service guidelines for the management of health-care worker exposures to HIV and recommendations for postexposure prophylaxis. 1998. *Morbidity and Mortality Weekly Report* 47 (RR-7): 1–28.

Recommendations for prevention and control of hepatitis C virus (HCV) infection and HCV-related chronic disease. 1998. *Morbidity and Mortality Weekly Report* 47 (RR-19): 1–39.

Tereskerz, P.M., and Jagger, J. 1997. Occupationally acquired HIV: The vulnerability of health care workers under workers' compensation laws. *American Journal of Public Health* 87: 1558–1562.

Tokars, J.I. et al. 1998. National surveillance of dialysis associated diseases in the United States, 1995. *ASAIO Journal* 44: 98–107.

LEGAL CITATIONS

Case Examples

Bragdon v. Abbott, 118 S. Ct. 2196 (1998).

Supreme Court ruling that declared a dentist's denial of care to an asympotmatic HIV-infected patient to be a violation of the Americans with Disabilities Act (ADA). The patient claimed her HIV status constituted a disability that substantially impaired her major life activity of reproduction.

Mauro v. Borgess Medical Center, 137 F.2d 398 (1998).

A federal Court of Appeals declared that a hospital's decision to remove an HIV-infected surgical technician from his position was *not* a violation of the ADA, as the technician posed a direct threat and significant risk to surgical patients because of his direct contact with them.

Statutory Example

Americans with Disabilities Act, Pub. L. No. 101-336, 104 Stat. 327 (1990), codified at 42 U.S.C., Sec. 12101 et. seq.

Federal law that protects individuals with disabilities from discrimination in business and government services, employment, insurance, public accommodations and telecommunications. A health care provider's office is considered a public accommodation.

CASE 19

An Elderly Driver

Selma is an 80-year-old widow who is being treated by an internist for hypertension. She tolerates her medications well and is considered to be in good health. She has suffered progressive visual loss, however, and has been told by her ophthalmologist that she has macular degeneration. Her visual acuity is 20/200 in her right eye and 20/70 in her left.

Selma lives by herself in a suburban neighborhood. Her grown children live in another state. One of her friends, who is a patient of the same internist, has confided that Selma is still driving, and she wonders if that is a good idea, considering her poor vision.

At Selma's next visit to her physician, she is asked about her driving. "Of course I'm still driving," she says. "How can you survive without a car out here?" She is eager to point out that she has never been in an accident, she only drives to the store now and then, drives at "a snail's pace," and would "certainly be able to see a cow or an elephant." She assures the doctor that there are no small children around and that she will be careful. Besides, she asserts, her peripheral vision is "as good as ever."

ISSUES TO CONSIDER

- Medical fitness to drive
- Confidentiality and professional obligations

MEDICAL CONSIDERATIONS

1. Of what significance is Selma's macular degeneration in terms of her ability to drive?

A driver must be able to see and understand traffic signs and signals, detect and avoid hazards, and respond adequately in unanticipated situations. Certainly, uncorrected visual disorders, as well as disorders of cognition, behavior, and any medical disease that impairs function, can at

324 ETHICS IN CLINICAL PRACTICE

some time interfere with an individual's ability to drive. Corrected visual acuity of 20/40 is required in most states for an unrestricted license to drive a vehicle.

It is not the person's particular diagnostic label but rather her functional ability when driving that is important to determine. For example, being labeled "epileptic" may not indicate driving disability if treatment is adequate and the person is seizure free; indeed, a controlled epileptic may be a much safer driver than someone with undiagnosed substance abuse. Many ophthalmologists believe that licensing requirements should be more flexible, depending on individual medical judgments rather than arbitrary visual acuity limitations.

One small study comparing people with and without age-related macular degeneration suggested that risk taking rather than visual limitations was the major factor in predicting traffic accidents. In the study, subjects with macular degeneration actually had fewer accidents, and this was attributed to their compensating for their visual problem by avoiding driving in unfamiliar areas, driving at slow speeds, avoiding nighttime driving, and taking fewer risks while driving.[1]

This may not be the case for Selma. Although she believes she is limiting her driving to manageable situations, she may be making an incorrect assessment, or she may be denying her functional limitations. Despite her otherwise apparent good health, macular degeneration can severely impair central vision and she may be unaware of hazards that she has avoided up to now by sheer luck. It is possible that if she cannot be persuaded otherwise, there is a danger that she may not cease driving until after she has been responsible for an accident, potentially causing harm to herself or others.

2. What if Selma's visual acuity were adequate but she had Alzheimer's disease? A history of syncope? Alcoholism, but denied driving while intoxicated?

As in the case of poor vision, it is the patient's function that is important rather than a specific age or diagnostic label. Certain diseases have been associated with an increased risk of being involved in a motor vehicle accident, including diabetes, seizure disorders, heart disease, Parkinson's disease, and others. However, within each disease group there are insufficient data on which to base medical criteria to distinguish those who can drive safely from those who cannot.

A number of essential driving skills are impaired in Alzheimer's disease. Drivers with Alzheimer's disease are not invariably involved in motor vehicle accidents, partly because they, like other older drivers, drive more slowly and take fewer risks. These compensations notwithstanding, deteriorating cognitive abilities, reflected in mental status examinations, and deteriorating visual skills, such as visual tracking and other aspects of visual attention, are concomitants of Alzheimer's disease that correlate with deteriorating driving performance and increased crash risk.

In the case of syncope, it would be important to assess the risk that this could recur. This would require a specific evaluation of the particular patient, but the cause of syncope is only determined in a minority of cases. Although the laws governing syncope of various etiologies differ, an episode of seizure- or nonseizure-related syncope would seem to be associated with similar risk. From a medical point of view, the important issues would be to assess the risk of recurrence and to what extent a given treatment would prevent recurrence.

Alcohol consumption is implicated in more than 50 percent of all fatal accidents. It could be argued that an alcoholic who did not drive while intoxicated might be a safe driver, but it would be important for a physician to assess if there were associated behavioral, physical, or cognitive problems that might impair the patient's driving abilities. For example, older individuals are more sensitive to the effects of alcohol and other substances that impair alertness and reaction time.

3. What if Selma had no overt medical problems but had recently been involved in several minor accidents for which she was clearly at fault?

It would be important to identify any underlying disease states that could be responsible. Visual or hearing impairments could interfere and would need to be identified and corrected if possible. Early Alzheimer's disease, Parkinson's disease, or other chronic neurologic disorders could lead to slowness of response time or impaired visuospatial function or judgment. In these cases, driving ability would be expected to deteriorate and it would be important to cease driving before an accident occurred.

In addition to such detectable impairments, age-related physiologic changes could be contributing factors. For example, with advancing age, impairments in spatial resolution and nighttime visibility may develop. A reliable person might be able to overcome these subtle problems by avoiding night driving and limiting daytime driving to optimal road conditions. Still, there might be other subtle alterations in vision, perception, or cognition that would remain undetected but could increase crash risk.

One explanation frequently given for the increased accident risk among the elderly is slow reaction time. Reaction time slows gradually with age, beginning in early adulthood, but there is much variability in the extent of the change, especially among older adults. One study suggests that perception response time in older drivers is well within the criteria used in highway design for the estimation of necessary stopping distance.[2] Yet adequate reaction time under experimental conditions might not reflect driving conditions in all circumstances, such as darkness, glare, fatigue after prolonged driving, or the driver's medical problem or functional limitation.

4. What factors might be contributing to Selma's persistence in driving?

Her explanations as to why she continues to drive despite her impairment suggest that this formerly self-sufficient woman feels dependent and vulnerable. She may also be unable or unwilling to recognize the reality of her deteriorating eyesight and its impact on her activities of daily living. It is not uncommon for patients with atrophic macular degeneration or other causes of slowly progressive visual loss to adapt to their impairment or, when it comes to critical activities, to deny their deficit. In addition, Selma is aware that alternatives to driving are limited. There is a severe shortage of public transportation in many communities, making the inability to drive a serious impediment to carrying out activities of daily living and to having adequate social contact, which in itself may affect the health of many elderly people.

ETHICAL AND LEGAL CONSIDERATIONS

1. What limits or restrictions are in place that would prevent people like Selma or other impaired individuals from driving?

The standards for issuing and renewing drivers' licenses vary tremendously from state to state, as do the factors calling for physician involvement in the evaluation of driver ability. Restricted licenses can be obtained in a number of states for people with varying degrees of visual impairment, and, in a few cases, with severe impairment.[3] Nine states have no requirement for static visual acuity testing at renewal of unrestricted licenses. Moreover, the vision screening done in the motor vehicle bureau is generally a cursory test of static visual acuity, which fails to detect important but subtle parameters of vision, such as visual field, dynamic visual acuity, and motor perception. These parameters, when abnormal, are known to be associated with crash risk. Some states have recently considered switching to mail-in license renewal or are increasing the time before license expiration, perhaps for budgetary reasons; however, some states are also beginning to consider a broader functional approach to testing.

Whether or not a repeat driving test would actually be required on the basis of advanced age varies significantly among states. Approximately 17 jurisdictions in the United States require additional tests or documentation for people in the older age groups. An impaired driver should be advised that some insurance policies require the insured to voluntarily report to the company any factors that affect their driving ability. Failure to comply could limit or even release the company's obligation to pay in the event of an accident. All states require patients with epilepsy to report their condition to the motor vehicle bureau, although it has been estimated that up to 90 percent of affected individuals fail to comply with this requirement.[4] In general, visual impairments must be reported by patients as well.

Eight states require physicians to report certain medical conditions (most often epilepsy) to state authorities. Whether the driver's license is limited or revoked on the basis of that information is a decision of the state department of motor vehicles and is not within the authority of the patient's personal physician. Physician-reporting laws have been criticized because they discourage patients from reporting symptoms to the physician, hampering treatment and potentially increasing accident risk. Some states have revoked their laws for this reason. Another problem with disease-specific laws is that the restrictions are rather arbitrary. This is highlighted by the wide variation among states in the details of the restrictions. For example, an epileptic is restricted from driving based on a seizure-free interval that ranges from 0 to 18 months, depending on the licensing state. Although 85 percent of states impose such restrictions for seizure disorders, only 52 percent impose restrictions for nonseizure syncope and only 16 percent for arrhythmia.[5]

There is no legally enforceable right to drive. Obtaining a license to drive is a privilege, not a right. The state does have the authority to suspend or revoke a license if someone commits egregious acts, such as driving while intoxicated or driving with a serious medical impairment. Some states have also made available the option of limited or restricted licenses depending on the individual's current medical condition or previous driving history. A temporary, limited, or restricted license may be issued, which would allow the individual to accomplish certain basic daily needs of living, such as traveling to work or basic shopping, while limiting or eliminating nonessential driving. In this way, the individual is afforded some independence yet the state has minimized the risk to the public.

2. What is the physician's obligation if he believes Selma is no longer capable of driving?

Because of her poor visual acuity, Selma poses the threat of harm to both herself and others. It is not certain that she would qualify for a restricted license in her state or even if that would be advisable. At a minimum, her physician should strongly advise her to severely curtail her driving or perhaps cease driving altogether and to find alternatives. If, as Selma fears, there are few alternatives, it would be equally important for the physician to help the patient explore what is available. He should advise her to call a local agency such as an Office on Aging or a Center for Low Vision and encourage her to explore the opportunities available through friends, family, local church groups, and others. Communities that lack good public transportation may have independent or community-sponsored shuttle buses for senior citizens to allow them to shop independently while avoiding the need to drive themselves. In many communities, private individuals, such as social workers, can be employed on a short-term basis to explore these options with the patient. If feasible, Selma might wish to explore alternative living arrangements, where she would be closer to the necessary services and would have more social contacts.

The physician would have similar obligations to any driver without special medical impairments, but whose driving skills are nonetheless impaired. In a few limited cases, however, an aging driver might benefit from a remedial driving course followed by a repeat road test. If appropriate, the physician should refer such a patient to organizations like the American Automobile Association or the American Association of Retired Persons (AARP), which offer courses geared specifically toward the needs and limitations of older drivers. In some states, older drivers who participate in the AARP driver safety course, 55 Alive, will receive insurance discounts.

If Selma does not follow her doctor's advice and continues to drive, the question then becomes whether her "unreasonable" position creates obligations for her physician beyond the realm of this physician-patient relationship. That is, should her physician take steps to curtail further driving by Selma and if so, what steps could be ethically and legally justified?

The physician must comply with local law. If this particular jurisdiction has reporting requirements regarding visual acuity, there is no choice but to report Selma. When no such requirement exists, as in most states, the physician must recognize that the assurance of confidentiality allows Selma to confide in her physician and feel comfortable seeking help. On the other hand, this might be heavily countered by the benefit to be gained if her impairment were reported to someone who would prevent her from driving and causing a serious accident. Loss of license or cessation of driving might not even have a significant impact on Selma's independence because her low vision has already curtailed her driving. Selma may maintain or improve her current level of independence in other ways, by hiring a driver, identifying friends or neighbors to help, or investigating and utilizing community services.

A physician seeking to report an impaired driver such as Selma would confront a number of practical dilemmas. To whom would such information be given? Is any mechanism in place to report impaired drivers? Would there be any obligation on the part of the physician beyond alerting some state authority? Does the physician have an obligation to reveal other impairments of patients like Selma or her modestly impaired contemporaries? Is there an obligation to reveal impairments in other circumstances, for example, a taxi driver with syncope or unstable angina? Would the physician who was consulted for this problem have the obligation to warn the patient's employer, taxi commission, or police? What are the obligations of the physician to unknown third parties who might possibly be affected by the actions of an impaired patient? In short, does the physician have an obligation to the general well-being of society that might override the obligations to an individual patient?

There are certain circumstances in which the benefits of confidentiality are outweighed by society's need to protect others from unknown dangers. These would include the vulnerable, such as a victim of possible child abuse; innocent third parties, such as those at risk of being exposed to a communicable disease; or individuals who are in such imminent or probable danger that breach of confidentiality in order to warn that individual is warranted and justifiable. Regulations and case law that apply to these situations have been discussed in Case 16 ("A Married Man Contracts Syphilis").

Selma's case also does not fall neatly into any of these categories. There are no identifiable third parties who could conceivably be warned about

Selma's impaired driving, given the randomness of her driving. Her actions do not constitute deliberate or determined threats against any one individual, or even any particular class of individuals. Presumably, the doctor could contact the local police or the state motor vehicle agency, but it is unlikely that coercive measures could be taken against Selma unless and until she demonstrated actions that clearly violated the law or endangered the welfare of others.

One potentially analogous situation is the company physician who finds out that an employee's health might jeopardize customers of the company—the impaired bus driver, for example. Unlike Selma's case, however, in this situation the physician has obligations not only to the patient but also to the company and its customers. As such, the nature of the relationship between patient and physician differs and presumably would lead to a different understanding between them. In contrast, a community-based physician presumably has no other obligations that would so strongly conflict with the demands of the physician-patient relationship apart from those few specified in the law. While Selma's physician, as a citizen, probably feels obligated to follow the law, there are usually no clear mandates in this kind of case, although the potential for harm is evident.

Ultimately, for Selma's physician, a decision as to how to proceed would depend on a sense of moral obligation to both patient and society, as well as a balancing of the likely risk of harm by breaching versus the harm of maintaining confidentiality. One may argue that by alerting appropriate authorities, the physician is not really breaching confidentiality; after all, the fact that Selma has poor vision is not really a secret. Yet it is not the usual role of the physician to consider himself an agent of the state and to make it his business to report a patient to a public agency such as the motor vehicle bureau or the police.

As the population ages, and the abilities of increasing numbers of drivers are questioned, there may be reason to broaden the currently limited relicensing requirements for older individuals. This would fall within the responsibility of state authorities rather than individual, private physicians, who are not agents of the state. The burdens that reporting requirements would place on physicians, in terms of sheer numbers as well as the harm caused to the physician-patient relationship, would be significant. Some argue that, rather than penalizing the elderly by revoking their licenses, highway design should be improved to fit the changing highway demography. Roads have been designed with young male drivers in mind, and signs and signals could be significantly improved to adapt to the changing needs.

It has been pointed out that elderly drivers as a group may be no more dangerous than others and probably are less dangerous than 18-year-old male drivers. Although the crash risk per mile driven is highest for the elderly, older licensed drivers on the average drive far fewer total miles than do members of other age groups and are responsible for far fewer accidents. Accidents caused by elderly individuals are at lower speeds, produce less damage, and lead to fewer pedestrian fatalities than those caused by youthful drivers. Eighty-year-old male and female drivers produce only about one-half the number of fatal accidents as their 20-year-old counterparts of the same sex, and 80-year-old female drivers produce only one-ninth as many fatal accidents as 20-year-old men. Although these statistics might argue against a sweeping decree to restrict older drivers as a group, they cannot be used to support the continued driving of someone known to be accident prone.

The ideal course for Selma's physician would arguably be to persuade Selma that her driving poses a substantial risk to herself and others. It is likely that it is also a legal requirement for her to report this impairment in her state. As her motivation for driving appears not to be stubbornness but rather fulfillment of legitimate needs, some reasonable compromise might be adopted to permit Selma to remain as independent as possible. It would be to everyone's benefit if Selma's needs could be met without the risk incurred by her own driving. Yet for physicians to act as "safety agents," reporting patients with questionable driving ability to the authorities, raises serious concerns about the integrity of the physician-patient relationship. It is not the physician's role, but the state's, to ensure the safety of the road.

REFERENCES

1. J.P. Szlyk et al., "A Comparison of Driving in Older Subjects with and without Age-related Macular Degeneration," *Archives of Ophthalmology* 113 (1995): 1033–1040.
2. P.L. Olson and M. Sivak, "Perception-Response Time to Unexpected Roadway Hazards," *Human Factors* 28 (1986): 91–96.
3. G. Fonda, "Legal Blindness Can Be Compatible with Safe Driving," *Ophthalmology* 96 (1989): 1457–1459.

4. A. Krumholz et al., "Driving and Epilepsy. A Review and Reappraisal," *Journal of the American Medical Association* 265 (1991): 622–626.

5. S.A. Strickberger et al., "When Should Patients with Lethal Ventricular Arrhythmia Resume Driving? An Analysis of State Regulations and Physician Practices," *Annals of Internal Medicine* 115 (1991): 560–563.

SUGGESTED READINGS

Associated Press. 1997. States consider limits on elderly drivers, 6 April.

Fitten, L.J. et al. 1995. Alzheimer and vascular dementias and driving. A prospective road and laboratory study. *Journal of the American Medical Association* 273: 1360–1365.

Fox, G.K. et al. 1997. Alzheimer's disease and driving: Prediction and assessment of driving performance. *Journal of the American Geriatrics Society* 45: 949–953.

Fozard, J.L. et al. 1994. Age differences and changes in reaction time: The Baltimore longitudinal study of aging. *Journals of Gerontology* 49: P179–P189.

Johnson, C.A., and Keltner, J.L. 1983. Incidence of visual field loss in 20,000 eyes and its relationship to driving performance. *Archives of Ophthalmology* 101: 371–375.

Levy, D.T. et al. 1995. Relationship between driver's license renewal policies and fatal crashes involving drivers 70 years or older. *Journal of the American Medical Association* 274: 1026–1030.

Lyznick, J.M. et al. 1998. Sleepiness, driving, and motor vehicle crashes. Council on Scientific Affairs, American Medical Association. *Journal of the American Medical Association* 279: 1908–1913.

Office of the Assistant Secretary for Transportation Policy. 1997. *Improving transportation for a maturing society.* U.S. Department of Transportation (see Appendix A).

Owsley, C. et al. 1998. Visual impairment, eye disease, and injurious motor vehicle crashes in the elderly. *Ophthalmic Epidemiology* 5: 101–113.

Perryman, K.M., and Fitten, L.J. 1996. Effects of normal aging on the performance of motor-vehicle operational skills. *Journal of Geriatric Psychiatry and Neurology* 9: 136–141.

Retchin, S.M., ed. 1993. Medical considerations in the older driver. *Clinics in Geriatric Medicine* 9: 279–490.

Reuben, D.B., and St. George, P. 1996. Driving and dementia—California's approach to a medical and policy dilemma. *Western Journal of Medicine* 164: 111–121.

Stutts, J.C. 1998. Do older drivers with visual and cognitive impairments drive less? *Journal of the American Geriatrics Society* 46: 854–861.

Taylor, J. et al. 1996. Risk of accidents in drivers with epilepsy. *Journal of Neurology, Neurosurgery, and Psychiatry* 60: 621–627.

Trobe, J.D. et al. 1996. Crashes and violations among drivers with Alzheimer disease. *Archives of Neurology* 53: 411–16.

LEGAL CITATION

Case Example

Praesel v. Johnson, WL-170067 (Tex. 1998).
The Texas Supreme Court held that physicians do not have a duty to warn patients with epilepsy not to drive, and do not have a duty to report the patient's condition to the state authorities. The lawsuit was brought by relatives of a deceased victim killed in a car crash caused by another man suffering a grand mal seizure. Physicians in Texas are permitted, but not mandated, to report the names of epilepsy patients to the State department of Public Health.

CASE 20

A Difficult Patient and the Limits of Provider Obligations

Arlene is a 26-year-old woman addicted to heroin. She has no steady source of income and no fixed address. For years she has used intravenous heroin and now has end-stage renal disease (ESRD).

Despite the constant recommendations by her doctors, and repeated attempts at in-patient drug rehabilitation and methadone maintenance, Arlene is either unwilling or unable to put an end to her drug use. When confronted with the probability that this has led to her kidney failure, she stated, "My kidneys are already shot." She has also refused a trial of corticosteroids because she found that her boyfriend, also a drug user with kidney disease, accepted such treatments and became "much sicker." Over the past year, Arlene has not adhered to medical regimens and has refused hemodialysis when it was recommended, however, she presents in a state of fluid overload in the local municipal hospital's emergency room approximately once a month, usually in the early morning hours, creating stress for the staff and chaos for the morning schedule of regular dialysis patients. On more than one occasion, she has been so critically ill that other patients have been bumped from the schedule.

At the request of the nephrologists, psychiatrists have examined Arlene several times and have diagnosed her behavior as "opioid abuse," and "antisocial personality disorder." They have also consistently stated that she "is competent to make decisions."

Recently, Arlene's behavior has become even more disruptive. The hospital's renal unit received a phone call from a nearby hospital stating that "your patient" was currently in its emergency room but would subsequently be transferred once her condition was stabilized. When Arlene did arrive at the municipal hospital, she was especially dirty and unkempt, used vulgar language with the staff, and exposed her genitals to other patients. Following her dialysis, she was admitted to a medical bed for further treatment, but as usual she insisted on leaving the hospital. After consulting with the Office of Risk Management, her doctors told her she could leave but would have to sign out "A.M.A." (against medical advice). They also informed her that the unit no longer wished to be responsible for her treatment, and they handed her a list of alternative dialysis centers in the area. The social worker offered to arrange for a transfer of her care to any of these facilities that would be willing to take her on as a patient.

ISSUES TO CONSIDER

- Decision-specific capacity
- Limits of provider obligations
- Allocation of expensive resources
- Transfers of emergency room patients

MEDICAL CONSIDERATIONS

1. Is Arlene correct when she asserts that no matter what she does now, her kidneys are "shot?"

Heroin addicts have a high rate of renal disease, which can be due to a number of conditions with varying prognosis. The most common form of heroin nephropathy, focal glomerulosclerosis (GS), generally progresses to end-stage renal disease (ESRD) within four years, depending on the severity at presentation. There is some evidence that the disease will progress more slowly in patients who completely abstain, however, progression often occurs despite discontinuation of the abused substance. Furthermore, there is no convincing evidence that corticosteroids or other immunosuppressive agents halt the course of the disease, and they are rarely used today. Thus, while Arlene's choice to refuse the corticosteroids was not necessarily one that was fully informed, she was correct in determining that the benefits would have been limited at best, and her refusal probably leaves her in no worse shape than she is in currently.

The prognosis of most other forms of chronic renal failure in heroin abusers is somewhat more favorable, assuming drug use stops in time. Drug abuse, in particular, subcutaneous injections ("skin popping"), may produce systemic amyloidosis with renal failure. This form of renal damage, thought to be the result of chronic or recurrent suppurative skin infections, occurs much later in the course of addiction, and abstinence should theoretically reduce risk. Other preventable causes of nephropathy in heroin addicts include endocarditis-associated glomerulonephritis and acute renal failure due to rhabdomyolysis.

Medicinal use of commercially available opioids (e.g., for chronic pain syndromes) does not cause renal failure. Illicit intravenous drug use may cause renal failure as a result of HIV infection (HIV-associated nephropathy), and hepatitis B (HBV) and C (HCV), which can cause membranoproliferative glomerulonephritis or cryoglobulinemia. Many intravenous heroin abusers abuse other illicit drugs as well, and these can lead to renal failure. Notable among these agents is cocaine, which can cause renal failure due to hypertension or rhabdomyolysis. Although early treatment of renal disease related to infectious agents, including HIV, may slow and possibly even arrest progression, there are currently no medical treatments that reverse ESRD.

Symptomatic treatments in the course of chronic renal failure, such as diuretics or dietary and medical treatments to control hyperkalemia, can reduce the need for dialysis, however, it is difficult for even highly motivated individuals with sufficient supports in the community to comply with this strict regimen.

Frequent dialysis lessens morbidity and long-term mortality of patients with ESRD. Arlene's erratic use of this necessary treatment is likely to be harmful to her. Thus, although she may be correct in believing that specific regimens will not restore kidney function, she will be incorrect if she asserts that adherence to her doctors' recommendations will not improve her health or life span. Furthermore, continued drug abuse will expose her to an array of superimposed illnesses.

Although Arlene's kidneys are "shot," her health could improve or at least be maintained, if she were willing and able to have continuing medical care. In particular, given the persistently high incidence of HIV and HCV infection among intravenous drug abusers (IVDAs) in certain municipalities (despite national declines), the availability of effective antiretroviral treatment, progress in the treatment of HCV infection, universal availability of hemodialysis, and entitlement programs for the poor and other at-risk groups, Arlene's health could benefit significantly. Unfortunately, convincing her to avail herself of these resources and guiding such a complex individual through the bureaucratic intricacies involved poses an immense challenge.

2. Are there any alternatives to offer Arlene, such as kidney transplant?

Given Arlene's current lifestyle, she would not be considered for kidney transplant. A successful transplant would eliminate the need for dialysis, but this patient would be at high risk of graft rejection. Although donor-recipient incompatibility would be the most likely cause of acute graft rejection, this recipient's probable failure to adhere to the posttransplant medical regimen would perhaps be the most important single contributing factor to late rejection.

Another question that sometimes arises in discussions about renal transplant for IVDAs is possible coinfection with HBV, HCV, or HIV. Patients infected with HCV prior to transplant may do no worse than uninfected patients in terms of graft survival and overall mortality. Likewise, there is currently no evidence that renal transplant worsens the prognosis of HIV-infected individuals, although transplants are currently rare among such patients. This is likely due to physician concerns (possibly unfounded) that immunosuppression would exacerbate HIV and HIV-related infections, as well as reluctance to use scarce resources in patients with a potentially fatal illness. HIV and renal disease are discussed further in Case 18 ("Surgical Delay in a Patient Infected with HIV").

ETHICAL AND LEGAL CONSIDERATIONS

1. Can an opioid abuser be capable of making health care treatment decisions?

Those whose role it is to determine decisional capacity are often placed in a difficult position. It is well known that craving for a substance such as heroin powerfully conditions judgment. Despite Arlene's psychiatric diagnoses, the determination of her decisional capacity must be made in the context of the specific decision to be made at the time in question, as is discussed in Case 2 ("Determining if a Patient Has Decisional Capacity"). Her impairment in certain aspects of her thinking (as manifested by her poor judgment concerning her lifestyle) may not compromise her ability to consider and weigh the risks and benefits of the treatment options available to her. For example, Arlene's decision to refuse the corticosteroids might have included an evaluation that a small benefit would not be worth the risk of the side effects that she observed in her boyfriend. It appears that the psychiatrists involved in Arlene's care recognized the crucial distinction between a diagnostic label and the ability to make specific medical decisions. Although frustrating for physicians, Arlene's case again illustrates how patient autonomy, supported by decisional capacity, must ultimately prevail even when the decision conflicts with beneficent intentions of physicians, whose wish to serve the medical best interest of the patient may conflict with the law's role as protector of the citizens' civil rights. The key is recognizing those cases in which capacity is intact despite obvious behavioral problems or thought impairment.

2. What are the physicians' legal and moral obligations to Arlene, given her treatment refusal?

Ideally, physicians should attempt to develop a relationship with the patient so they can establish what her goals are and, through open and honest discussion of treatment options, how those goals might best be achieved. The doctor is obligated to maintain patient confidences and to fully inform the patient about the diagnosis, treatment options, and prognosis. These obligations to the patient rest on the notion of promoting the patient's well-being, as defined by the patient. The doctor is not a "medical agent" of society, charged with enforcing a prescribed health care regimen.

In most circumstances, the limits of the doctor's authority are defined by the willingness of the patient to comply with the advice given. Nothing can be imposed on a patient against his or her will except when the refusal puts others at risk (see Case 16, "A Married Man Contracts Syphilis," and Case 17, "A House-Bound Woman with Tuberculosis") or if the patient lacks decisional capacity and the refusal arises out of the inability to comprehend the decision.

With a patient such as Arlene, the physician's beneficent instincts and training are tested to the limits. If Arlene were found to lack decisional capacity and her choices were allowed to stand, this would constitute patient abandonment rather than respect for patient autonomy. If the patient has decisional capacity, has been sufficiently informed, and yet refuses beneficial care, there may be little more the physician can do other than to be accessible and to encourage continuous dialogue. For example, it would be incumbent on Arlene's physicians to make certain that she understood the dangers of erratic dialysis and the need to adhere to a strict regimen and to attempt to connect her to a social support system so that she would have ready access to care. Establishing an ongoing, continuous relationship with a primary care physician in the community would also be an important source of support for Arlene's adherence to a dialysis treatment regimen. Despite these options, Arlene has the right to make "wrong" choices about her health care, as long as she understands the consequences to herself.

3. Given Arlene's erratic behavior, are there limits that her providers can ethically or legally impose on the course of her care?

Limits to the provision of care would depend on the circumstances. When the patient presents herself in true emergency circumstances, either at the hospital where a relationship has already been established or in an unfamiliar emergency room at another facility, treatment would have to be provided. Facilities (whether public, voluntary, or private) with emergency services have created the expectation in the minds of the public of the availability of emergency assistance. The facility cannot then pick and choose which emergencies it wishes to respond to and which it does not.

Under federal legislation, an emergency department must respond to and treat a medical emergency until the patient's medical condition has stabilized and the threat of a further emergency has ceased. The Emergency Medical Treatment and Active Labor Act (EMTALA) was intended to ensure that all patients who arrive at an emergency department, no matter what their medical condition or psychosocial background, receive an appropriate medical screening exam and treatment for their emergency condition, prior to being discharged from the hospital or transferred to another facility. It was originally designed to combat the "dumping" of poor or uninsured patients out of emergency departments, and today provides protection for a full range of discrimination concerns for any patient who arrives at a hospital seeking emergency treatment. For patients such as Arlene, whose reputation, demeanor, or lifestyle might lead some facilities to eject her from their facility, EMTALA would ensure that she be screened and that all emergency conditions be stabilized prior to her discharge or transfer. Under EMTALA, hospitals are also forbidden from checking the patient's insurance status or from seeking prior authorization from a managed care organization prior to initiating the medical screen and provision of necessary emergency services. Thus, as unpleasant as Arlene may be, the hospital emergency room to which she presented herself would have no choice but to evaluate her and address any emergency conditions, even if the hospital informed Arlene ahead of time that it no longer wished to continue caring for her.

Legitimate exceptions to this general principle of emergency accessibility do exist and are particularly pertinent to emergency care in crowded urban settings. The first exception has to do with the actual resources of the emergency room. If the demands of emergency care truly overwhelm the available resources, such that continued admission of emergency room patients would pose a threat to current patients and lead to inadequate attention to new ones, it would be justifiable for a diversion mechanism to be put into place to send incoming patients to area facilities more capable of handling that patient at that particular time. Such a diversion scheme would be for a limited time, and measures would have to be employed to make certain that diversion criteria rested on sound medical judgments rather than more insidious, prejudicial criteria, such as an unpopular or communicable disease (e.g., delirium tremens, AIDS, TB) or socioeconomic status. Hospitals that utilize diversion mechanisms must do so only in accord with formal hospital policies, in compliance with any applicable state and federal regulations.

A second exception to this principle reflects the lack of primary care that faces many who consequently utilize emergency rooms as walk-in clinics. If attention to a walk-in patient with a nonemergent problem would divert scarce resources from true emergency cases, it would be justifiable for providers to postpone the nonemergent situation until emergencies are handled and, if need be, to reschedule the patient for follow-up care in an outpatient routine care setting. If a patient such as Arlene made a regular habit of showing up at the emergency room *before* the onset of an emergency because she preferred to receive treatment at her own convenience, it would be justifiable for the emergency room to decline to initiate treatment once it was clearly established that she had no immediate needs. (Under EMTALA, however, the emergency department would still be obligated to conduct an appropriate medical screening exam and to make a formal determination that no emergency condition existed prior to declining to offer her services in the ER). Arlene may have the right to refuse or accept specific treatments, but she does not have the right to receive treatment at her own convenience, particularly if such demands impinge on the more urgent needs of other patients. Once it was determined there was no immediate crisis, Arlene's demands would then properly have limits placed on them, as providers and facilities have obligations to patients with true emergency conditions in the emergency department.

Further, providers need not suffer verbal or physical abuse by a patient. Providers and facilities have every right to impose limits on freedom of behavior in the clinical setting if that behavior infringes on their delivery of care and the well-being of third parties. Health professionals must be trained to expect certain types of risks, however, such as a violent patient with schizophrenia, delirium, or other confusional states. These risks are intrinsic to the profession and need to be anticipated so that harm can be avoided.

Thus, while it could be argued that Arlene has the right to limit the intervention that providers wish to offer, so too can her providers draw limits to their involvement with Arlene if she displays behavior that is unjustifiable and disruptive to the clinical setting, or, if after open dialogue, no mutually acceptable arrangement can be found. Criteria would have to be established to ensure that these limits were prompted not by mere dislike of the patient or her lifestyle but by concern over the legitimate harm and threat she posed to the caregiving environment and other patients.

As Arlene's doctors and facility cannot simply abandon her, some other alternative must be found. With difficult patients, it is not uncommon for doctors to develop a "contractual" relationship, literally drafting an agreement of understanding concerning the terms and conditions of treatment. If the patient violates the contract in some significant and meaningful way, the provider might then begin to sever the relationship, although still having the obligation to assist her in finding access to sufficient care elsewhere, if it exists. Any decision to terminate a relationship with a patient must be done according to a formal protocol, so as to ensure the termination has a legitimate and acceptable basis. Clinicians also need to ensure that the patient has been given reasonable notice of the termination, in order to gain access to other services should subsequent need arise. This, of course, may not solve the problem for the community because Arlene might well continue her erratic behavior at other health care facilities. Ultimately, the facilities in the community might attempt to arrive at a joint resolution to this problem.

4. Should the expensive resource of hemodialysis be available for a patient in Arlene's circumstances?

Given the current policies and perspectives in the United States, Arlene is entitled to receive hemodialysis if it is medically indicated. This entitlement does not extend to unlimited access whenever or wherever she chooses, but it does reflect unlimited access to dialysis regardless of age, disease, prognosis, socioeconomic status, and other factors that limit access in other countries. Universal access to dialysis for patients with ESRD is unique to the United States. In the United Kingdom, for example, budget allocations of the National Health Service can never be exceeded. Strict adherence to policy in the UK and other countries likely leads to de facto rationing of dialysis, and in fact, the United Kingdom has one of the lowest treatment rates for ESRD in the Western world. Explicit treatment selection criteria include consideration of the patient's quality of life and age. Unlike the United States, patients in the United Kingdom are not automatically entitled to treatment because of their clinical condition.[1]

In the United States, an explicit policy decision to pay for anyone in need of chronic hemodialysis was put into effect through the federal Medicare system in 1973. The impetus for this policy decision was due to the ad hoc, often discriminatory manner in which patients were selected for dialysis in the early days of its availability. The cost to Medicare of the ESRD program in 1995 was approximately $8.9 billion,[2] far greater than initial estimates. This cost explosion is in part due to the changing demography of patients, who are currently much older and sicker than previous estimates projected. It has created disincentives for the government to pay for any other class of patients as defined by their specific disease.

Currently, most dialysis facilities are for-profit ventures. Facilities may determine whether or not they wish to enroll patients based on ability to pay in excess of what is covered by Medicare. Thus, although the government pays for dialysis, this does not mean that any dialysis patient can go to any facility and demand treatment. For patients such as Arlene, the only recourse to ongoing care may be through public facilities, which cannot turn anyone away and which may be less comfortable or desirable than private treatment centers. Likewise, simply because a facility obtains Medicare reimbursement, a private physician with privileges there is not required to take on any and all patients. Because government funds pay for dialysis, there is access, but one must have medical need and may not be able to select the treatment center of one's choice.

For patients such as Arlene, whose lifestyle and behavior may be repugnant to many in society, the Medicare funding provides access. That guaranteed access may not diminish the personal feelings of some providers that Arlene ought not to have this access. Some of those perspectives are based on biases unrelated to the patient's specific medical condition. For example, a desire to limit Arlene's access to dialysis because she is a homeless person or suffers from an illness that might be categorized as "self-induced" would be unethical and unsupportable. Social disadvantages and other adverse circumstances, such as a history of abuse in childhood or exposure to parents who abused harmful substances, may lead to situations like Arlene's. Moreover, there is increasing evidence that behavioral problems such as substance abuse and personality disorders have a genetic basis (see Suggested Readings). A system that does not deny care to patients who have smoked excessively or who have eaten unhealthy foods should not deny care to Arlene because of the possibility that her disease is self-induced or self-perpetuating.

Nevertheless, if there were doubt as to the efficacy of a particular treatment option for a patient with ESRD who continued to use drugs, the treatment might be legitimately withheld unless she demonstrated a consistent change in her behavior that would increase the likelihood of its efficacy. Kidney transplant would be a case in point. Although dialysis keeps her alive and relatively well despite her lifestyle, a kidney transplant might fail under these circumstances. In contrast to hemodialysis, which is expensive but widely available, renal transplant is a costly, and scarce, resource. In such cases, criteria have been employed concerning who ought to have access to this resource. The criteria ought to include the utility of the intervention, the suitability of the candidate from a medical standpoint, the ability of a patient to adhere to a posttransplant treatment regimen, and the likelihood of its medical success, but ought not to include the patient's value to society.

REFERENCES

1. J.K. McKenzie, "Dialysis Decision Making in Canada, the United Kingdom, and the United States," *American Journal of Kidney Disease* 31 (1998): 12–18.
2. S. Garella, "The Costs of Dialysis in the USA," *Nephrology, Dialysis, Transplantation* 12 (Supp. 1)(1997): 10–21.

SUGGESTED READINGS

Adams, J., and Murray, R. 1998. The general approach to the difficult patient. *Emergency Medicine Clinics of North America* 16: 689–700.

American Medical Association, Office of the General Counsel, Division of Health Law. Ending the patient-physician relationship (see Appendix A).

Baker, C.H., and Goldsmith, T.M. 1998. From triage to transfer: HCFA's update on EMTALA. *Health Law Digest* 26: 3–14.

Baldwin, D.S. et al. 1997. Nephrotoxicity secondary to drug abuse and lithium use. In: *Diseases of the Kidney,* ed. R.W. Schrier and C.W. Gottschalk, 1203–1230. Boston: Little, Brown and Company.

Bleyer, A.J. et al. 1999. An international study of patient compliance with hemodialysis. *Journal of the American Medical Association* 281: 1211–1213.

Des Jarlais, D.C. et al. 1998. Declining seroprevalence in a very large HIV epidemic: Injecting drug users in New York City, 1991 to 1996. *American Journal of Public Health* 88: 1801–1806.

Friedman, E. 1996. End-stage renal disease therapy: An American success story. *Journal of the American Medical Association* 275: 1118–1122.

Groves, J.E. 1978. Taking care of the hateful patient. *New England Journal of Medicine* 298: 883–887.

Inglehart, J.K. 1999. The American health care system—Medicaid. *New England Journal of Medicine* 340: 403–408.

Johnson, C.C. et al. 1996. Working with noncompliant and abusive dialysis patients: Practical strategies based on ethics and the law. *Advances in Renal Replacement Therapy* 3: 77–86.

Lerner, B.H. et al. 1998. Rethinking nonadherence: Historical perspectives on triple-drug therapy for HIV disease. *Annals of Internal Medicine* 129: 573–578.

Nissenson, A.R., and Rettig, R.A. 1999. Medicare's end-stage renal disease program: Current status and future prospects. *Health Affairs* 18: 161–179.

Orenlicther, D. 1991. Denying treatment to the noncompliant patient. *Journal of the American Medical Association* 265: 1579–1582.

Port, F.K. 1992. The end-stage renal disease program: Trends over the past 18 years. *American Journal of Kidney Disease* 20 (Suppl. 1): 3–7.

Plomin, R. 1994. The genetic basis of complex human behaviors. *Science* 264: 1733–1739.

Quaid, K.A. et al. 1996. Issues in genetic testing for susceptibility to alcoholism: Lessons from Alzheimer's disease and Huntington's disease. *Alcoholism: Clinical and Experimental Research* 20: 1430–1437.

Rettig, R. 1996. The social contract and the treatment of permanent kidney failure. *Journal of the American Medical Association* 275: 1123–1126.

Rounsaville, B.J. et al. 1991. Psychiatric disorders in relatives of probands with opiate addiction. *Archives of General Psychiatry* 48: 33–42.

Sledge, W.H., and Feinstein, A.R. 1997. A clinimetric approach to the components of the patient-physician relationship. *Journal of the American Medical Association* 278: 2043–2048.

Spital, A. 1998. Should all human immunodeficiency virus-infected patients with end-stage renal disease be excluded from transplantation? The views of U.S. transplant centers. *Transplantation* 65: 1187–1191.

Weingart, S.N. et al. 1998. Patients discharged against medical advice from a general medicine service. *Journal of General Internal Medicine* 13: 568–571.

LEGAL CITATIONS

Case Examples

Brown v. Bower, No. J86-0759 (b) (S.D. Miss. Dec. 12, 1987).
Hospital mandated to continue providing treatment to a disruptive dialysis patient. Treatment could not be denied if denial was unrelated to patient's medical needs.

Burditt v. United States Department of Health and Human Services, 934 F.2d 1362 (5th Cir. 1991).
Hospital cannot transfer an uninsured female patient with high blood pressure during labor. Patients in labor are considered "unstable" under federal legislation, which requires the stabilization of a patient's condition before she may be transferred out of an emergency room.

In re Baby K, Nos. 93-1899, 93-1923, 93-1924, 4th Cir. (Va. Feb. 10, 1994).
Federal court upheld the obligation of an emergency department to provide resuscitative support to an anencephalic infant whose mother repeatedly sought emergency room treatment for the child. This obligation was supported by the mandates of the federal EMTALA legislation.

Payton v. Weaver, 131 Cal. App. 3d 38, 182 Cal. Rptr. 225 (1982).
Case similar to *Brown v. Bower,* although termination of treatment ultimately was upheld because of sufficient notice and the patient's continued lack of cooperation.

Statutory Example

Consolidated Omnibus Budget Reconciliation Act of 1985 (COBRA), Pub. L. No. 99-272, Sec. 9121, 100 Stat. 164-167 (1986) (codified at 42 U.S.C.A. Sec. 1395dd (1994 and West Supp. 1998)).
Federal law known as EMTALA (Emergency Medical Treatment and Active Labor Act), which requires all hospitals participating in Medicare to conduct appropriate medical screening exams for all patients who arrive at the facility requesting emergency services, to ascertain whether the patient has an emergency condition, and to stabilize the patient prior to discharging the patient or transferring the patient to another facility.

CASE 21

"Do Everything": Physician Obligations in the Face of Family Demands

Evelyn is an 86-year-old widow with multi-infarct dementia and severe ischemic cardiomyopathy. She lives in a nursing home, where she has been bedridden for a year. She occasionally speaks and follows some commands but does not communicate in a consistent fashion. It is uncertain if she recognizes any of her loved ones or those who take care of her.

Evelyn developed increasing shortness of breath and was transferred to the local hospital, where she was treated for pneumonia and congestive heart failure (CHF). Despite resolution of the pneumonia and aggressive medical treatment of the heart failure, her condition remains grave. She has dyspnea, a heart rate of 110, and bilateral pleural effusions. Her ejection fraction is 18 percent. Thoracentesis was performed and 200 mL of transudative fluid was removed. The patient appears to have tolerated the procedure well but her clinical condition has not improved significantly. Pulse oximetry reveals that she has an oxygen saturation of 70 to 80 percent while receiving oxygen by face mask.

Recognizing that the patient's short- and long-term prognosis is poor, Evelyn's physician has decided to address her resuscitation status with her family, in accordance with the hospital's do-not-resuscitate policy. The patient's daughter and granddaughter become extremely upset, stating that they want "everything done" for the patient. The patient's grandson, a dermatologist who does not live in town, is in contact via telephone and he says, "Do whatever you have to do to keep her alive." He insists that the physician obtain cardiology and pulmonary consultation, that the patient be presented to the intensive care unit (ICU) for transfer, that a second thoracentesis be performed so that the effusions are completely drained, and that chemical pleurodesis be performed to prevent fluid reaccumulation or a drum catheter inserted so that fluid can be withdrawn as needed. Evelyn's physician hesitates, pointing out that the fluid will reaccumulate, she may require mechanical restraints to prevent her from pulling out any devices that are inserted, and pleurodesis would be painful and possibly unsafe. If she had a cardiac or respiratory arrest, which is almost certain to occur soon, cardiopulmonary resuscitation would likely fail to revive her; if she were revived, she might have to face uncomfortable days on a respirator before her death. The family remains adamant, stating that "nothing is worse than death." They also admit, however, that Evelyn did not previously express treatment wishes.

When the ICU attending physician is approached about admitting Evelyn to the unit, he refuses to consider it, noting that "the family is totally crazy." He suggests to Evelyn's physician that he avoid doing a blood gas because a poor result will give the family "more ammunition."

ISSUES TO CONSIDER

- Defining the goals of treatment interventions
- Physician obligations in the face of family demands
- Access to intensive care units for patients with poor prognosis
- Medical futility

MEDICAL CONSIDERATIONS

1. What is the prognosis for a patient with advanced congestive heart failure who is 80 years old?

Evelyn has intractable, chronic CHF and has New York Heart Association Class IV symptoms (severe functional limitation due to heart disease). Cardiac mortality is highest in patients with ejection fraction below 20 percent and marked functional limitation (low age–adjusted peak oxygen consumption during exercise), and increases with advancing age.

A variety of predictive models have been used to determine prognosis and survival in patients with life-threatening illness, including the Acute Physiology and Chronic Health Evaluation (APACHE) scores, the Karnofsky Performance Status, and others (see Suggested Readings). These models may have applicability in estimating prognosis in groups of patients, but they are not sufficiently accurate to make precise decisions in individual cases, especially in the extreme cases, as insufficient numbers of patients in the extreme cases are tallied. Moreover, there is subjectivity in interpretation and use of these scales, which leads to poor inter-rater reliability. It may be that subjective factors are in the end more often applied in individual cases than objective scales.

In people of Medicare age the prognosis of CHF is limited, with six-year survival following first hospitalization for this condition approximately 13 to 25 percent.[1] The Medicare population includes patients considerably younger and less impaired than Evelyn. Evelyn, who is very elderly, functionally impaired, and has intractable symptoms of heart failure, satisfies all National Hospice Organization prognostic criteria for early mortality in heart disease,[2] and has a grave prognosis. If she were to have an asystolic cardiac arrest and undergo cardiopulmonary resuscitation (CPR), there is virtually no chance that she would be discharged alive, even if her heart rhythm were initially restored (see Case 12, "Resuscitation Decision in a Patient with Lung Cancer").

2. What benefit could Evelyn derive if she were admitted to an ICU?

Patients with severe heart failure generally are admitted to an ICU for close observation and administration of treatments that cannot be administered without monitoring devices, including a pulmonary artery (Swan-Ganz) catheter. Such treatments might include continuous intravenous inotropic agents or vasopressors, or mechanical assist devices such as intra-aortic balloon counterpulsation to maintain blood pressure. Such treatments are not intended for use in chronic CHF, but for patients who are expected to recover or as a bridge to surgery or cardiac transplant. Oral medications used for CHF, such as digoxin and ACE inhibitors, would not provide enough benefit for Evelyn.

Although Evelyn would not be a candidate for transplantation given her advanced age and poor overall function, there are no specific age limitations placed on potential transplant recipients. The poorer survival of heart transplant recipients over 65 is one factor that is considered when making decisions about allocation of such a scarce resource. The demand for donor organs has increased steadily; currently, the ratio of available donor hearts to potential recipients is approximately 1 to 10.

There is probably no palliative advantage to an ICU admission. It is doubtful that Evelyn would achieve any additional symptomatic improvement if she received inotropic agents. In fact, invasive treatments, noisy monitoring devices, frequent monitoring, and the overall environment of the ICU might reduce her comfort level. Likewise, it is not possible to determine the extent to which her life would be prolonged by ICU treatment. If her life were prolonged during the hospital stay, she would be at high risk of nosocomial pneumonia, catheter-related sepsis, or other iatrogenic infections. Increasingly, nosocomial, hospital-acquired infections are caused by organisms with a high degree of resistance to broad-spectrum antibiotics, further complicating the clinical situation. In short, admission to an ICU for the purposes of sophisticated treatment would be very unlikely to provide any sort of clinical benefit.

3. What would be the value of a drum catheter or chemical pleurodesis?

A procedure to prevent fluid accumulation might produce some temporary and partial palliation but would be of no long-term benefit in the face of this incurable illness. If the added comfort were sufficient to outweigh the risks and discomfort, these interventions might be justified as part of a palliative care plan. In this situation, however, the procedures could possibly lead to discomfort that outweighed any prolonged benefit. In the case of pleurodesis, some discomfort might be expected, and there is the danger of further respiratory compromise; continuous or repeated removal of transudative fluid that is dependent on hemodynamic factors generally is unsuccessful if the underlying cause is not corrected and may lead to further hemodynamic compromise.

If the goal is to maximize the patient's comfort with a minimum of risk, the most logical approach is probably to use standard pharmacologic management of the heart failure and to give oxygen by nasal cannula or face mask. Adjunctive treatment with morphine might be helpful not only in terms of the heart failure but because it might reduce dyspnea. The use of morphine and other sedatives in palliative treatment of incurable illness is discussed in Case 2 ("Determining if a Patient Has Decisional Capacity") and Case 3 ("Urgent Surgery in a Stuporous Patient").

4. What would be the rationale for performing an arterial blood gas (ABG)?

The obvious rationale is to determine the need for intubation. Because of this patient's poor cardiac output, pulse oximetry cannot reliably assess this need. Although arterial blood drawing is painful and not without risk, it can be performed swiftly and safely when done by an experienced person, and the risks are minor compared to the benefit that Evelyn might derive from the availability of accurate diagnostic information.

If the ABG result demonstrated respiratory failure, the next logical step would indeed be endotracheal intubation, and repeated ABGs or an intra-arterial line would be required to assess the patient's ongoing status. One cannot say with absolute certainty that such a patient could never be weaned from a respirator, but it is certain in this case that ventilatory support would not address her underlying disease, heart failure. Thus, even a simple blood gas, if viewed purely from a medical point of view, might inexorably lead to a succession of uncomfortable, and not clearly beneficial, treatments.

Another rationale for performing an ABG is that it could supply important information about the patient's prognosis. Such information might better define how to proceed, assuming that there was agreement over the goals of care. Because there is disagreement in this case, the physician might be reluctant to do the test because he knows a poor ABG result might further fuel the family's demands. The test result cannot be read in isolation; it is but one of many factors used to determine what, if any, additional measures should be initiated on behalf of the patient. What needs to be defined in a frank and open dialogue with the patient's family are the goals of treatment intervention at this point in the patient's disease process. This would clarify for them what "everything that can be done" actually means in the context of this type of illness—which interventions, if any, provide relief of symptoms or restoration of function, and which, instead, merely prolong her dying, and may in fact cause discomfort in the process.

ETHICAL AND LEGAL CONSIDERATIONS

1. How should discussions proceed with this family?

At this point in the decision process, it is clear that a frank and comprehensive discussion with the patient's family needs to be held. A family meeting with the key involved family members, as well as with critical members of the health care team, would be essential to convene at this point. In some hospitals, ethics consultation or mediation resources might be available to assist with such a meeting, particularly if prior attempts to work with the family have been unsuccessful (see Case 11, "A Teenager with Prolonged Unconsciousness").

The involved physicians should explain to this family objectively and in understandable language the patient's current clinical status, her short- and long-term prognosis, and the options available to address her symptoms, as well as the benefits, risks, and burdens of these options. If the physicians are recommending specific options, it would be important for them to explain why they are recommending them, for example, that clinical experience has shown that patients in Evelyn's condition generally survive for only a few days or weeks. Finally, it would be important to clarify the motivation behind the family's demands that "everything be done." Do they place heavy emphasis on the sanctity of life, based on religious or other personal beliefs, that will lead them to continue making treatment requests, regardless of the costs to the patient? Do they feel that Evelyn would wish to remain alive until an important family milestone is reached, such as a wedding or birth? Have they been given inadequate or inaccurate information from another member of the team about Evelyn's condition? Are their expectations simply unrealistic? Are they responding to their own psychological or emotional needs, which may be obscuring both the reality of the situation and, more importantly, the best interests of the patient?

At the moment, this family finds itself in a position that appears, on the surface, to give them control over whether their relative lives or dies. It must be made clear to them that although they may see a cause and effect relationship between their decisions and what happens to Evelyn, she is in fact dying no matter what treatment is rendered. The role of this family is not to prevent Evelyn from dying (something beyond their control) but rather to help determine Evelyn's interests in the process of dying and to illuminate as best as possible what Evelyn would want for herself, given her fatal condition (see Case 4, "Management of Life-Threatening Illness"). If Evelyn's value system included comfort in the face of incurable illness rather than exhaustive efforts at life prolongation, it would be important for the family to acknowledge this. The family, in fact, might find it more comfortable to acknowledge Evelyn's fate and accept a more palliative approach to care at this point if they were able to conclude that the patient herself would prefer this.

It is essential to make certain that the family comprehends the broad picture for this patient. While there are specific interventions that may demand their informed consent or refusal, isolated discussions of discrete medical interventions will present a fragmented picture. These different options should be placed in a larger context for the family: How does each intervention being discussed fit into the total picture of what can reasonably be expected for Evelyn? Such a discussion is a fact-based one, with the goal of ensuring that their understanding of Evelyn's condition and their expectations are in line with the reality of the patient's situation. It is also important that the family be given a consistent message from all providers in language they understood and with a communication process that acknowledges their own emotional needs as Evelyn's fate becomes more clear. Sometimes the communication context in hospital settings, with its attendant time pressures and numerous caregivers, can create challenges for families who earnestly want to arrive at the best decision for their loved one.

All critical members of Evelyn's family should be part of this communication process. If it is impractical to involve everyone in the discussions, then the family should designate one or two key individuals to receive information and convey it to the others. Although the grandson appears to have an authoritative voice for this family, it should not be assumed that because he is a physician he automatically understands the patient's condition and prognosis. The fact that his specialty lies in a different area of practice does not make him *less* likely to understand, but, like any other family member with an emotional stake in a relative's health, he may be unable to objectively view the circumstances. If a factual understanding can be achieved between the clinicians and the family, attempts should then be made to define the overall goals of care for this patient. If the source of the impasse is a fundamental and unremitting disagreement as to *how* to proceed, it should at least not be based on any factual misunderstanding or miscommunication concerning the patient's condition.

At this point, the nature of the discussion will shift to a more subjective evaluation of what *meaning* should be ascribed to the facts of Evelyn's situation. The physicians will need to honestly probe what is motivating their own recommendations in this case. Are they recommending a course of treatment based only on what is medically achievable (an objective perspective), or is their recommendation also influenced by the value that they place on this patient's circumstance (a subjective perspective)? Do these physicians believe that the treatment requested by the family is futile? If so, they must carefully consider what meaning they ascribe to this term and whether it is universally shared. They must also consider what, if any, policies exist within the hospital regarding the issue of medical futility (see Case 12). It is likely that these physicians believe that the quality of Evelyn's life, and the pain and suffering she may be experiencing, are more important to consider than her life's exact duration, but they may understand the nature of the dilemma better if they acknowledge the role of such values and that the family's value system and perhaps the patient's may be different from their own.

Likewise, it is important for the family members to probe their own motivation; this may lead them to reconsider what the *patient* would have wanted, or what would serve *her* interests, rather than their own emotional concerns. While it does not appear that the patient had a written advance directive, it is possible that among family members or with caregivers or other residents of the nursing home, Evelyn, prior to her loss of capacity, may have voiced preferences regarding her end of life care. The family's requests, ultimately, may not only be in conflict with the patient's own values, but could also bring harm to her. Involved clinicians should try to help family members balance the benefits to be achieved for Evelyn from various treatment options versus the burdens she would experience as a result.

2. Are the physicians obligated to follow the demands of this family?

It is unclear whether the family's demands are based on their own wishes or an understanding of what the patient would have wanted in this situation. Although they admit that she herself never explicitly spoke to this issue, it is possible that they are interpreting what her wishes *would* have been. As discussed in earlier cases, when a patient's surrogate attempts to assert the patient's right to *refuse* care (a negative right), this usually deserves respect. The question remains, whether there is an equally valid right to *obtain* treatment (a positive right), worthy of the same response from providers.

Assuming that the facts of the case are clarified and well understood by all, Evelyn's physicians are under no obligation to accede to either patient or family demands for treatment that is useless in the context of the patient's illness.[3] Physicians cannot be forced to provide treatment they believe is outside of the accepted standard of care under the circumstances. Such a determination, however, should derive from the physician's medical expertise, not from his or her personal value system. Evelyn's physicians appear to be following the standard of care for a patient with heart failure; this consists of correction of treatable causes and palliation of symptoms, as, short of heart transplant, there is no cure for this patient's condition. It might be argued that there is an evolving, if not already established, standard that interventions that can neither restore function nor provide palliation should not be offered.[4] If the interventions demanded by this family do not conform to this standard, then there is no obligation to accede to their specific demands.

The problem in such cases, however, is that there may be a disagreement not over medical facts but over *values,* and whose values should have authority—the patient (or surrogate) or the physician. This clash of values, more than disagreement over facts, was the basis for a major court suit brought by physicians in Minnesota *(In re Wanglie).* Physicians and the hospital challenged the authority of family members to insist on aggressive measures for Helga Wanglie, an 87-year-old woman in a persistent vegetative state, who also had lung disease and could not be weaned from a respirator. It was clear that she would never regain physical or cognitive function, but her husband and adult children insisted that aggressive measures be continued despite numerous discussions with the physicians, who had explained the realities of the patient's medical condition. It was unclear whether the family's demands represented their knowledge of the patient's wishes or rather their own interpretation of what the interests of the patient were.[5] Nonetheless, the impasse led to the unprecedented situation in which the providers, not the family or patient, initiated litigation to stop treatment.

The focus of the providers' case was twofold: First, they wished to have the family removed as the decision makers for the patient, arguing that the family was unable to make decisions in Mrs. Wanglie's best interests. Second, once a new surrogate decision maker was appointed, they wished the court to clarify what their obligations to the patient were— whether or not they were obliged to continue treatment that was not technically futile in the strictest interpretation of the word but which the physicians nonetheless adjudged to be of no benefit to the patient.

Only the first aspect of the case was considered by the court. The court ruled that there was no reason to remove the family as decision makers for the patient. The *implication* was that the providers were obligated to follow the wishes of the family, although this was never explicitly addressed by the court. Ironically, three days after this litigation ended, Mrs. Wanglie died, despite continued aggressive interventions.

From a legal perspective, the *Wanglie* decision has little formal influence or precedential value, because it was a trial-level, state court decision that was not appealed. No other court is legally bound to follow it. The *Wanglie* case did, however, bring an important issue to light, and, as in Evelyn's case, represents a murky and evolving area in law. Physicians always have the option of transferring care of a patient whose family demands are not in accord with their own view of good medical practice, but in difficult cases, it is often impossible to find a physician or facility to accept the patient. The inability of the providers in the *Wanglie* case to transfer her care illustrates this dilemma. Although one cannot be forced to practice against one's conscience, one also cannot walk away from a patient with medical needs.

What if the physician's in Evelyn's case, or in the *Wanglie* case, chose to act on their own opinions of the patient's best interests and bypassed the involvement of family members? Such unilateral decisions by physicians or health care institutions might reflect an application of their personal perspectives of an acceptable quality of life rather than their professional opinions based on medical expertise. This could lead down a slippery slope and ultimately to situations in which potentially treatable patients were allowed to die. Given the tremendous authority that physicians have over medical resources, it would be dangerous, in this argument, if the subjective, value-based decisions by physicians were allowed to determine unilaterally how resources are allocated. A counterargument might be that a physician is a moral agent who has rights, including the right to avoid participating in treatment that violates his or her professional integrity. As in the *Wanglie* case, the physicians caring for Evelyn have the right to attempt to transfer the care of the patient, but in a truly difficult situation they might well have difficulty in finding a physician who would accept her. Moreover, if the physicians felt that Evelyn's family was acting against her best interests, it would perhaps be more important to avoid transferring her care and instead to continue to advocate for what they believed was in her medical best interests.

Another consideration in a case such as Evelyn's is the use of expensive resources, including access to an intensive care bed, given her debilitated condition and poor prognosis. Most intensive care units have admissions criteria that consider prognosis and current clinical status to determine whether ICU admission would be appropriate for the particular patient. Broader considerations of the use of technologically sophisticated and expensive resources for a patient of Evelyn's age and poor health condition are discussed in the references.[6]

REFERENCES

1. J.B. Croft et al., "A Poor Prognosis for an Emerging Epidemic in the Medicare Population," *Archives of Internal Medicine* 159 (1999): 505–510.

2. B. Stuart et al. *Medical Guidelines for Determining Prognosis in Selected Noncancer Diseases*, 2nd ed. (Washington, DC: National Hospice Organization, 1996), 6–9.

3. A.S. Brett and L.B. McCullough, "When Patients Request Specific Interventions," *New England Journal of Medicine* 315 (1986): 1347–1351.

4. S.H. Miles, "Medical Futility," *The Journal of Law, Medicine and Health Care* 20 (1992): 310–315.

5. S.H. Miles, "Informed Demand for 'Non-Beneficial' Medical Treatment," *New England Journal of Medicine* 325 (1991): 512–515.

6. Callahan, D. *Setting Limits. Medical Goals in an Aging Society* (New York: Simon & Schuster, 1987).

SUGGESTED READINGS

Alpers, A., and Lo, B. 1992. Futility: Not just a medical issue. *The Journal of Law, Medicine and Health Care* 20: 327–329.

Angell, M. 1991. The case of Helga Wanglie: A new kind of "right to die" case. *New England Journal of Medicine* 325: 511–512.

Cantor, N.L. 1996. Can healthcare providers obtain judicial intervention against surrogates who demand "medically inappropriate" life support for incompetent patients? *Critical Care Medicine* 24: 883–887.

Council on Ethical and Judicial Affairs, American Medical Association. 1999. Medical futility in end-of-life care. Report of the Council on Ethical and Judicial Affairs. *Journal of the American Medical Association* 281: 938–941.

Cranford, R., and Gostin, L. 1992. Futility: A concept in search of a definition. *The Journal of Law, Medicine and Health Care* 20: 307–309.

Criteria Committee of the American Heart Association, New York City Affiliate. 1994. Classification of functional capacity and objective assessment of patients with diseases of the heart. Nomenclature and criteria for diagnosis of diseases of the heart and great vessels. 9th ed. Boston: Little, Brown and Co.

Daniels, N. 1989. *Just health care*. New York: Cambridge Univesity Press.

Glance, L.G. et al. 1998. Intensive care unit prognostic scoring systems to predict death: A cost-effectiveness analysis. *Critical Care Medicine* 26: 1842–1849.

Hunt, SA. 1998. Current status of cardiac transplantation. *Journal of the American Medical Association* 280: 1692–1698.

Jecker, N.S., and Schneiderman, L.J. 1995. When families request that "everything possible" be done. *Journal of Medicine and Philosophy* 20: 145–163.

Knaus, W.A. et al. 1992. The APACHE III prognostic risk system. Risk prediction of hospital mortality for critically ill hospitalized adults. *Chest* 100: 1619–1636.

Levine, C., and Zuckerman, C. 1999. The trouble with families: Toward an ethic of accommodation. *Annals of Internal Medicine* 130: 148–152.

Neijer, C. et al. 1998. Bioethics for clinicians: 16. Dealing with demands for inappropriate treatment. *Canadian Medical Association Journal* 159: 817–821.

Swigart, V. et al. 1996. Letting go: Family willingness to forgo life support. *Heart and Lung* 25: 483–494.

Schneiderman, L.J. et al. 1996. Medical futility: Response to critiques. *Annals of Internal Medicine* 125: 669–674.

LEGAL CITATIONS

Case Examples

In re Wanglie, No. PX-91-283 (4th Dist. Ct., Hennepin City, Minn., July 1, 1991).
Hospital sought court permission to withdraw ventilator support from an 87-year-old woman in a vegetative state, believing that the support was futile under the circumstances. Her husband did not want the respirator withdrawn, and the court held that the husband was the appropriate surrogate decision maker for the patient. The patient died three days after the court decision.

Gilgunn v. Massachusetts General Hospital, Mass. Super. Ct., No. 92-4820, Verdict 21 (1995).
Relatives of a patient unsuccessfully sought damages against a hospital for the hospital's decision to refuse to accede to the relative's demand that resuscitation measures be applied to the patient.

CASE 22

A Man with Alcoholic Cirrhosis Wants a Liver Transplant

Larry is a 40-year-old advertising executive who has used alcohol heavily for 20 years. He has recently had several hospitalizations for complications of cirrhosis, believed to be due to chronic alcoholism. He now has ascites, esophageal varices, and is recovering from hepatic encephalopathy.

Following his most recent hospitalization he resolved to quit drinking and has not drunk alcohol for two months since discharge. He has been followed by an outpatient alcohol rehabilitation program and is said to be doing well. This contrasts with frequent recidivism prior to his serious illness, when, he says, "I never took it as seriously as I do now." Larry began regular use of alcohol in his teens. In recent years, he has drunk at least one pint of vodka every day and began to have frequent absences from his work, until his illness forced him to leave his job.

Larry's older brother is a physician with many connections in the medical community. He feels that Larry would be a good candidate for a liver transplant and has spoken to some of his colleagues, who have put him in touch with a local transplant center but have advised him to list his brother in two other states where the supply of donor livers is greater relative to potential recipients.

Except for alcohol-related illness, Larry has never been hospitalized. He has hypertension but was previously noncompliant with his medication regimen.

ISSUES TO CONSIDER

- Allocation of scarce resources
- Organ donation

MEDICAL CONSIDERATIONS

1. What is Larry's prognosis if he has a liver transplant, assuming he does not drink alcohol again?

Overall three-year survival rate among liver transplant recipients is approximately 71 percent (graft survival 62 percent), with the greatest patient death and graft failure rate occurring within the first year.[1] One-year patient survival rate of liver transplant recipients is approximately 85 percent, compared to 80 percent one-year survival of nonrecipients with hepatic cirrhosis and with ascites, encephalopathy, or other serious complications. Median survival of such patients, however, is less than two years with no transplant.

2. How does Larry's history of alcohol consumption affect his prognosis?

There is evidence that the prognosis is similar to that of nonalcoholic recipients of liver transplant.[2] Patients with acute hepatic necrosis, cholestatic disease, or biliary cirrhosis have a lower risk of long-term graft failure, but malignant neoplasms confer a six times greater risk compared to cirrhosis, and direct comparisons with such a disease magnify the difference.

Cirrhotic patients with a history of chronic alcohol use not infrequently suffer from coexisting liver disease, such as chronic hepatitis, or may suffer from other illnesses that produce liver failure. In one series, the histology in 20 percent of explanted livers demonstrated that non–alcohol-related liver disease was the actual underlying illnesses leading to transplant.[3] Alcohol use does not seem to increase the risk of noncompliance with immunosuppressive medications.

Probably only a minority resume pathologically severe drinking leading to acute illness that can be directly attributed to alcohol use. Likewise, serial biopsies generally do not show changes typical of alcohol toxicity. Alcohol toxicity is possible, however, and it is important to consider that resumption of alcohol use can lead to extrahepatic alcohol-related illness as well as liver disease.

3. What is the likelihood that someone with Larry's alcohol history will stop drinking?

Liver transplantation for patients with alcohol-related liver failure is controversial. Data from studies on liver transplant patients show that approximately 30 percent resume some degree of alcohol use within three years following transplant.[3] These data may be skewed, however, by reluctance to refer patients perceived by physicians as high risk for recidivism, and preferential listing of patients scoring well on these predictive scales. As many as 95 percent may return to alcohol use when followed on the long term, using sensitive interview methods of detection.[4]

Despite these statistics, it is not possible to predict on an individual basis, and in the alcohol abusing population in general, restoration of a controlled pattern of drinking is believed to be rare.

4. Given the uncertainties of long-term harm to a liver graft, is Larry a candidate for a liver transplant?

Approximately 19 percent of liver transplants are performed in the United States in patients believed to suffer from alcohol-related liver disease.[5] Although alcohol as an etiology is not considered a contraindication, someone who has abstained from alcohol consumption for only two months is unlikely to be placed on a waiting list for a transplant. Satisfaction of criteria and placement on a waiting list imply that the center would be willing to perform the transplant immediately; it does not mean the patient can be on the list merely to acquire a graft at some unspecified time in the future if the need arose. Most liver transplant programs currently require six months of abstinence, although there are exceptions to a fixed requirement. Likewise, most programs require a favorable assessment by a substance abuse professional. The higher cost of treating a liver transplant recipient whose underlying cause of liver failure was alcohol related could lead individual centers to reevaluate their criteria.[6]

Six months of abstinence is desirable from a medical point of view (as well as a resource allocation standpoint) because of the possibility that a patient could recover from the acute toxic effects of alcohol (alcoholic hepatitis), eliminating the need for transplant. Larry's recurrent decompensations were very likely related to the acute effects of alcohol superimposed on chronic cirrhosis.

Specific medical criteria for listing have been developed,[2] but these criteria are rarely fixed because there may be extenuating circumstances that would be deemed important by the local transplant program's selection committee. Listing criteria relevant to other organs have been promulgated by the United Network for Organ Sharing (UNOS), Richmond, Virginia.[5]

ETHICAL AND LEGAL CONSIDERATIONS

1. Should Larry's history of alcoholism influence or affect his ability to obtain a new donor liver?

Donor organs suitable for transplantation are one of the few truly *scarce* resources in our current health care delivery system. As transplant techniques and pharmacological interventions have improved the success rates of organ transplantation, and as the range of potential donor organ recipients has expanded, demand for such organs now vastly exceeds supply, creating a situation of true rationing among those in need of an organ transplant to survive. Recent statistics paint a stark portrait of this dire situation: As of January 1999, more than 64,000 patients were listed on organ donation waiting lists for such organs as hearts, kidneys, livers, and lungs. The most recent data on the number of organs donated per year show that in 1997, a little more than 9,000 organs were recovered for donation. Each year, more than 4,000 individuals listed on waiting lists die before they have the opportunity to receive a donor organ. Thousands more never even become eligible to be listed on waiting lists owing to a variety of reasons, including their inability to meet medical criteria, their lack of insurance to pay for this expensive technology, or their lack of a social support structure to permit them to undergo the rigorous regimen often necessary to support the new organ and ward off rejection following the surgery. It is thus clear that donor organs are a vital and scarce resource, requiring proper stewardship of their collection and distribution.

The current collection of donor organs is completely reliant on the voluntary and altruistic motives of donors and their families. Respecting the individual autonomy of patients and their loved ones to determine whether or not to donate viable organs, the current system of organ collection is a fragile one whose integrity is critical for maintaining and nurturing continued organ contributions. If patients or their families should perceive gross inequities in the system, or should they lose their faith or trust in the motives of those who seek their organs for donation, the system could collapse, with devastating consequences for the thousands of patients whose survival necessitates new donor organs. Sharp debate has surfaced concerning strategies designed to increase organ donation and to distribute those organs in a fair and equitable manner. Thus, concerns have arisen as to whether patients in need of new livers as a result of chronic alcoholism should be singled out for special consideration of their status as potential organ recipients: that is, should the fact of a causal relationship between their alcoholism and their need for a new liver be factored into their eligibility? Should they be held accountable or in some way blameworthy, and perhaps therefore not be entitled to receive such a scarce and expensive resource? Will the public lose faith in an organ allocation system that provides new organs to patients whose own actions contributed to their deteriorated and life-threatening conditions? Is it fair to single out such patients for special scrutiny?

There are many ethical arguments both to support and reject special consideration of alcoholics as potential organ recipients. Given the truly scarce nature of available transplantable livers, many have argued that it is justifiable to consider how the actions of the patients contributed to their dire medical condition. Since we simply cannot meet the demand of all potential liver recipients, a system of rationing must be put in place, and many believe it ethically justifiable to consider the patient's own actions in such situations. This argument is particularly advanced as there are demonstrated methods to assist alcoholic patients in efforts to combat their illness, well before it leads to the irreversible destruction of their livers. In this line of reasoning, their inability to seek out and accept help to combat their alcoholism should not then be rewarded by making available a new donor liver. Moreover, given the concern for recidivism even in patients who pledge abstinence in order to receive a new liver, many argue that the scarcity of the resource justifies this heightened scrutiny and even rejection of their candidacy for a new donor organ. Finally, there is concern that families will find it unacceptable to donate the organs of their loved ones if they were implanted into patients whose own actions led to their demise (although there is no evidence to support that notion to date).

Taking into consideration patients' blameworthiness for access to effective treatment for their conditions raises highly provocative questions. Our tradition of medical care has not been to place blame with attendant consequences for a patient's health condition as a way to manage access to health care. For example, patients whose diabetes is out of control because of excess weight or whose lung cancer is thought to be the result of years of heavy smoking have not been denied treatment despite the connection between their poor health habits and resulting illness. A standard of the "virtuous" patient as a measure of entitlement to care has never been incorporated into our system of delivery. Moreover, it is debatable whether a history of alcoholism and resulting liver disease is totally the result of a failure of will on the patient's part. There is evidence to suggest that both genetic and environmental factors may contribute to alcoholism and that lack of treatment may stem from factors well beyond a lack of will, including such concerns as lack of access to care because of health insurance problems or other socioeconomic factors that cause treatment delays or denials for a range of conditions.

While the scarcity of the resource does demand stringent, objective criteria to ascertain appropriate allocation of donor organs, most commentators believe it is not justifiable to categorically deny access to the list merely because of one's prior history of alcoholism. While medical criteria are not uniformly standardized across transplant programs, such programs usually consider factors such as medical condition and prognosis, likelihood of benefit from the transplant, and ability to sustain posttransplant regimens necessary to ward off organ rejection. Undoubtedly, such factors are not completely objective and more subjective factors inevitably influence access as well, but categorical denial of consideration based on alcoholism status does not appear warranted. For example, some programs have developed abstinence criteria and recidivism data to help determine the potential eligibility of such candidates. Many programs incorporate psychiatric consultation and evaluation to help determine the patient's and family's ability to adhere to the strict demands of the transplant protocols. Such adherence is vital to the long-term success of the procedure.

Given that patients with end-stage liver disease have no alternative for long-term survival if organ transplant is not available, and given that data have now been accumulated to suggest liver transplant success with patients who have a history of alcoholism, equity would seem to demand that such patients be considered potential candidates along with other patients. This is not to say that their history of alcoholism cannot be factored into the larger picture of their transplant candidacy, but merely that it should not categorically disqualify them from consideration. For a patient such as Larry, his ability to sustain his abstinence and to adhere to posttransplant protocols would heavily influence his eligibility for a donor organ. If those criteria were satisfied, there would be no justification to deny him access to the waiting list if all other medical criteria were met.

2. Why has Larry been advised to register on out-of-state lists?

Given the continuous scarcity of available donor organs, the current waiting list system for allocating organs is highly sensitive and has been the focus of much debate over the last several years. The need to ration organs has necessitated ongoing reexamination of the fairness and ethical justification for the current allocation systems.

The current system of organ allocation has its roots in the Uniform Anatomical Gift Act of 1968, which was premised on the notion that patients have the autonomy and freedom to determine and make known in advance whether they wish their organs to be donated upon their deaths. Creation of this legal framework was intended to stimulate and encourage organ donation given medical advances. All states adopted legislation similar to this Act, and it became routine for individuals to make known their desire to donate organs through the drivers' license systems in each state.

In 1984, the federal National Organ Transplant Act was passed both to ban the sale of donor organs and to create the infrastructure for a national, not-for-profit organ retrieval and allocation system. The United Network for Organ Sharing (UNOS)[5] became the entity responsible for this national system, and a series of regional collection and distribution areas were created to facilitate this process. Two years later, in 1986, additional federal legislation put into place the current "required request" system, whereby hospitals participating in Medicare and Medicaid were required to develop policies to identify potential organ donors in order to ensure that families were made aware of the option to donate their loved one's organs. Virtually all states passed their own legislation in support of this required request system.

Over the years, despite the fact that many potential organ donor candidates still remain unidentified, and despite the fact that in a significant percentage of cases families are still reluctant or unwilling to donate organs, this system has led to some improvements in organ retrieval, particularly as the eligibility of potential donors has broadened to include older donors.

Nonetheless, shortages of available organs are still acute, and dramatic variations occur from one region to another. This is due to many factors, some of which may be amenable to change. The current UNOS allocation system is heavily focused on a local and regional strategy, whereby attempts are made to distribute organs locally, or if necessary regionally. Allocation beyond the region is only available if no eligible recipients can be identified in the local region. Because of various eligibility criteria and donation patterns, this means that waiting list lengths and waiting times can vary dramatically from one region of the country to another. In one region a patient might have to wait hundreds of days, risking continued deterioration as a result, while in another region a patient with the same profile may wait less than a hundred days. These vast differences have led to sharp inequities in certain cases. For example, money has a significant influence on which lists, and how many lists, patients register for. In order to be listed on a waiting list, patients must to be able to demonstrate their ability to pay for the procedure. Some potential candidates have no insurance or have insurance that will not cover the costs of the transplant, and thus may not gain access to any waiting lists, despite medical need. For other patients, insurance will only pay for the procedure in their own regions. For patients with significant personal financial resources, who do not need to rely on insurance to cover the costs of the transplant, they can then gain access to lists outside of their region, even to the point of targeting those regions with the shortest wait. Thus, while personal resources have no role in the system of *retrieving* organs, they do play a role in who actually *receives* the donor organs.

Some patients have also been excluded from waiting lists not because of ability to pay or because of their medical condition per se, but because of other underlying conditions that appear to taint their eligibility from a "social worth" perspective. For example, recent debate centered around one program's denial of waiting list status to a patient whose medical history included Down syndrome. While this patient ultimately was listed and did receive a transplant, her situation spotlighted the still subjective and potentially discriminatory system that leads to waiting list referrals in the first place. Lack of access to primary care and inadequate or absent insurance coverage has meant that many minority and other vulnerable populations may be referred less frequently for transplant, or they may be referred at a point when their conditions are much more perilous, thus making the risks of waiting once on the waiting list that much more critical.

While some states have attempted to redress certain inequities by, for example, banning multiple registrations, these have not been effective in eliminating many serious criticisms of the current system. In recent years the federal government has tried to mandate a system that would be more equitable and that would look to provide organs to those most in need, regardless of their geographic location. This mandate has met with significant resistance at the state level, particularly as many small transplant programs believe a national distribution system might put them out of business. Some states have begun to pass legislation that bans the distribution of organs received from state residents outside of the state. There are additional concerns that the current voluntary donor system might be damaged if donor families grew concerned that organs were being given to unknown recipients well outside their community. This is of particular concern as it has been difficult to stimulate donations from minority communities. For minority populations, there is particular sensitivity to making donations when they may not have equal access as recipients for transplant organs.

Thus, given Larry's resources and connections in the medical community, he may be personally able to improve his chances for an organ through his multiple registrations. Yet this ability precisely illustrates many of the inequities of the current organ allocation system.

REFERENCES

1. H.M. Lin et al., "Center-Specific Graft and Patient Survival Rates. 1997 United Network for Organ Sharing (UNOS) Report," *Journal of the American Medical Association* 280 (1998): 1153–1160.
2. M.R. Lucey et al., "Minimal Criteria for Placement of Adults on the Liver Transplant Waiting List: A Report of a National Conference Organized by the American Society of Transplant Physicians and the American Association for the Study of Liver Diseases," *Liver Transplant Surgery* 3 (1997): 628–637.
3. M.R. Lucey et al., "Alcohol Use after Liver Transplantation in Alcoholics: A Clinical Cohort Follow-Up Study," *Hepatology* 25 (1997): 1223–1227.
4. L. Howard et al., "Psychiatric Outcome in Alcoholic Liver Transplant Patients," *Quarterly Journal of Medicine* 87 (1994): 731–736.
5. United Network for Organ Sharing (UNOS), Richmond, VA (see Appendix A).
6. J. Showstack et al., "Resource Utilization in Liver Transplantation," *Journal of the American Medical Association* 281 (1999): 1381–1386.

SUGGESTED READINGS

Alexander, G.C., and Sehgal, A.R. 1998. Barriers to cadaveric renal transplantation among blacks, women, and the poor. *Journal of the American Medical Association* 280: 1148–1152.

Anonymous. 1998. Organ donors increased substantially during 1998. *New York Times,* 18 April, 30.

Cohen, C., Benjamin, M., and the Ethics and Social Impact Committee of the Transplant and Health Policy Center Ann Arbor, Michigan. 1991. Alcoholics and liver transplantation. *Journal of the American Medical Association* 265: 1299–1301.

Council on Ethical and Judicial Affairs, American Medical Association. 1995. Ethical considerations in the allocation of organs and other scarce medical resources among patients. *Archives of Internal Medicine* 155: 29–40.

Eckhoff, D.E. et al. 1998. Race: a critical factor in organ donation, patient referral and selection, and orthotopic liver transplantation? *Liver Transplant Surgery* 4: 499–505.

Glannon, W. 1998. Responsibility, alcoholism, and liver transplantation. *Journal of Medicine and Philosophy* 23: 31–49.

Hung-Mo, L. et al. 1998. Center-specific graft and patient survival rates. 1997 United Network for Organ Sharing (UNOS) report. *Journal of the American Medical Association* 280: 1153–1160.

Klapheke, M.M. 1999.The role of the psychiatrist in organ transplantation. *Bulletin of the Menninger Clinic* 63, no. 1: 13–39.

Moss, A.H., and Singer, M. 1991. Should alcoholics compete equally for liver transplantation? *Journal of the American Medical Association* 265: 1296–1298.

Quaid, K.A. et al. 1996. Issues in genetic testing for susceptibility to alcoholism: Lessons from Alzheimer's disease and Huntington's disease. *Alcoholism: Clinical and Experimental Research* 20: 1430–1437.

Schmidt, V.H. 1998. Selection of recipients for donor organs in transplant medicine. *Journal of Medicine and Philosophy,* February: 50–74.

Stolberg, G.G. 1999. Fight over organs shift to states from Washington. *New York Times,* 11 March, 1(A).

White, A.J. et al. 1998. The effects of New York state's ban on multiple listing for cadaveric kidney transplantation. *Health Services Research* 33: 205–222.

Zetterman, R.K. et al. 1998. Age and liver transplantation: a report of the liver transplantation database. *Transplantation* 66: 500–506.

LEGAL CITATION

Statutory Example

National Organ Transplant Act (1984).
Federal legislation outlawing the sale of donor organs and facilitating the development of a nationwide organ retrieval and allocation system.

CASE 23

Genetic Testing in a Woman with a Family History of Breast Cancer

Rachel, a 40-year-old woman, is concerned because there is a history of breast cancer in her family and she heard at her synagogue that genetic testing for breast cancer is now available and would like to pursue this option. The doctor tells her that genetic testing is only available at the University Medical Center, which is located 100 miles away.

The patient's mother died of breast cancer at the age of 55, and her older sister recently developed breast cancer at the age of 48. Her 38-year-old sister is healthy, as are her 18-year-old daughter and 16-year-old son. Her maternal grandmother died in Poland during the war, and there are no other close female relatives.

ISSUES TO CONSIDER

- Testing for genetic illness in adults
- Genetic counseling
- Disclosure of genetic test results to third parties
- Susceptibility versus disease genes

MEDICAL CONSIDERATIONS

1. What information will genetic testing for breast cancer provide that will help Rachel make health care decisions?

BRCA1 and *BRCA2* are germ-line susceptibility genes that confer an elevated risk of breast cancer, as well as ovarian, colon, and prostate cancer. Enhanced risk exists in individuals who carry additional, though less common alleles, and other genes may contribute to risk by other mechanisms.

Although approximately 5 to 10 percent of breast cancer cases are hereditary, and although about two-thirds of familial breast cancers are due to these genes, the positive and negative predictive value of testing for these genes is not precisely known. For example, the prevalence of *BRCA1* in groups of patients who have breast cancer ranges widely, depending on racial or ethnic group and strength of family history of breast or ovarian cancer.

While a positive test would be cause for concern, particularly in the highest susceptibility groups, a negative test might confer a false sense of security. Methodology has not been perfected and many gene carriers may remain undetected by current methods. Other genes have been associated with breast cancer, especially in women with strong family histories, and other as yet unknown genes might confer similar or higher risks. Finally, nongenetic factors are believed to increase the risk of breast cancer.

The risk of ovarian cancer in gene carriers is also high, with cumulative risk greater than 26 percent by age 70, and possibly as high as 85 percent. Risk of prostate cancer is increased in male carriers, and colon cancer in both sexes, raising issues of importance for Rachel's son.

2. If Rachel is *BRCA*-positive what strategies exist to reduce her risk of developing cancer?

Regardless of whether or not Rachel is *BRCA*-positive, her strong family history of breast cancer in first-degree relatives confers an increased risk of breast cancer and possibly other cancers. Therefore, she should receive counseling about breast cancer prevention, take steps to diagnose it early, and prevent it if possible.

There are no separate strategies known to reduce the risk specifically in *BRCA* carriers, however, using standard (nongenetic) risk profiles, a recent multicenter, placebo-controlled trial has demonstrated that tamoxifen reduces but does not eliminate the likelihood of developing breast cancer in at-risk women, mostly white.[1] No separate studies have evaluated specific methods of risk reduction in women with *BRCA* genes. An added long-term benefit of tamoxifen might be a reduction in the risk of osteoporotic fractures, but potential problems are elevated risk of endometrial cancer, deep vein thrombosis, and pulmonary embolus.

Although the relative risk reduction for someone like Rachel might be no greater than 56 percent, Rachel would be a candidate for tamoxifen prevention. Current information is based on follow-up of five years, and it is likely that she would want to know about lifelong protection. Research is underway to determine if raloxifene, a newer selective estrogen receptor modulator, can reduce the risk of breast cancer.[2]

A more dramatic and costly preventive maneuver is prophylactic mastectomy, which has recently been shown to significantly reduce the likelihood of developing breast cancer in women with a family history.[3] In this retrospective study, the risk profile did not include assessment of genetic markers, and in one estimate, approximately 97 percent of that group of women undergoing prophylactic mastectomy probably would have survived without the surgery.[4] Breast cancer has developed in residual breast tissue in some women undergoing prophylactic mastectomy. The risk reduction in women who are *BRCA1*- or *BRCA2*-positive is not known as of this writing but estimates are that gains in life expectancy are possible among young women undergoing this procedure, but not among those 60 years of age or older. Regardless of her choice of treatment, Rachel should be counseled to have regular mammography, do regular self-examination, and visit her physician regularly.

Early detection of ovarian cancer is more difficult. Strategies include bimanual pelvic examination, transvaginal ultrasound, and measurement of tumor antigen CA-125. Unfortunately, the latter two methods are associated with a high false-positive rate, and physical examination with a high negative rate. The efficacy of prophylactic oophorectomy remains uncertain.[5] Colon cancer screening by regular sigmoidoscopy or colonoscopy is far more reliable, with early treatment conferring a nearly 100 percent cure rate.

3. What benefit would this information have for Rachel's son?

There is little or no data on which to base specific recommendations for prevention in male carriers (of any age) of *BRCA* mutations. Since the risk of prostate and colon cancer in *BRCA* mutation carriers appears to be higher than for the general population, such individuals should at least follow standard recommendations for cancer screening. Rachel's son should probably have screening with fecal occult blood and sigmoidoscopy, although it is uncertain at what age this should begin and how frequently it should be performed. Prostate and colon cancer in the general population begin to increase in incidence only in midlife.

Although the efficacy of colon cancer screening is well accepted, there is persistent controversy surrounding prostate cancer screening, since early treatment is not necessarily associated with reductions in morbidity or mortality. Continuing research has begun to classify subgroups of patients who would stand to benefit from early treatment based on age and histological type.[6] Further study would be needed to determine if male

BRCA carriers would be at risk earlier than age 50. These issues are discussed further in several selections in the Suggested Readings.

4. How might the clinical options differ for other genetic diseases, such as Huntington's disease, Alzheimer's disease, and others?

In contrast to Huntington's disease genetic mutations, *BRCA1* and *BRCA2* are susceptibility genes, which interact with other genetic and environmental factors in causing the disease; modifiable risk factors have been identified, and preventive strategies may exist. Huntington's disease, a progressive neurologic condition with usual age of onset between age 30 and 40, is caused by a disease gene, which is the sole factor determining the disease state. Recent evidence indicates that the genetics of Huntington's disease are far more complex than previously believed. The Huntington's disease gene exhibits "anticipation," in which the mutation expands with succeeding generations, so that older generations may not exhibit the disease until late life, if at all, but their children and grandchildren would have a greater likelihood of developing clinically apparent disease. Thus, the sensitivity and specificity of genetic testing have not been fully clarified. There appear to be no cofactors increasing susceptibility that could be avoided, and, more important, no specific treatments exist that could benefit a patient if the diagnosis were made in the preclinical stage.

Heritability of Alzheimer's disease is also complex. Alzheimer's disease is the most common cause of dementia and usually becomes clinically apparent in late life. A minority of cases are clearly familial, may have an earlier onset, and have been associated with disease genes. Late onset cases are associated with susceptibility genes, of which apolipoprotein E (APOE) has been studied as a possible candidate. The *APOE* epsilon 4 allele is more common among patients with Alzheimer's disease than among the general population, but is not present in at least 40 percent of cases and is common among individuals who do not develop the disease. Cofactors, including head trauma, have been identified, but much research is needed to better clarify sensitivity and specificity of genetic screening and risk conferred by other factors. Prospective trials of Alzheimer's disease prevention are in progress, including estrogen and antiinflammatory agents, but no reliable preventive maneuvers have yet been identified.

An increasing number of adult-onset diseases have been associated with disease and susceptibility genes and this is a field of active research.[7] Early developments have led to promotion of genetic testing that may be premature in terms of its application, and, given the rapidity of medical advances in this field, inappropriate recommendations are likely to occur with increasing frequency.

ETHICAL AND LEGAL CONSIDERATIONS

1. Given the uncertainties about the test and the test results, how should Rachel be counseled? What issues should she consider as she makes her decision?

Rachel's concern that she is at increased risk for breast cancer, given her family history and ethnic origins, appears well founded. After skin cancer, breast cancer is the most common cancer diagnosis in women, and a strong family history of breast cancer is the strongest risk factor for an individual patient being diagnosed with breast cancer. Therefore, her interest in possible genetic testing, in order to better understand her breast cancer risk, seems, at first glance, appropriate and supportable.

Testing for *BRCA* mutations, however, involves a complex set of risks and benefits for the patient being tested. In order for a patient such as Rachel to make an informed, autonomous decision as to whether or not testing is desirable, she should be aware of a range of psychological, social, familial, and economic considerations. Unlike other tests she may have had in the past, genetic testing for *BRCA* mutations will not provide definitive information regarding her health status, and it will leave her with a range of quandaries that may have significant implications not only for herself, but also for her children and other members of her family. Thus, a thorough informed consent process is essential before a patient consents to *BRCA* testing. Moreover, potential testing recipients must be provided with both pretest and posttest counseling by qualified medical geneticists or genetic counselors, who will be able to provide accurate, up-to-date information about the test, as well as support and guidance about test result implications, for both the patient and her family.

As with any informed consent process, Rachel must be provided with information concerning the purpose of the test, benefits from testing, its limitations, the health implications of test results (whether positive or negative), other potential risks that may accompany a positive test result, her alternatives to testing, and, given the nature of the information, what levels of confidentiality attach to the results. There may also be financial implications for this test, including the real possibility that her insurance may not pay for the costs of the test. Rachel may decide that the benefits of testing outweigh the risks for her, but before making this choice she should be fully cognizant of what she will learn from the test and how that information might help or harm her.

Regarding the benefits of testing, Rachel will need to understand that the test results will give her a better sense of her *risk* for being diagnosed with breast or ovarian cancer, though this information is of a probabilistic, rather than deterministic, nature. A negative test result will not mean that she could never get breast cancer, only that she does not have certain genetic mutations associated with increased risk of breast cancer. Positive test results will confirm her suspicions that her family history leaves her at increased risk of breast or ovarian cancer, and she will then need to understand her options regarding proactive monitoring or even prophylactic interventions to lessen her chances of actually being diagnosed with these diseases. By becoming more aware of her risk for breast cancer, enhancing her monitoring activities, or even employing prophylactic intervention measures, Rachel may ultimately save her life. Despite diagnostic advances, for many women, breast cancer is not diagnosed until it has already reached an advanced stage. In fact, out of all specialties, the most common reason for malpractice litigation is delayed breast cancer diagnosis.

While the test poses no physical risk, the informational risks of the test are substantial. First, there may be a significant psychological effect on Rachel if her test results are positive. For example, women have reported heightened anxiety following positive test results, as well as guilt of potentially passing on such mutations to their children. Experienced genetic counselors will probe such issues with patients prior to testing in order to ascertain whether they might suggest testing is not appropriate at this time or to give the patient the time and skills to consider how she might respond to a positive test result. How confidential the results will be may also have significant impact on Rachel's family relationships as well as on her eligibility for various types of insurance or other potential discriminatory acts, including problems in the workplace. Just how confidential the test results will be, and who may have access to these results, must be discussed with Rachel prior to any testing.

Much of this information will take time to carefully consider and integrate into her own personal values and life circumstances. Written materials to supplement a counseling session should be provided to Rachel. This decision to be tested may very well be one that she wishes to discuss and consider with other loved ones. To the extent possible, it is recommended that this informed consent process be patient centered, that is, one that explores and provides information of particular interest to the individual patient. Patients seek out genetic testing with various sets of expectations and understandings. Given the imprecise nature of the test results, and the quandary of options that may surface as a consequence, it is essential that Rachel take the time and receive the informed guidance necessary to truly consider how this test may benefit her, and whether those benefits outweigh the burdens that may follow for herself and her family, should the test results be found positive.

2. If Rachel's test results come back positive for *BRCA* mutations, would she be obligated to share this information with her family?

The confidentiality of genetic test results is one of the most troublesome aspects of current endeavors in genetic testing. Genetic test results can have profound implications for both individual patients as well as the larger group of blood relatives who may share their genetic makeup. Furthermore, because test results may be predictive of future health status, they may have enormous negative implications for one's access to health, life, or disability insurance, as well as potential impact on employment opportunities or other fundamental life activities, including decisions about marriage and procreation. Such results may be used to categorize, stigmatize, or ostracize patients today for events that may or may not ever happen in their future. Particularly when treatment options are limited in response to test results, patients may experience negative consequences based on that information, without opportunity to therapeutically benefit with the test results in hand.

As to whether or not Rachel would have an obligation to disclose her test results to her children, sister, or other blood relatives, there currently is no specific legal obligation on the part of the patient to disclose such test results, but some ethicists and other scholars have suggested a moral obligation to disclose genetic test results to others who may share their genetic traits, at least in certain defined circumstances. Such circumstances might depend upon the seriousness of the disease tested for, how treatable the disease might be, especially if caught in early stages, and how the gene might be transmitted. Failure to disclose such information may have significant impact on other relatives, as opportunities for proactive interventions may be lost. Disclosure itself might also carry risks, however, including the same sort of psychological, social, and economic risks that the original patient may face. In fact, some might argue that relatives would have a right not to know if they so chose. Some may not be ready to hear the news or act upon it, in the way the patient has. These dilemmas clearly underscore how important and valuable it would be, in advance of testing, for the patient to consider whether and to whom she would disclose a positive test result. Relatives might even be canvassed in advance of testing, not for their permission for the testing itself to proceed, but rather concerning their own desire to know if a genetic predisposition surfaces. In a sense, the information that results from genetic test results is more than individual; its implications may reverberate throughout the family. Given the strong family history, particularly if Rachel is also found to have a *BRCA* mutation, she may feel a strong desire to disclose her status to her sister, her daughter, or even her son, who also may be at risk for the mutation. How they then choose to act upon this information will be their own decision.

While some ethicists have suggested that Rachel might be morally obligated to disclose this information to other close relatives who are also at risk, she herself currently has no *legal* obligation to disclose such information. Unlike situations involving communicable disease (see Case 16, "A Married Man Contracts Syphilis"), for example, Rachel herself is doing nothing to put third parties at any increased risk. She herself poses no direct threat to anyone at this point, and the information that she may come to possess, while perhaps relevant to other family members, does not in and of itself directly contribute specific information about their own health status. These other family members can themselves determine their own *BRCA* status if they so wish.

Some have sought to analogize this to a situation like the *Tarasoff* case, in which identifiable third parties were put at risk due to the actions of the patient (also see Case 16). While the analogy probably fails in this case, given the fact that the patient is doing nothing to increase the risk to the third parties, nor is there a cause and effect relationship between the actions of the patient and the risk these third parties may already face due to their genetic makeup, there has been at least one judicial case where a court has declared that *physicians* may have a legal duty to warn children that a parent's illness is genetically transmissible, and that they, too, may also be at risk. While this is an isolated case in just one jurisdiction, it does portend that a duty to warn, and limitations on confidentiality, are likely to be of increasing concern as more is learned about the genetic origins of illness and how prophylactic actions may lessen or eliminate the risks incurred following the disclosure of genetic mutations.

3. If Rachel is found to be positive for *BRCA* mutations, would this have any affect on her insurance status or her activities in other areas of daily living, including the workplace?

There is no doubt that fear of discrimination based on one's genetic traits is a very real concern to many people, and surveys have shown that individuals are either inhibited from such testing because of these concerns or believe they have experienced discrimination as a result of genetic tests.[8] The actual occurrence of such discrimination is very hard to measure, but this fear and anxiety are ever present and have fueled a recent flurry of legislative initiatives to try to limit the use of genetic test results in the workplace and in insurance issuance.

In the employment arena, individuals fear that because of genetic traits that may make them more susceptible to future illness, or that may leave them at enhanced risk of illness due to exposure to substances in the workplace, they may therefore not be offered employment at all, or not be offered insurance coverage through their employment, which is the largest source of insurance coverage in this country. The Equal Employment Opportunity Commission (EEOC) has stated that the Americans with Disabilities Act (ADA) prohibits employers from discriminating based on genetic test results (see Case 18, "Surgical Delay in a Patient Infected with HIV"), but this pronouncement has never been tested in court, and the extent of its protection is therefore unclear.

What is more worrisome for many people is the potential effect of a genetic test result on their access to health insurance. While there may be therapeutic benefit to such genetic testing, many fear the results could also disqualify them for coverage of the disease for which they are at genetic risk, or that coverage would be prohibitively expensive as a consequence of their test results. In 1996, Congress passed the Health Insurance Portability and Accountability Act, which included provisions to address concern about genetic discrimination. The statute prohibits group plans from using genetic information to limit eligibility from insurance coverage or to consider a genetic predisposition as the equivalent of a preexisting condition. As with most legislation, however, much is left unaddressed or uncovered by this Act. For example, it provides no protections for individuals who purchase their own health insurance on an individual basis or for individuals who are covered through their employment by self-insured plans. The Act also does not prohibit insurers from requesting genetic tests, even if they are prohibited from using the information in a discriminatory way.

Some 24 states have separately considered or enacted legislation to try to address loopholes in the federal law, but these actions as well leave many gaps in their scope of coverage. For example, many state legislative initiatives focus specifically on the concrete results of a particular genetic test, yet leave uncovered actions based on family history. So, while an insurer many not be able to use a test result in a discriminatory fashion, it may be able to consider a family history of a disease prevalence as influential in its decision to either issue coverage or set a particular rate. Many critics of the current system have suggested that only comprehensive federal legislation addressing the larger realm of medical privacy can remedy the current set of loopholes and patchwork coverage that exists around the country. Given the strong array of interests in these issues, including those of the insurance industry, as well as the strong concerns of the business community in health care expenditures, such comprehensive legislative efforts have to date been unsuccessful.

If Rachel does decide to be tested and receive test results indicating a *BRCA* mutation, she may be obligated to disclose this information if she subsequently applies for health, life, or disability insurance. If she were tested as part of a research protocol, so that the costs of the tests would be covered by the research institution, then she might not need to submit for insurance coverage of the test costs. Not all insurers currently pay for *BRCA* testing, and while a few commercial laboratories now offer the test to consumers outside of a research protocol, the costs of the test can vary enormously, from several hundred to even several thousand dollars. Furthermore, while Rachel may have insurance coverage for the costs of the tests, others in her family may not if they decide to seek testing as a result of her own test results. All of these issues raise enormous complications and require serious consideration prior to a decision to embark upon testing. Therefore, once again, the importance of pretest counseling by qualified and knowledgeable counselors becomes critical.

REFERENCES

1. B. Fisher et al., "Tamoxifen for Prevention of Breast Cancer: Report of the National Surgical Adjuvant Breast and Bowel Project P-1 Study," *Journal of the National Cancer Institute* 90 (1998): 1371–1388.

2. S.R. Cummings et al., "The Effect of Raloxifene on Risk of Breast Cancer in Postmenopausal Women: Results from the MORE Randomized Trial," *Journal of the American Medical Association* 281 (1999): 2189–2197.

3. L.C. Hartmann et al., "Efficacy of Bilateral Prophylactic Mastectomy in Women with a Family History of Breast Cancer," *New England Journal of Medicine* 340 (1999): 77–84.

4. A. Eisen and B.L. Weber, "Prophylactic Mastectomy—The Price of Fear," *New England Journal of Medicine* 340 (1999): 137–138.

5. D. Schrag et al., "Decision Analysis—Effects of Prophylactic Mastectomy and Oophorectomy on Life Expectancy among Women with *BRCA1* or *BRCA2* Mutations," *New England Journal of Medicine* 336 (1997): 1465–1471.

6. P.C. Albertsen et al., "Competing Risk Analysis of Men Aged 55 to 74 Years at Diagnosis Managed Conservatively for Clinically Localized Prostate Cancer," *Journal of the American Medical Association* 280 (1998): 975–980.

7. D. Ravine and D.N. Cooper, "Adult-Onset Genetic Disease: Mechanisms, Analysis and Prediction," *Quarterly Journal of Medicine* 90 (1997): 83–103.

8. E.V. Lapham et al., "Genetic Discrimination: Perspectives of Consumers," *Science* 274 (1996): 621–624.

SUGGESTED READINGS

American College of Physicians. 1997. Screening for prostate cancer. *Annals of Internal Medicine* 126: 480–484.

American Society of Clinical Oncology. 1996. Statement of the American Society of Clinical Oncology: Genetic testing for cancer susceptibility. *Journal of Clinical Oncology* 14: 1730–1736.

American Society on Human Genetics Social Issue Subcommittee on Family Disclosure. 1998. ASHG statement: Professional disclosure of familial genetic information. *American Journal of Human Genetics* 62: 474–483.

Benkendorf, J.L. et al. 1997. Patients' attitudes about autonomy and confidentiality in genetic testing for breast-ovarian cancer susceptibility. *American Journal of Medical Genetics* 73: 296–303.

Burke, W. et al. for the Cancer Genetics Studies Consortium. 1997. Recommendations for follow-up care of individuals with an inherited predisposition to cancer. II. *BRCA1* and *BRCA2. Journal of the American Medical Association* 277: 997–1003.

Chodak, G.W. 1998. Comparing treatments for localized prostate cancer—Persisting uncertainty. *Journal of the American Medical Association* 280: 1008–1010.

Deftos, L.J. 1998. The evolving duty to disclose the presence of genetic disease to relatives.
Academic Medicine 73: 962–968.

Durfy, S.J. 1998. Testing for inherited susceptibility to breast cancer: A survey of informed
consent forms for *BRCA1* and *BRCA2* mutation testing. *American Journal of Medical
Genetics* 75: 82–87.

Freedman, T.G. 1998. Genetic susceptibility testing: Ethical and social quandaries. *Health
and Social Work* 23: 214–222.

Geller, G. et al. 1997. "Decoding" informed consent: Insights from women regarding breast
cancer susceptibility testing. *Hastings Center Report* 27, no. 2: 28–33.

Geller, G. et al. 1997. Genetic testing for susceptibility to adult-onset cancer: The process
and content of informed consent. *Journal of the American Medical Association* 277:
1467–1474.

Geller, L.N. et al. 1996. Individual, family and societal dimensions of genetic discrimination: A case study analysis. *Science and Engineering Ethics* 2: 71–88.

Grady, C. 1999. Ethics and genetic testing. *Advances in Internal Medicine* 44: 389–411.

Green, R.M., and Thomas, A.M. 1997. Whose gene is it? A case discussion about familial
conflict over genetic testing for breast cancer. *Journal of Genetic Counseling* 6: 245–
254.

Jacobsen, P.B. et al. 1997. Decision making about genetic testing among women at familial
risk for breast cancer. *Psychosomatic Medicine* 59: 459–466.

Khovidhunkit, W., and Shoback, D.M. 1999. Clinical effects of raloxifene hydrochloride in
women. *Annals of Internal Medicine* 130: 431–439.

Kodish, E. et al. 1998. Genetic testing for cancer risk: How to reconcile the conflicts. *Journal of the American Medical Association* 279: 179–181.

McNaughton Collins, M. et al. 1997. Medical malpractice implications of PSA testing for
early detection of prostate cancer. *The Journal of Law, Medicine, and Ethics* 25: 234–
242.

Nance, M.A. 1996. Huntington Disease—Another chapter rewritten. *American Journal of
Human Genetics* 59: 1–6.

National Society of Genetic Counselors. 1997. Predisposition genetic testing for late-onset
disorders in adults. *Journal of the American Medical Association* 278: 1217–1220.

Newman, B. et al. 1998. Frequency of breast cancer attributable to BRCA1 in a population-
based series of American women. *Journal of the American Medical Association* 279:
915–921.

Phillips, K.A., and Glendon, G. 1999. Putting the risk of breast cancer in perspective. *New
England Journal of Medicine* 340: 141–144.

Pokorski, R.J. 1997. Insurance underwriting in the genetic era. *American Journal of Human
Genetics* 60: 205–216.

Rhodes, R. 1998. Genetic links, family ties, and social bonds: Rights and responsibilities in the face of genetic knowledge. *Journal of Medicine and Philosophy* 23: 10–30.

Rothenberg, K. et al. 1997. Genetic information and the workplace: Legislative approaches and policy challenges. *Science* 275: 1755–1757.

Rubinsztein, D.C. et al. 1996. Phenotypic characterization of individuals with 30-40 CAG repeats in the Huntington disease (HD) gene reveals HD cases with 36 repeats and apparently normal elderly individuals with 36–39 repeats. *American Journal of Human Genetics* 59: 16–22.

Slooter, A.J.C., and van Duijn, C.M. 1997. Genetic epidemiology of Alzheimer's disease. *Epidemiologic Reviews.* 19: 107–119.

Spencer, C.P. et al. 1999. Selective estrogen receptor modulators: Women's panacea for the next millenium? *American Journal of Obstetrics and Gynecology* 180 (3 pt. 1): 763–770.

Stolberg, S.G. 1998. Concern among Jews is heightened as scientists deepen gene studies. *New York Times*, 22 April, 24(A).

Weaver, K.D. 1997. Genetic screening and the right not to know. *Issues in Law and Medicine* 13: 243–281.

Wilfond, B.S. et al. 1997. Cancer genetic susceptibility testing: Ethical and policy implications for future research and clinical practice. *The Journal of Law Medicine, and Ethics* 25: 243–251.

LEGAL CITATIONS

Case Examples

Safer v. Pack, N.J. Super. Ct. App. Div. A-2234-94T2 (July 11, 1996).
 Court ruling that physicians may have a duty to warn the children of patients who have a genetically transmissable condition. This case involved a lawsuit brought by the daughter of a patient, who died of polypopsis, against her father's oncologist, after she, too, was diagnosed with multiple polypopsis. The daughter claimed she should have been warned of her father's disease so she could have sought out early detection and treatment.

Tarasoff v. Regents of University of California, 17 Cal. 3d 425, 551 P.2d 334, 131 Cal. Rptr. 14 (1976).

Statutory Examples

Health Insurance Portability and Accountability Act, Pub. L. No. 104-191 (1996).
 Federal law that provides some protection to limit the use of genetic information by group health insurers to deny insurance coverage.

Wisconsin Stat. Sec. 48.432 (1994).

Statutory obligation of child-placing adoption agencies to notify adoptees over the age of 18, or guardian/adoptive parents of adoptees under 18 if they receive information that a birth parent or subsequent child of the birth parent has or may have a genetically transmissable disease.

CASE 24

Assisted Reproduction in a Woman with Strong Religious Beliefs

Jessica is a 33-year-old teacher who has been unable to become pregnant after trying to conceive for the last five years. For the past two years she has been performing a series of tests for urinary luteinizing hormone (LH) every month in order to time sexual intercourse. She and her husband Ted have an 8-year-old daughter and are anxious to have another child, so they decided to be evaluated at a nearby infertility center that was recommended by Jessica's gynecologist.

After both Jessica and Ted were fully evaluated, they were told that no apparent cause of infertility can be found in either, and that theirs is a case of "unexplained infertility" in Jessica, who is nine years older than when she conceived her first child. It is possible that Jessica will respond to medications that stimulate her ovaries and increase her chances of conception. The doctor explained that she is not too old to have a successful pregnancy, but the older she gets the less likely she will be able to conceive, even with the latest methods.

At the infertility clinic, Jessica often chats with other patients in the waiting room and has befriended another woman, who is a practicing Catholic like Jessica. Both women are opposed to abortion and discuss the possible religious objections they might encounter regarding infertility treatment. Jessica has spoken to her priest, who told her that the church had no objection to medications that stimulate ovulation, but that most other methods, such as in vitro fertilization (IVF), or "test tube babies," were not permitted. He did caution her about the possibility of multiple births if she became pregnant, and that the issue of reducing the number of embryos might arise. This, he said, is strictly forbidden, because it is tantamount to abortion.

Concerned about her "biological clock," Jessica was anxious to proceed as soon as possible. She was offered a course of gonadotropins to induce "superovulation," and she agreed enthusiastically. It was explained to her that after a baseline pelvic ultrasound, she would need to give herself a daily injection of recombinant follicle-stimulating hormone (FSH) for a week or more, and would require from five to seven visits to the office in the first month to monitor hormone levels in the blood and receive additional ultrasound examinations.

When sufficient mature follicles are noted on the ultrasound, Ted will have to give her a precisely timed, intramuscular injection of human chorionic gonadotropin (HCG) in the buttocks. This will trigger ovulation and, about two days later Jessica would have to return to the office where her husband's prepared sperm would be inserted into the uterus via the cervix. Jessica agreed to everything, but had religious objections to the unnatural method of artificial insemination. The physician says they can use the "natural method" (coitus), but adds that she should also have artificial insemination the next day, because this will improve the precision of the timing and circumvent any unidentified problem with the cervix, such as problems with the cervical mucus. Still, Jessica rejected that option.

During her first cycle, ultrasound and blood tests revealed a suboptimal response, and Jessica did not become pregnant during that cycle. She became discouraged because she expected the great expense and considerable inconvenience associated with the regimen to yield success. Three months later, her husband persuaded her to return to the infertility center for another round. This time she was told, she would receive a higher dose of FSH to increase her chances of becoming pregnant.

This time Jessica had a vigorous response and ultrasound revealed multiple mature follicles. Although at first delighted, Jessica and her husband are dismayed about the options they are now given. The options include forgoing the HCG injection ("canceling the cycle") and waiting until the next month when the response might be less vigorous; to "coast," or wait for the estrogen levels to decline before giving HCG, although the likelihood of pregnancy would be lower; or to receive HCG, and attempt to become pregnant. Unfortunately, because Jessica's estrogen levels are quite high, she has an enhanced risk of developing the ovarian hyperstimulation syndrome (OHSS) if she selects the last option. In addition, the physician explains, there is a very real possibility of multifetal pregnancy. If this were to occur, multifetal reduction would be strongly recommended, and this is not permitted according to Jessica's religious beliefs.

All of these options are troubling to Jessica and her husband. While she thinks they may have been described to her before she began the process, she is now faced with a stark set of considerations. Jessica is most keenly aware that the likelihood of pregnancy and delivery will decline rapidly as the months go by. She decides she wants to complete this cycle, saying that whatever happens she is in God's hands. She is willing to take the risk, citing a highly publicized case of healthy septuplets that she had seen on television.

ISSUES TO CONSIDER

- Assisted reproduction
- Survival and morbidity in very low-birth-weight infants
- Directive versus nondirective counseling

MEDICAL CONSIDERATIONS

1. At the outset, what were the chances that Jessica would become pregnant and have a live baby? What are they now?

Approximately 5 percent of women of Jessica's age who have infertility (defined as the inability to conceive after three years of regular intercourse) become pregnant spontaneously each cycle. The pregnancy rate after induction of superovulation with gonadotropins would thus need to be seen in that light. Recent data from a multicenter study showed that, overall, the chances of a live birth after superovulation and intrauterine insemination were approximately 22 percent (15 percent for intracervical insemination), for women 40 years of age and younger, often after multiple cycles.[1] The likelihood of pregnancy and live birth, regardless of the method, declines steadily after age 35, even in someone like Jessica who had one successful pregnancy nine years earlier. Likewise, the pregnancy rate is dependent upon the actual sperm count of the partner. Transcervical or intrauterine insemination of the donor's (in this case, Jessica's husband) sperm into the uterus conveys an overall rate of live birth of 25 percent. In contrast to natural intercourse, this method would circumvent any cervical factor contributing to infertility, such as abnormalities in cervical mucus, although there is evidence that sperm ejaculated during intercourse is of higher quality.

If she were to develop a multifetal pregnancy, this would not necessarily increase her chances of having a live baby, because of the risk of miscarriage (see below). Likewise, multiple pregnancy with three or more fetuses confers a risk of morbidity and mortality greater than the risks of fetal reduction performed by an experienced team.

Pooled national data from infertility centers using a variety of assisted reproductive technologies (mostly IVF) show that women under 35 years of age have approximately 29 percent chance of having a live birth.[2] This proportion varies widely, depending on the center reporting, the age of the woman, the cause of infertility in either parent, and other methodological and statistical factors. For a woman 40 years of age or older, the live birth rate after IVF is only 9 percent.

2. What are the risks of infertility treatments to Jessica?

The main risks are related to the risks of multiple pregnancy, which occur far more frequently among women undergoing infertility treatments that involve ovarian stimulation. Multiple pregnancy is associated with an enhanced risk of preterm labor and the attendant risks of forestalling delivery, which may require prolonged bedrest, hospitalization, administration of intravenous fluids and medications to reduce uterine contraction, and possible medical complications that these interventions entail. Multiple pregnancy is also associated with a greater risk of maternal hemorrhage and use of cesarean section and also increases the risk of gestational diabetes and hypertension.

A relatively uncommon but potentially serious side effect of Jessica's treatment is the ovarian hyperstimulation syndrome (OHSS), which is related mostly to the use of gonadotropins, such as human menopausal gonadotropin (hMG) or purified or recombinant follicle stimulating hormone (FSH). The resulting superovulation is believed to lead to OHSS when excessive amounts of estradiol are produced by each follicle. Symptoms of OHSS include pelvic pain, marked fluid retention, third spacing and dehydration, pleural or pericardial effusion, hypovolemia resulting in renal failure, and hypercoagulable state that can lead to potentially life-threatening thromboembolic phenomena.[3] OHSS may be worsened by pregnancy. The risk is lower in women receiving in vitro fertilization because follicular fluid can be extracted prior to transfer of the embryo to the uterus.

Concerns have been raised that ovarian stimulation can increase the risk of ovarian cancer. This concern derives from the observation that nulliparity and delayed childbearing are associated with an increased risk, suggesting that repeated ovulation is the key contributing factor. Infertility alone is also a risk factor, however, and there is no convincing evidence that induction of ovarian superovulation in women with infertility further increases the incidence of ovarian cancer beyond that conferred by the other risk factors, and this issue remains controversial.

3. What are the risks of multiple pregnancy to Jessica's baby or babies?

Multiple pregnancy, whether as the result of infertility treatments or spontaneous conception, is associated with an increased risk of premature delivery. On the average, the duration of pregnancy is 35 weeks for twins, 33 for triplets, and 29 for quadruplets, as compared to 39 weeks for singletons. Pregnancies that occur as the result of ovulation induction have an elevated rate of premature delivery, even with singletons. This is related to administration of hormones that ripen the cervix, and the risk is increased in multiple pregnancy, probably because of uterine overdistension.

Newborns of multiple pregnancy often have low birth weight with its attendant risks. Virtually all quadruplets (mean gestational age 31 weeks), and approximately 90 percent of triplets (mean gestational age 33.5 weeks) are born prematurely. Birth weights of such preterm infants is approximately 1500 to 1700 grams.

Overall survival of low-birth-weight infants decreases with decreasing weight at birth, decreasing gestational age (if it can be gauged), and with associated maternal factors. Unfortunately, premature infants may develop severe morbidity, such as bronchopulmonary dysplasia, neurologic damage, or blindness. Although survival rate and incidence of severe morbidity among very-low-birth-weight (VLBW) infants ($\leq$ 1500g) have improved steadily over the years, along with strides in perinatal and neonatal care, risks of major morbidity and the length of hospital stay remain substantial. This is particularly marked for infants in the lowest birth weight categories. Overall outcomes of very-low-birth-weight singletons are summarized in Table 7–24.1.

Very-low-birth-weight infants who survive are at increased risk of developing a variety of disabilities. The majority of premature infants of less than 35 weeks gestational age develop respiratory distress syndrome (RDS) and many require mechanical ventilation, at least in the short term. Nearly all infants under 1,000 grams at birth or less than 27 weeks gestational age have RDS. RDS is due to lack of pulmonary surfactant, a substance produced by the mature infant lung that prevents alveolar collapse. Pneumonia, patent ductus arteriosus, and other problems associated with prematurity may coexist. Long-term ventilation may lead to bronchopulmonary dysplasia, which in turn can lead to chronic lung disease. Availability of exogenous pulmonary surfactant has reduced

Table 7–24.1 Outcomes among Very-Low-Birth-Weight Singletons

Birth Weight (g)	Number (%)	Survival to Discharge (%)	Hospital Length of Stay among Survivors (days)	≥1 Major Morbidity among Survivors (%)
501–750	999 (22)	49	122	48
751–1000	1047 (23)	85	87	34
1001–1250	1130 (25)	93	59	15
1251–1500	1417 (31)	96	43	10

Source: Data from D.K. Stevenson et al., Very Low Birth Weight Outcomes of the National Institute of Child Health and Human Development Neonatal Research Network, January 1993 through December 1994, *American Journal of Obstetrics and Gynecology,* Vol. 179, pp. 1632–1639, © 1998, Mosby-Year Book, Inc.

but not eliminated morbidity and mortality among preterm infants with RDS.

Periventricular-intraventricular hemorrhage occurs shortly after birth in 35 to 45 percent of infants of less than approximately 32 weeks gestation; these hemorrhages are related to vascular fragility and fluctuations in cerebral blood pressure, the latter partly due to respiratory distress and accompanying ventilatory treatments. Although the majority of these hemorrhages are mild and are not believed to be associated with lasting problems, severe hemorrhage is associated with a high incidence of severe neurologic sequelae in survivors. The tiniest babies are most likely to have hemorrhages and these are frequently severe.

Another potentially serious complication is retinopathy of prematurity (ROP). Fortunately, retinal disease in premature infants often reverts to normal, but when retinal scarring occurs, blindness results in 25 percent of cases. Overall, for those under 1,000 grams, the risk of blindness is approximately 5 to 11 percent. The tiniest infants may have a particularly high risk of developing scarring retinopathy. Other long-term complications of ROP include poor visual acuity, strabismus, and high-grade myopia.

4. What are the risks and benefits of fetal reduction for the mother? The surviving newborns?

Multifetal reduction, which involves ultrasound-guided placement of a needle through the abdominal wall or vagina during the mother's first trimester of pregnancy, is associated with a small risk of infection or bleeding, but overall the risks are less than carrying three or more fetuses to term. The needle is passed into the uterus and potassium chloride is injected into the fetus, which is then observed for asystole.[4] Selection of the fetus or fetuses to be reduced is generally based on size or position, or estimates of likelihood of viability if possible. Generally fetal number is reduced to two (three usually at the request of the parent and one usually for twin pregnancies where medical indications suggest one will not survive).

Between 6 and 18 percent of pregnancies during which fetal reduction is undertaken are lost, that is, the mother miscarries all remaining fetuses before 24 weeks gestation, and the likelihood of this happening increases with the number of fetuses present prior to reduction. Because pregnancy loss may occur several weeks after the procedure it is not possible to know if it is a direct result of the procedure or if it happens spontaneously, as miscarriage occurs frequently in multiple pregnancy. In one study of 140 women with triplet pregnancies (132 the product of assisted reproduction), 9 percent of those undergoing fetal reduction to twins had spontaneous miscarriage, compared to 21 percent of those attempting to carry the triplet pregnancy to term.[5] Since most multiple pregnancies now are the result of assisted reproduction, other factors related to the mother, fetus, or ovarian stimulation cannot be ruled out as the cause of this high rate of fetal loss.

Emotional consequences of fetal reduction may be significant. These are often added to the stresses of undergoing prolonged, taxing, and costly infertility treatments. Mothers who have undergone fetal reduction mourn the loss of the fetus, but often resolve these emotional reactions after several months, and when surveyed, generally would undergo the same procedure again. Some parents, however, have lingering feelings of guilt and sadness. Pregnancy loss after a long period of unsuccessful and complicated infertility treatments can be devastating. Often the loss occurs after 24 weeks of gestation.

If the child or children are born prematurely, there are additional stresses involved in potentially prolonged hospitalization and in some cases the emotional and financial toll of raising a handicapped child.

There is no evidence of an enhanced risk to surviving newborns who are the products of assisted reproduction, above and beyond the risks associated with multiple pregnancy.

5. What are the medical consequences of multiple pregnancy for children?

The major consequences are low birth weight and prematurity. Neonates with very low birth weight tend to develop more slowly than their peers. Many functional impairments can subside, but others may not become apparent for many years. Although functional outcomes have improved in recent years, long-term studies of late outcome of these children (based on experience with children born approximately one decade ago) suggest that VLBW infants have a much higher chance of developing specific medical conditions in childhood, such as asthma, cerebral palsy, and epilepsy, and have a higher rate of mental retardation, than children of moderately low or normal birth weight. Very-low-birth-weight children, in addition, are at higher risk of having functional impairments that limit their performance of activities of daily living. While factors such as maternal IQ and socio-economic status tend to determine IQ in most children, IQ may be less than 85 in nearly 50 percent of infants with extremely low birth weight (1,000 grams or less), independent of these factors. Even infants who weigh 1,000 to 1,500 grams at birth have substantially worse academic performance in school than normal-birth-weight children of the same IQ levels.

Functional impairments may be on the decline for infants larger than 800 grams, but for the smallest infants there has been little or no change and impairments tend to be more severe than for larger VLBW infants.

6. If Jessica has a miscarriage and wishes to continue infertility treatments, are there alternative methods that might be acceptable to her?

Religious proscriptions with regard to assisted reproduction tend to be highly variable, not only because of variability among formal religious doctrines, but perhaps because of variability in their interpretation among clergy and the individual. For example, Jessica felt that ejaculation should only occur during intercourse, thus preventing the option of intrauterine insemination. Since IVF has been forbidden, she could perhaps discuss the option of gamete intrafallopian transfer (GIFT) with her priest. In this method, she would undergo ovarian stimulation as before, and her eggs would be retrieved and mixed with sperm externally, but not cultured. The egg and sperm would be placed directly into the fallopian tube where fertilization could occur. The acceptability of GIFT over IVF derives from the fact that fertilization itself occurs inside the body, rather than "in a test tube." Unfortunately, GIFT is more invasive and costly than IVF, but it may in fact have an overall higher success rate. Other methods of assisted reproductive technology are discussed in the references.[6]

ETHICAL AND LEGAL CONSIDERATIONS

1. Could some of the dilemmas now facing Jessica and her physician have been considered during an informed consent process?

The decision to utilize assisted reproductive technologies (ART) is a momentous one for a patient and her family, given the physical, psychological, and financial demands that are often placed on a family as a result of pursuing this medical option. As ART is essentially elective and there are many other ways that a patient could address her problems with infertility, a thorough informed consent process, exploring all available options (both medical and nonmedical), their risks and benefits, alternatives and other essential information, becomes critical to the integrity of the process. Furthermore, given the highly emotional and personal nature of this treatment path, it is essential for providers to clearly understand the values and expectations of patients who wish to make use of such options. Patients seeking ART often do so after long and arduous attempts to otherwise conceive a child. They may be emotionally fragile and vulnerable, raising the specter of concern that informed consent to potentially risky procedures may not be as informed or voluntary as one might hope. The informed consent process, then, needs to be part of a larger ongoing dialogue between providers and the patient, so that all are fully aware of the treatment and decision-making parameters and implications, before embarking on this path with an individual patient. This is truly a situation in which informed consent must be more than a paper process or signed consent form. In Jessica's situation, that seems not to have happened.

At a minimum, patients contemplating various ART techniques should be informed of the risks and benefits of the specific treatment they might be contemplating, both for themselves, their families, and their potential fetuses. As discussed earlier, the various medications and interventions are each accompanied by the potential for serious side effects, with limited chances of success in many cases. Whether or not certain potential risks are worth undergoing for certain potential benefits is usually a personal decision for the patient to determine, but in order for her to weigh the risks and benefits, she must have accurate, up-to-date, individually relevant information. Therefore, a patient such as Jessica should have had extensive conversations with her providers about such matters as the risks of the medications on which she was placed (including the potential for multiple follicle maturity), the chances for successful pregnancy for a patient with her profile, and the program's broader success rates and experiences with this technique.

For many programs, success may be defined as achieving a pregnancy, even if the patient ultimately doesn't carry to term. All ART programs are now required to report various statistics and outcomes to the Centers for Disease Control (CDC) so that patients will be able to discern the experience and success of various clinical programs in a manner that permits them to make objective comparisons of their options. The CDC has cautioned, however, that reported statistics might reflect selection bias, in that individual centers might treat various subgroups of patients who are likely to have different outcomes. In addition, some clinics might promote success rates based on methods deemed inappropriate by current standards (i.e., transferring larger numbers of embryos in IVF than recommended).[2]

Perhaps most importantly, the potential for a multifetal pregnancy and the risks and potential options in response ought to have been addressed prior to initiating the ovary stimulation. In particular, Jessica's strong religious convictions and her willingness to consider options should not come as a surprise to her care providers, and in fact, should have been an integral consideration to the decision to initiate ART and the choice of treatment selected. For example, for this patient GIFT might have been appropriate. Mentioned briefly above, GIFT is a process whereby extracted oocytes are mixed with sperm and then placed directly into the fallopian tube where fertilization is hoped to occur. This procedure is sometimes acceptable to people whose religion proscribes IVF, since GIFT fertilization occurs inside the body. It requires a surgical procedure with general anesthesia and is associated with higher risk than IVF. Clearly, a two-way dialogue concerning risks, benefits, and values, both of the providers and of the patient and her family, should be an essential component to the decision to pursue ART. While patients and physicians are free to disagree about acceptable risks and options, such disagreements ought to be surfaced well in advance of the point when actions are irrevocable or unchangeable. The potential for multiple fetuses and the implications of this is certainly one area that should be seriously discussed in advance.

Beyond informed consent, a broader process of counseling ought to be available to patients and their families throughout the ART process. Decision points are certainly vulnerable times when patients and their families may need supportive guidance in evaluating options within the context of their individual lives. In particular, patients often need extensive counseling in order to fully understand, prospectively, where various decisions may lead them in this process. Given the vulnerability of patients in this circumstance, the pressure they perceive due to the time and costliness of this process, and the impact such treatment decisions have on the patient and on the broader family construct, supportive counseling is critical. Whether such counseling should be directive, that is, intended to steer patients in a certain direction, is a matter of debate and probably varies depending upon the individual philosophies of the program providers. For some programs, concern about the risks of multiple fetal pregnancies means that patients must be willing to consider the option of selective reduction as a response. For patients whose chances of a successful outcome are very slim, some programs will provide counseling to place their expectations in a very realistic framework, including counseling them not to pursue this path. Other programs are more willing to accept even the unlikeliest of candidates or are willing to abide by whatever decisions the patient makes. Regardless of the directiveness of the counseling, however, there is no excuse for not having full, frank, and informed discussions, responsive to patient concerns and expectations, articulating the programs' philosophies concerning the various techniques, and reflective of real risks and implications, prior to beginning the ART path with the patient.

2. Is selective reduction an ethically justifiable response to the dilemma of a multifetal pregnancy?

The incidence of multifetal pregnancy and multiple births has risen dramatically in the last 20 years, much of this attributable to the use of ART. Statistics from 1995 show that 37 percent of pregnancies achieved through ART involved multiple births, whereas the incidence of multiple births in the general population is 2 percent (Table 7–24.2). Moreover, between

Table 7–24.2 Rate of Twin and Triplet Pregnancy

Ovarian Cycle	Twin Pregnancy	Triplet Pregnancy	Quadruplet (or more) Pregnancy
Natural	1%	.01%	extremely rare
Gonadotropin	25%	5%	uncommon

Source: Data from I. Souter and T.M. Goodwin, Decision Making in Multifetal Pregnancy Reduction for Triplets, *American Journal of Perinatology,* Vol. 15, pp. 63–71, © 1998, Thieme Medical Publishers, Inc.

1974 and 1994, the rate of triplet and higher order multiple births increased fourfold, with two-thirds of this increase attributable to ART.[6] In many ways this is a remarkable testament to the success of ART, yet it comes with significant cost and the potential for wrenching ethical dilemmas when such techniques result in multifetal pregnancies.

While there is debate about the ethical justification for selective reduction in multifetal pregnancy, there is little debate in theory about the obligation to proactively avoid this result if at all possible. Physicians providing ART clearly have an ethical obligation to minimize the potential for such an outcome, yet this obligation seems to be only sporadically respected, given the continued prevalence of multiple births. In this situation, preventive ethics would dictate that in circumstances of ovarian stimulation, when multiple mature follicles are detected, the injection of HCG be withheld. In situations involving IVF, the transference of a limited number of embryos will help avoid a multifetal pregnancy. In some countries, such as England, legislation mandates how many embryos can be transferred per IVF cycle (no more than three in England). In the United States, no state or federal legislation exists to mandate a specific number, though professional organizations such as the American Society for Assisted Reproduction have set out various guidelines depending on the patient profile. The dilemma is that every patient is somewhat different, the technology is evolving, and the certainty of the process is never known in advance. Coupled with this are the expectations that patients bring to this process—their perspectives formed by happy media stories of successful multiple births, the pressures they feel emotionally and psychologically because of financial constraints or time delays, and their willingness to court risk given the potential for a long-sought benefit. Moreover for ART programs, success rates are critical to the viability of the program. The more embryos implanted the more likely the chance of success. All of these pressures present real challenges to the obligation to avoid the multifetal pregnancy if at all possible.

As previously described, serious risks confront both patients and their fetuses when multifetal pregnancies go forward. Not only is the mother's health put at significant risk, but the potential for growth retardation or preterm delivery, with resulting physical and mental impairments of the fetuses, is a real concern. The risk of perinatal mortality also increases with a higher number of fetuses. Thus, when confronted with a multifetal pregnancy, patients and their providers face three choices: to end the pregnancy in its entirety through abortion, an option that for many is not possible or desirable, given the tremendous efforts undertaken to reach such a stage; to continue the pregnancy as is, with its real attendant risk of harm to the mother and fetuses; or to selectively reduce the pregnancy, using a procedure that will terminate the lives of some of the fetuses for the potential of improving the chances of the surviving ones. From a medical perspective, while this option is clearly not one that should be casually employed or routinely utilized, it does offer the potential for limiting risks and improving the chances of a healthy and successful pregnancy.

The choice of selective reduction carries its own risks. From a physical perspective, it does create some risks for the remaining fetuses and the success of the pregnancy. Psychologically, parents often experience grief as a result, and there is never assurance of the quality of the lives preserved versus the potential quality of life of the fetuses terminated. Perhaps most difficult are the many serious ethical concerns that arise from this process. Many see this as tantamount to abortion, which for many, including Jessica, is not an acceptable option. Some believe that while abortion is acceptable in certain circumstances, selective reduction goes beyond acceptability, as it is the purposeful destruction of an intentionally created life. Still others believe that the "use" of some fetuses for the "benefit" of others violates basic moral tenets of human life as an end in itself, not a means to something else. Yet others see this as a regrettable yet justifiable way to achieve the best outcome possible in a tragic circumstance. For some, it is no different than abortion, viewed as a private and ethically justifiable decision between a woman and her provider.

The array of opinions in this ethically challenging circumstance certainly suggests at a minimum that this is an issue for ART programs and potential patients to consider (and try to avoid) well in advance of its actual occurrence. Certainly the potential for a multifetal pregnancy should be an essential aspect of the ART informed consent process. Programs must clearly enunciate their philosophy and policy on such an issue and patients should be given the opportunity to consider and express their own views, prior to any agreement to proceed with ART. It is would even be advisable, if possible, to come to agreement on the number of embryos to be transferred, or the number of mature follicles to be acceptable, in order for the patient to be supported in her pursuit of pregnancy.

3. What financial pressures may influence the choices of patients undergoing ART?

ART is an extraordinarily expensive response to the problem of infertility, thereby placing it beyond the means of many couples desiring, but unable, to conceive a child. Depending on the types and number of procedures employed, patients can spend tens if not hundreds of thousands of dollars, without ever being sure that they will achieve a successful outcome. Such a circumstance places enormous pressure on the patient and her family from a financial perspective, and it places enormous pressure on ART programs to achieve a successful outcome for the patient.

By and large, few patients have insurance that covers even a portion of this tremendous expense. While some insurance programs pay for certain procedures associated with infertility, such as semen analysis, surgical opening of tubes or clomiphene for ovary stimulation, very few programs pay for the newer, more sophisticated options such as IVF. Several years ago, litigation arose in several states against insurers who did not explicitly exclude coverage for such procedures and some of these suits were successful, but currently, most policies explicitly exclude ART from insurance coverage. While eight states currently mandate insurance coverage for at least certain aspects of infertility treatment, including IVF, self-insured or self-funded insurance programs provided through corporate employers are excluded from these state mandates, under the federal ERISA program (see Case 14, "Suicide Risk in a Managed Care Patient"). State Medicaid programs by and large do not cover infertility treatments. More recently, the Supreme Court declared that reproduction is a fundamental life activity, so that inability to reproduce would be considered a disability under the Americans with Disabilities Act (see Case 18, "Surgical Delay in a Patient Infected with HIV"). Whether or not this would then mean that patients could force their employers to accommodate their infertility through the provision of insurance coverage for ART, however, has not yet been litigated.

There are data to support that insurance coverage for ART would only slightly increase premiums of managed care organizations, yet few seem motivated to date to provide such coverage. ART programs, therefore, often require payment up front from patients out of fear that once services are provided, patients may then not be able or willing to follow through on the financial commitment they have made. Perhaps the most controversial aspect of this payment process has been the institution by some programs of a "money-back guarantee," whereby patients meeting a certain profile will be refunded some of the costs of their ART treatments if the process is ultimately unsuccessful. Many critics, including the American Medical Association, have argued against such programs, claiming it is unethical to suggest that certain outcomes in medicine can be guaranteed and that patients may not be able to make a truly informed decision in such a coercive context. Others suggest that this may be a way to allow ART to be available to patients and families who otherwise could not afford to gamble what perhaps may amount to their life savings on a process that may yield no success, and that may then prevent them from pursuing other options such as adoption. While no state has yet legislated against these money-back programs, there is certainly concern that consumers are informed of and fully understand the implications of these guarantees (which often have many restrictions and limitations) prior to going forward.

REFERENCES

1. D.S. Guzick et al., for the National Cooperative Reproductive Medicine Network, "Efficacy of Superovulation and Intrauterine Insemination in the Treatment of Infertility," *New England Journal of Medicine* 340 (1999): 177–183.
2. Centers for Disease Control, "1996 Assisted Reproductive Technology Success Rates," *National Summary and Fertility Clinic Reports* (see Appendix A).
3. J.G. Schenker, "Prevention and Treatment of Ovarian Hyperstimulation," *Human Reproduction* 8 (1993): 653–659.
4. R.L. Berkowitz et al., "The Current Status of Multifetal Pregnancy Reduction," *American Journal of Obstetrics and Gynecology* 174 (1996): 1265–1272.
5. S. Lipitz et al., "A Prospective Comparison of the Outcome of Triplet Pregnancies Managed Expectantly or by Multifetal Reduction to Twins," *American Journal of Obstetrics and Gynecology* 170 (1994): 874–879.
6. The New York State Task Force on Life and the Law, *Assisted Reproductive Technologies. Analysis and Recommendations for Public Policy* (New York, 1998).

SUGGESTED READINGS

Alexander, J.M. et al. 1995. Multifetal reduction of high order multiple pregnancy: Comparison of obstetrical outcome with nonreduced twin gestations. *Fertility and Sterility* 64: 1201–1203.

American Medical Association, Council on Ethical and Judicial Affairs and Council on Scientific Affairs. 1996. Report 70: Joint report on issues of ethical conduct in assisted reproductive technology. *Code of Medical Ethics* 6, no. 2: 2.

American Society for Reproductive Medicine. 1997. Practice Committee Reports: Guidelines on number of embryos transferred; Elements to be considered in obtaining informed consent for ART, June (see Appendix A).

Berkowitz, R.L. 1998. Ethical issues involving multifetal pregnancies. *Mount Sinai Journal of Medicine* 65, no. 3: 185–190, 215–223.

Committee on Ethics, American College of Obstetricians and Gynecologists. 1999. Nonselective embryo reduction: Ethical guidance for the obstetrician-gynecologist. *ACOG Committee Opinion No. 215,* April.

Escobar, G.J. et al. 1991. Outcome among surviving very low birthweight infants: A meta-analysis. *Archives of Disease in Childhood* 66: 204–211.

Evans, M.I. et al. 1996. Ethical issues surrounding multifetal pregnancy reduction and selective termination. *Clinics in Perinatology* 23: 437–451.

Hidlebaugh, D.A. et al. 1997. Cost of assisted reproductive technologist for a health maintenance organization. *Journal of Reproductive Medicine* 42: 570–574.

Horbar, J.D. et al. 1993. Predicting mortality risk for infants weighing 501 to 1500 grams at birth: A National Institutes of Health Neonatal Research Network report. *Critical Care Medicine* 21: 12–18.

Hunter, D.G., and Mukai, S. 1992. Retinopathy of prematurity: Pathogenesis, diagnosis, and treatment. *International Ophthalmology Clinics* 32: 163–184.

Jobe, A.H. 1993. Pulmonary surfactant therapy. *New England Journal of Medicine* 328: 861–868.

Klotzko, A.J. 1998. Medical miracle or medical mischief? The saga of the McCaughey septuplets. *Hastings Center Report* 28, no. 3: 5–8.

McCormick, M.C. 1992. The health and developmental status of very low birth-weight children at school age. *Journal of the American Medical Association* 267: 2204–2208.

McCormick, M.C. 1993. Has the prevalence of handicapped infants increased with improved survival of the very low birth weight infant? *Clinics in Perinatology* 20: 263–277.

McIntire, D.D. et al. 1999. Birth weight in relation to morbidity and mortality among newborn infants. *New England Journal of Medicine* 340: 1234–1238.

Mosgaard, B.J. et al. 1997. The impact of parity, infertility and treatment with fertility drugs on the risk of ovarian cancer. *Acta Obstetrica et Gynecologica Scandinavica* 76: 89–95.

Papiernik, E. et al. 1998. Should multifetal pregnancy reduction be used for prevention of preterm deliveries in triplet or higher order multiple pregnancies? *Journal of Perinatal Medicine* 26: 365–370.

Peabody, J.L., and Martin, G.I. 1998. From how small is too small to how much is too much. Ethical issues at the limits of neonatal viability. *Clinics in Perinatology* 23: 473–489.

Society for Assisted Reproductive Technology and the American Society for Reproductive Medicine. 1996. Assisted reproductive technology in the United States and Canada:

1994 results generated from the American Society for Reproductive Medicine/Society for Assisted Reproductive Technology Registry. *Fertility and Sterility* 66: 697–705.

Souter, I., and Goodwin, T.M. 1998. Decision making in multifetal pregnancy reduction for triplets. *American Journal of Perinatology* 15: 63–71.

LEGAL CITATIONS

Statutory Examples

Fertility Clinic Success Rate and Certification Act of 1992, 42 U.S.C.A. Sec. 263a-1 et seq. Federal legislation that mandates that all Assisted Reproductive Technology (ART) programs annually report their success rates to the Centers for Disease Control and Prevention (CDC), which will then publish clinic-specific success rates. The intent of this legislation is to ensure that the general public has access to accurate, uniformly reported information concerning infertility services.

Two states have passed legislation mandating specific disclosure requirements for the informed consent process of ART:

Virginia Code Ann. Sec. 54.1 - 2971.1 (1997).

New Hampshire Rev. Stat. Ann. Sec. 168-B: I (1995).
New Hampshire also mandates that couples receiving a donor embryo, IVF, or participating in a surrogacy contract first undergo implications counseling, in order to assess their ability to deal with the implications of the procedure. The couple must also provide the physician conducting the procedure with proof of the counseling. (New Hampshire Rev. Stat. Ann. Sec. 168-B:13, 168-B:18 (1995)).

CASE 25

Prenatal Counseling of a Pregnant Woman at Risk for HIV Infection

Lisa is a 27-year-old woman who has recently become pregnant. She has begun to attend a prenatal clinic in a large public hospital, where her medical expenses are covered by Medicaid. The gynecology resident at the clinic has determined that Lisa is at approximately 10 weeks gestation and has assessed her risk of HIV infection and other sexually transmitted diseases (STDs). Lisa's chart indicates that she had previously attended a substance abuse clinic in the hospital. Lisa's husband is still in treatment at that clinic and has "tested positive."

Because the prevalence of HIV infection is high in the population of intravenous drug users using that clinic, the resident counsels Lisa about HIV infection and the risks it would pose to her and her unborn child and asks her if she has been tested for HIV. She says she has not and expresses reluctance to be tested because she "wouldn't want to know." The resident continues to explain the importance of her being aware of her HIV status and that the information would be kept confidential. He then presents her with an informed consent form that she needs to sign prior to having the HIV blood test. "I'm not signing anything," she says. She adds that her husband and she have "safe sex," and she is "not worried."

ISSUES TO CONSIDER

- Prenatal counseling regarding HIV
- Reducing risk of vertical transmission of HIV to newborns

MEDICAL CONSIDERATIONS

1. How effective are "safe sex" practices in reducing the risk of HIV transmission between heterosexual partners?

Although it is difficult to ascertain the actual practices of study subjects, epidemiologic evidence as well as laboratory evidence looking at the efficacy of condoms and other barrier methods of preventing HIV transmission suggest that "safe sex" practices reduce the risk of HIV transmission. Specifically, regular condom use has been shown to effectively prevent transmission of HIV in heterosexual intercourse.[1] If Lisa's sexual contact has been limited to her husband, this has precluded completely "safe sex," as it is not possible to conceive and be certain of avoiding transmission of STD. However, it has been estimated that conception is much more likely per sexual exposure than transmission of HIV. It would be important to know what Lisa's understanding of "safe sex" was—whether this meant the avoidance of what she perceived as unsafe (e.g., anal intercourse) or the regular and correct use of a condom during all sexual encounters.

Recent optimism regarding newer and highly active antiretroviral treatment (HAART), and knowledge that HAART has markedly reduced mortality, could reduce adherence to safe sex practices. Evidence of this has been found in the recent increase in rectal gonorrhea coupled with reduction in condom use in gay men, especially 25 to 34 year olds, raising concerns that HIV incidence could increase as well. Safe sex practices are summarized in the references.[2,3]

2. What are the risks to an HIV-infected mother who goes to term untreated?

Pregnancy is associated with decreased levels of *CD4+* lymphocytes. This leads to a decline in cell-mediated immunity, a resulting "immune tolerance," which presumably is an important factor in enabling the pregnancy to proceed normally. There is controversy over whether this natural decline in *CD4+* cell count accelerates the course of HIV infection and increases maternal mortality. Conflicting studies may reflect differing outcomes related to socioeconomic status, residence in a developing country, or other factors that could affect medical care of HIV. A marked decline in *CD4+* count, which might occur as a result of HIV infection, would be associated with the risk of opportunistic infection (as in any HIV-infected individual), and the need for antiretroviral treatment (ART) and antimicrobial prophylaxis against these infections.

3. What are the short- and long-term risks to her child if she is HIV infected and remains untreated?

There is no conclusive evidence that asymptomatic HIV infection per se results in adverse outcomes of a pregnancy, such as perinatal mortality, premature birth, spontaneous abortion, or low birth weight, although there may be a higher risk in developing countries for reasons stated above. Nonetheless, in subgroups of infants, such as those infected in utero early in the first trimester, there may be a higher risk of growth retardation, malformations, and fetal loss. Treatment of an infected mother to reduce opportunistic infections might require use of potentially teratogenic agents, such as trimethoprim, pentamidine, ganciclovir, ketoconazole, or others.

The most important risk is that of maternal-fetal transmission of HIV. Among infants born in the United States, the overall risk is approximately one in three without antiviral treatment. Maternal-fetal transmission of HIV is believed to occur as the result of transplacental infection or neonatal contact with maternal blood or secretions during parturition. HIV also appears in breast milk and can be transmitted from mother to infant during nursing.

The consequences of untreated antepartum or intrapartum HIV infection are profound. In the United States, the cause mortality of HIV-infected infants has been as high as 15 percent at one year and 50 percent at five years. The five-year mortality is as high as 85 percent in some developing countries. In a 1989 Florida study, symptomatic infection developed in children with perinatally acquired HIV at a median age of 8 months and the median survival from time of diagnosis was 38 months.[4] These figures are likely to change with prenatal prophylaxis and HAART.

In addition to the risks of HIV infection, a child of infected parents, even if born uninfected, would face the possibility of being orphaned at a relatively early age. The consequences of this would depend on the availability and quality of alternate caretakers.

4. How might HIV testing be of benefit to Lisa?

If she were found to be HIV negative, one could be optimistic about the outcome of her pregnancy, although standard HIV testing is sometimes associated with false negative results, especially if exposure was recent. Lisa would then need to be counseled about safe sex techniques in the future. Conception would not be advised, but if she and her husband chose not to take this advice, they would need to be counseled to limit unprotected sexual exposure by use of ovulation detection kits (available without prescription). They would also need to be evaluated and treated for other STDs, which would significantly increase susceptibility to HIV in the noninfected partner and increase viral shedding and thereby infectivity of the infected partner. STDs can also increase HIV viremia, which could accelerate disease progression.

If she were found to be HIV infected, early treatment would be of great benefit for her and her unborn child. Among women with early infection, antiretroviral treatment (ART) during pregnancy and delivery decreases the risk of perinatal transmission by approximately two-thirds, from 22.6 percent to 7.6 percent.[5] A recent study demonstrated that in utero exposure to zidovudine (AZT) produced no adverse effects in HIV-uninfected children born to HIV-infected women when they were followed as long as 5.6 years.[6] Elective cesarean section may further lower the risk of transmission[7]; in patients with early infection, combined elective cesarean section and prenatal, intrapartum, and neonatal ART, it is possible to lower the rate of vertical transmission to 2 percent. There is evidence that ART might produce equal benefit in mothers with more advanced HIV disease. In these women, however, there are other factors to consider, such as potential risks of fetal exposure to antimicrobial agents that prevent opportunistic infections, or unknown fetal risk of combination ART regimens that are currently standard treatment for HIV-infected adults with low *CD4+* cell counts or high viral load. Nonpharmacologic methods to reduce perinatal transmission include avoidance of cigarette smoking and unprotected sex with multiple partners, and, for postnatal care, the avoidance of breast-feeding. Additional advances in preventive ART have recently been reported (see Appendix).

Finally, both Lisa and her infant, if indicated, could receive close follow-up of *CD4+* count and viral load, antimicrobial prophylaxis against opportunistic infections, and other standard therapy, including special immunization schedules for infections of childhood.[8] Lisa should be made aware that HIV treatment is reimbursed by Medicaid and certain other entitlement programs.

5. How does HIV testing differ from other prenatal screening that will be offered to this patient?

Prenatal testing can help guide treatment. Rh status will determine if the mother should receive immune globulin (Rho-GAM) on the birth of an Rh-positive infant, in order to prevent hemolytic disease in a subsequent Rh-positive infant. Active syphilis infection can be treated in order to prevent maternal morbidity and congenital syphilis in the newborn. Rubella titers will determine if the mother is immune; if not, she can be monitored for active infection, and pregnancy termination can be offered if she is infected during a critical time. For a woman who is not yet pregnant, rubella immunization can be given and pregnancy avoided for the few weeks required for immunity to be achieved. Infants of mothers who are hepatitis B virus carriers can receive early treatment with hyperimmune globulin and hepatitis vaccine, substantially reducing the likelihood of subsequent infection. Knowledge of the mother's and her partner's carrier state for autosomal recessive genetic disease, such as sickle-cell or Tay-Sachs disease, might prompt genetic counseling. If the patient is already pregnant, she might want to consider amniocentesis or chorionic villus sampling, if predictive testing is available for the disease in question. The goal might be pregnancy termination if the fetus is found to be affected by the disease (see Case 27, "Tracheoesophageal Fistula in a Newborn with Down Syndrome"), however, continuing advances in medical genetics and assisted reproductive technology are likely to affect such reproductive choices in the future.[9]

HIV testing would likewise provide important medical information, as outlined earlier. Because proper treatment currently reduces but does not eliminate the risk of vertical transmission (and has thus far been validated only in cases when the mother is mildly infected), Lisa might wish to have the pregnancy terminated. This might be a greater consideration if she also were found to have a low *CD4+* cell count and high viral load, a situation in which risk of transmission is greater and safety and efficacy of recommended treatment is less certain.

More than with other forms of testing (with the possible exception of hepatitis B), disclosure of the mother's positive HIV results might lead to employment, housing, insurance, or health care discrimination. Such discrimination has been limited due to judicial rulings and the enactment of laws and regulations in many jurisdictions (see Case 18, "Surgical Delay in a Patient Infected with HIV"). In all states, a separate written informed consent must be obtained from a patient prior to the implementation of an HIV blood test, as was as initiated in this case.

6. When her child is born, he or she will be offered screening for sickle-cell disease, hypothyroidism, phenylketonuria, and other derangements of amino acid metabolism, as mandated by the state; should the child also be tested for HIV?

From a medical perspective, it would be important to know the HIV status of any at-risk newborn. Precise information cannot always be readily obtained, however. Virtually all babies born of HIV-infected mothers carry maternally transmitted immunoglobulin G (IgG) for HIV, and this cannot be distinguished from actual infection for at least 12 to 15 months, when maternal antibody wanes and is lost. Immunoglobulin M determination of HIV infection is not reliable or sensitive at the present time. Viral culture of infant (not cord) blood is sensitive and specific, but culture techniques are laborious, expensive, and generally performed only in large hospitals or academic centers. A highly specific and more rapid determination is the identification of viral DNA sequencing in infant blood using the polymerase chain reaction (PCR), but this technique also requires a highly sophisticated laboratory to ensure accuracy.

If the mother is known to be HIV infected, prophylaxis against maternally acquired HIV should be instituted in the newborn immediately. However, when the mother's HIV status is not known, the most practical approach is to test the newborn for the presence of HIV antibody. If the test is positive, antiretroviral therapy can be initiated, as a positive test indicates maternal infection and the risk of peripartum transmission. Follow up PCR testing would then be done to determine the infant's infection status. Repeat PCR testing might be needed in the first one to four months of life, as viral replication might have been insufficient at birth to be detected in serum.

Currently, mandatory HIV testing of all newborns occurs in one state (New York), and in a few other states (e.g., Indiana) HIV testing of newborns without parental consent is permissible in certain defined circumstances.

ETHICAL AND LEGAL CONSIDERATIONS

1. How aggressively should this patient be counseled regarding the option of being tested for HIV infection?

As the gynecologist has begun to explain, there is a strong possibility that Lisa herself is infected. Thus, there is a significant risk that her current pregnancy could result in an HIV-infected child, who will face serious illness, continuous contact with the medical system, and limited life span, among other tragedies. Is this a risk that Lisa should be permitted to take for her unborn child, particularly given the dramatic decrease in HIV transmission that accompanies the use of ART and other proactive measures in HIV-infected pregnant women?

The incidence of HIV infection in women continues to rise, especially in impoverished urban settings, where a large proportion of residents are members of racial or ethnic minority groups. In some places, AIDS is a leading cause of death among women between the ages of 15 and 47 years, the years of childbearing. Thus, the question of reproductive rights in this infected population has taken on great importance, both in terms of social policy and in terms of the practical consequences of dealing with children who could be infected or could become orphaned.

Counseling women who fit this epidemiologic profile or who are actually pregnant raises some historic concerns, given the racial and socioeconomic makeup of the infected populations. The very women among whom AIDS is most prevalent are those who have historically undergone discrimination because of race or socioeconomic status and suffered coercion regarding their reproductive rights. The ability of women to reproduce has historically been used as justification for controlling their actions, limiting their opportunities, and applying force to their most intimate bodily decisions, such as decisions related to childbearing. For example, in the United States, black women were historically subjected to forced sterilization, and these programs were under way when the eugenics movement was in fashion. The genocidal associations of forced sterilization have thus not been lost on these patient populations, and there is widespread suspicion among many individuals that efforts to influence reproductive decisions among poor and minority women still carry immoral goals.

In general, there are two schools of thought concerning the nature of counseling that should be given to pregnant women regarding genetic or other types of tests that may have implications for their newborns. One school of thought asserts that counseling should be value neutral, or nondirective. Nondirective counseling would provide the woman with as much accurate information as possible concerning her risks, her options, and the implications of her choices, so that whatever decision she makes will be the result of a fully informed consent process. No one will try to make the decision for the patient; the ultimate decision will be the woman's. Arguments in favor of nondirective counseling are based on advances in genetic screening possibilities, which often carry uncertain implications, coupled with legal and social policy recognition of a woman's right to control her own reproductive decisions.

Directive counseling, in contrast, would provide the woman with the same sort of information that she would receive during nondirective counseling, but it would incorporate persuasive reasoning concerning what direction the woman should take. Directive counseling would suggest, even strongly recommend, specific options to the patient based on the counselor's judgment that certain outcomes are undesirable, such as a possible one-in-three risk of transmitting HIV to the fetus if the pregnant woman is not treated for her HIV. Although directive counseling is not coercive in the sense that it could not force a woman into a specific course, there is concern that the lines between persuasion and coercion are sometimes difficult to draw, particularly for vulnerable populations who may not even realize that the choice is ultimately theirs to make. Arguments in favor of directive counseling cite the long-term public health advantages of eliminating perinatal transmission HIV, particularly given recent medical advances.

Due to the dramatic changes in HIV treatment options that have developed over the last several years, and the ability to markedly reduce the risk of HIV transmission from mother to child, the decisional framework concerning testing for HIV during pregnancy has been sharply altered as well. Federal guidelines now recommend *universal* counseling for HIV testing of all pregnant women, regardless of their geographic, ethnic, or socioeconomic background. In fact, it is now considered to be part of the standard of prenatal care to counsel all pregnant women about the benefits of HIV testing, given the enormous opportunity to lessen if not eliminate perinatal HIV transmission. A recent report from the Institute of Medicine even goes so far as to recommend that HIV testing become a routine part of the panoply of testing utilized for all pregnant women, so that women should be advised that HIV testing is now routine and the norm for pregnant women. While women would still have the option to refuse such testing, the burden would fall on them to do so, rather than presenting them with the more value-neutral option to consider the possibility of HIV testing for themselves.

Such strong, directive counseling is a dramatic departure from the practices that were in place just a few years ago, prior to current understanding of the dramatic impact of new treatment options on both HIV transmission and containment of viral load and infection. In this case, the push for strong, directive counseling, even to the incorporation of such testing as part of standard practice, has followed dramatic medical advances. While there is continued concern that women make an informed, voluntary decision to undergo HIV testing, given the potential implications that HIV infection may have for their own health and personal lives, there is felt to be clear justification to now strongly and persuasively convince pregnant women that the benefits of HIV testing during pregnancy outweigh the possible risks that may follow a positive test result.

Some studies show that a significant percentage of surveyed physicians so strongly favor prenatal HIV testing that they would support the mandatory implementation of such testing for all pregnant women. The American Medical Association has also endorsed mandatory HIV testing for all pregnant women. Few states, however, have legislated such a mandatory program, and it is unclear whether such mandatory testing would survive constitutional challenge, given the strong legal support women have attained over the years for reproductive freedom and nondiscrimination based on gender. Mandatory testing for all pregnant women would also have to survive scrutiny under a "least restrictive alternative" constitutional analysis (see Case 17, "A House-Bound Woman with Tuberculosis").

Thus, in this situation, the resident's actions to strongly counsel the patient regarding the benefits to be gained through HIV testing were probably justifiable and in accord with what is now considered standard of care for pregnant women. While the resident must ultimately accept Lisa's choice not to be tested, he most certainly would want to explore with her now, and in subsequent visits, why she "wouldn't want to know" her HIV status. It would be critical to ascertain that her refusal was informed and accurately reflected the potential risks she might face as a result of a positive test. Future clinic appointments would provide opportunity to continue to probe the issue, if necessary, though certainly prenatal care should in no way be contingent upon her desire to be tested or not.

From a legal perspective, the resident should carefully document the circumstances of the counseling and Lisa's refusal, as well as subsequent efforts to encourage her to be tested. While no case law yet exists, it is theoretically possible that a physician who failed to adequately counsel a patient, and whose patient ultimately gave birth to an HIV-infected baby, could face liability charges as a result. Certainly as counseling for HIV testing becomes routine practice in obstetric care, a physician who fails to provide such counseling would court some legal risks in the event an HIV-infected child was born.

2. What nonmedical factors might be contributing to Lisa's desire not to be tested?

While enormous benefit would accrue to Lisa's fetus if, by chance, Lisa were found to be HIV positive and began treatment during pregnancy, there continue to be certain risks associated with positive HIV test results.

For example, access to sensitive, timely care, particularly for pregnant women and especially in the context of possible substance abuse, is still problematic for many women. Such women may fear legal repercussions or discrimination in their receipt of care (see Case 26, "A Pregnant Woman Using Cocaine"). Despite assurances of confidentiality, Lisa may appropriately fear a positive test result could lead to discriminatory consequences in terms of housing, employment, or access to care. She might also fear the stigma that might be associated with her child's care if the child were known to be HIV positive.[10]

Furthermore, while the HIV status of Lisa's husband is unknown, it is possible that a determination that she is HIV positive could have significant, perhaps even harmful, consequences in her personal life. Partner notification and contact tracing is now the norm in the context of HIV in many states (see Case 16, "A Married Man Contracts Syphilis"), and Lisa may fear her husband's reaction to her HIV status. A correlation between substance abuse, HIV status, and physical violence has been substantiated in the literature. It is possible Lisa may fear for her physical safety. There may also be legitimate fears of abandonment or isolation as a result of HIV positivity, which would be particularly traumatic, given her pregnancy and concerns about her own health as well as that of the baby's.

Finally, given the often alien, chaotic, and time-pressured environment of a public clinic, as well as the lack of an established relationship with her care providers, Lisa may lack the trust and comfort necessary to support such a momentous decision as determining HIV status. In time, with individually sensitive counseling and support, she may come to determine that the benefits of testing to her fetus outweigh her concerns for herself following an HIV test.

3. Could Lisa prevent HIV testing of her child at birth?

Controversy surrounding HIV testing of newborns has heightened in recent years as federal legislation has created strong incentives for states to reduce perinatal transmission and medical advances have underscored the value of early intervention.

In 1996, federal legislation reauthorizing the Ryan White Act (providing states with millions of dollars to fund AIDS-related services) mandated that states must achieve certain outcomes by the date of March 2000, or risk losing such federal funds. Specifically, each state must demonstrate that it has done one of the following:

1. Reduced the level of new AIDS cases as a result of perinatal transmission by 50 percent of its 1993 rate;
2. Achieved an HIV testing rate of at least 95 percent among women receiving prenatal care in the state; or
3. Implemented mandatory HIV testing for all newborns whose mothers were not tested for HIV prenatally.

States unable to document any of these outcomes risk losing federal financial support for AIDS services.

Some states have already mandated newborn HIV testing. New York became the first state to implement mandatory HIV testing for all newborns, regardless of parental consent. By implication, this means that all new mothers in New York will receive notice of their own HIV status, whether or not they wish to be tested themselves. Other states are beginning to consider and implement similar mandates. For example, Indiana recently implemented a law that permits physicians to test newborns without maternal consent, within 48 hours of birth, if the physician believes it is "medically necessary." Such a discretionary option does leave open the potential that HIV testing will be implemented on a discriminatory basis.

Thus, depending on the state where Lisa gives birth, and her decision as to whether or not to be tested during pregnancy, it is possible that her baby might be tested, despite her refusal, after birth. For additional consideration of parental decision making concerning newborns, see Case 27.

Finally, if her baby were tested and found to be HIV positive, there is a theoretical risk that Lisa might be legally liable in some way for the resulting HIV infection in her newborn. While such liability has yet to be found for the transmission of HIV, there have been cases of criminal charges being filed, and liability found, for maternal use of illegal substances that results in the birth of a child with positive drug toxicologies. Case 26 that follows examines this arena of maternal responsibility and liability.

REFERENCES

1. I. DeVincenzi, "A Longitudinal Study of Human Immunodeficiency Virus Transmission by Heterosexual Partners," *New England Journal of Medicine* 331 (1994): 341–346.

2. Public Health Service Task Force, "Recommendations for the Use of Antiretroviral Drugs in Pregnant Women Infected with HIV-1 for Maternal Health and for Reducing Perinatal HIV-1 Transmission in the United States," *Morbidity and Mortality Weekly Report* 47 (RR-2)(1998): 1–30.

3. Z. Stein et al., "Safer Sex Strategies for Women: The Hierarchical Model in Methadone Treatment Clinics," *Journal of Urban Health* 76 (1999): 62–72.

4. G.B. Scott et al., "Survival in Children with Perinatally Acquired Human Immunodeficiency Virus Type I Infection," *New England Journal of Medicine* 321 (1989): 1791–1796.

5. R.S. Sperling et al., "Maternal Viral Load, Zidovudine Treatment, and the Risk of Transmission of Human Immunodeficiency Virus Type 1 from Mother to Infant," *New England Journal of Medicine* 335 (1996): 1621–1629.

6. M. Culnane et al., "Lack of Long-Term Effects of In Utero Exposure to Zidovudine among Uninfected Children Born to HIV-Infected Women," *Journal of the American Medical Association* 281 (1999): 151–157.

7. The International Perinatal HIV Group, "The Mode of Delivery and the Risk of Vertical Transmission of Human Immunodeficiency Virus Type 1—A Meta-Analysis of 15 Prospective Cohort Studies," *New England Journal of Medicine* 340 (1999): 977–987.

8. American Academy of Pediatrics. Committee on Pediatric AIDS, "Evaluation and Medical Treatment of the HIV-Exposed Infant," *Pediatrics* 99 (1997): 909–917.

9. K. Xu et al., "First Unaffected Pregnancy Using Preimplantation Genetic Diagnosis for Sickle-Cell Anemia," *Journal of the American Medical Association* 281 (1999): 1701–1706.

10. B.W. Levin et al., "Treatment Choice for Infants in the Neonatal Intensive Care Unit at Risk for AIDS," *Journal of the American Medical Association* 265 (1991): 2976–2981.

SUGGESTED READINGS

Armstrong, A. et al. 1993. Breast-feeding during primary maternal human immunodeficiency virus infection and risk of transmission from mother to infant. *Journal of Infectious Disease* 167: 441–444.

Bedimo, A.L. et al. 1998. Reproductive choices among HIV positive women. *Social Science and Medicine* 46: 171–179.

Chervenak, F.A., and McCullough, L.B. 1996. Common ethical dilemmas encountered in the management of HIV-infected women and newborns. *Clinical Obstetrics and Gynecology* 39: 411–419.

Condoms for prevention of sexually transmitted diseases. 1998. *Morbidity and Mortality Weekly Report* 37, no. 9: 133–137.

Dula, A. 1992. Yes, there are African-American perspectives on bioethics. In *African-American Perspectives on Biomedical Ethics,* eds. H.E. Flack and E.D. Pellegrino, 193–203. Washington, DC: George Washington University Press.

The European Collaborative Study. 1991. Children born to women with HIV-1 infection: Natural history and risk of transmission. *Lancet* 337: 253–260.

Faden, R.R., and Kass, N.E., eds. 1996. *HIV, AIDS, and childbearing: Public policy, private lives.* New York: Oxford University Press.

Indiana's newborn testing law, as cited. 1998. *Journal of Clinical Ethics* 9: 324.

Lester, P. et al. 1995. The consequences of a positive prenatal HIV antibody test for women. *Journal of Acquired Immune Deficiency Syndrome and Human Retrovirology* 10: 341–349.

Louvorn, A.E. et al. 1997. HIV testing of pregnant women: A policy analysis. *Journal of Public Health Policy* 18: 401–432.

Minkoff, H., and O'Sullivan, M.J. 1998. The case for rapid HIV testing during labor. *Journal of the American Medical Association* 279: 1743–1744.

Minkoff, L. et al. 1990. Pregnancy outcomes among mothers infected with human immunodeficiency virus and uninfected control subjects. *American Journal of Obstetrics and Gynecology.* 163: 1598–1604.

Nakashima, A.K. et al. 1998. Effect of HIV reporting by name on use of HIV testing in publicly funded counseling and testing programs. *Journal of the American Medical Association* 280: 1421–1426.

New York Department of Health, Maternal-Pediatric HIV Prevention and Care Program. 1997. *HIV counseling and testing of newborns as part of the Comprehensive Newborn Testing Program,* 97–102. Albany: New York Dept. of Health Maternal-Pediatric HIV Prevention and Care Program.

Panossian, A.A. et al. 1998. Criminalization of perinatal HIV transmission. *Journal of Legal Medicine* 19: 223–255.

Rogers, M.F. 1997. Epidemiology of HIV/AIDS in women and children in the USA. *Acta Paediatrica Supplement* 421: 15–16.

Rothenberg, K.H. et al. 1995. Domestic violence and partner notification: Implications for treatment and counseling of women with HIV. *Journal of the American Medical Women's Association* 50, nos. 3 and 4: 87–93.

Ryder, R.W. et al. 1989. Perinatal transmission of the human immunodeficiency virus type I to infants of seropositive women in Zaire. *New England Journal of Medicine* 320: 1637–1642.

Schneider, C.E. 1997. Testing, testing. *Hastings Center Report* 27, no. 4: 22–23.

Segal, A.I. 1996. Physician attitudes toward human immunodeficiency virus testing in pregnancy. *American Journal of Obstetrics and Gynecology* 174: 1750–1755.

Selton, D.L. 1966. Is it the time . . . to require that all pregnant women undergo HIV testing to protect their unborn children? Despite concerns over confidentiality and privacy, clinical advances seem to be pushing that way. *American Medical News,* 2 September.

Sprauve, NE. 1996. Substance abuse and HIV pregnancy. *Clinical Obstetrics and Gynecology* 39: 316–332.

St. Louis, M.E. et al. 1993. Risk for perinatal HIV-I transmission according to maternal immunologic, virologic, and placental factors. *Journal of the American Medical Association* 269: 2853–2859.

Stoto, M.A., ed. 1999. Reducing the odds: Preventing perinatal transmission of HIV in the United States. Washington, DC: National Academy Press (from the Committee on Perinatal Transmission of HIV, Institute of Medicine, and Board on Children, Youth, and Families, National Research Council).

Success in implementing Public Health Service guidelines to reduce perinatal transmission of HIV—Louisiana, Michigan, New Jersey, and South Carolina 1993, 1995, and 1996. 1998. *Morbidity and Mortality Weekly Report* 47, no. 33: 688–691.

Temmerman, M. et al. 1990. Infection with HIV as a risk factor for adverse obstetrical outcome. *AIDS* 4: 1087–1093.

Update: Perinatally acquired HIV/AIDS—United States. 1997. *Morbidity and Mortality Weekly Report* 46: 1086–1092.

U.S. Public Health Service recommendations for human immunodeficiency virus counseling and voluntary testing for pregnant women. 1995. *Morbidity and Mortality Weekly Report* 44 (RR-7): 1–15.

Zierler, S. 1996. Sexual violence against women living with or at risk for HIV infection. *American Journal of Preventive Medicine* 12: 304–310.

LEGAL CITATIONS

Case Example

Dunn v. White, 880 F.2d 1188 (10th Cir. 1989).
Mandatory HIV testing does not violate a prisoner's rights under the First or Fourth Amendment to the Constitution.

Statutory Example

U.S. Federal Law: 42 U.S.C. Sec. 300ff-34 (1996).
Federal law mandating that states must adopt the Centers for Disease Control (CDC) guidelines recommending HIV counseling and testing for all pregnant women. If federally set targets for the reduction of perinatal transmission are not then met, mandatory measures regarding HIV testing will ensue.

CASE 26

A Pregnant Woman Using Cocaine

Sandra, a young mother, habitually uses cocaine and has abused other illicit drugs in the past. She has now become pregnant and visits a local clinic where she receives prenatal care. On a recent visit, analysis of her urine revealed cocaine exposure even though she has stated that she is no longer using cocaine. Her obstetrician advised her to stop using cocaine because it will harm her fetus. Sandra mentioned that her other baby is "normal," and adds, "I hardly ever use cocaine."

A few weeks later Sandra takes her two-year-old son to the pediatric clinic at the same hospital to be treated for an ear infection. When the pediatrician becomes aware of Sandra's pregnancy, he calls the prenatal clinic. He urges the obstetrician in charge of Sandra's care to take action. A pregnant woman who is knowingly going to harm a developing fetus with cocaine use should be incarcerated, he says, and if this patient refuses to give up her habit, she should be reported to the district attorney's office. The obstetrician replies that he shares the pediatrician's concern but that they have no authority to do this, it would be a violation of patient confidentiality, and if "doctors went around reporting pregnant women, no one would seek out prenatal care."

ISSUES TO CONSIDER

- Conflicts between maternal and fetal interests
- Physician obligations in the context of illicit drug use

MEDICAL CONSIDERATIONS

1. What is the effect of a mother's cocaine use on the fetus?

Use of cocaine by a pregnant woman has a wide range of health consequences for the developing fetus. Cocaine is a powerful vasoconstrictor and this produces uteroplacental vasoconstriction, which reduces nutrient delivery to the fetus and produces fetal anoxia.

Although there is some disagreement among the various reported studies, maternal cocaine use appears to be associated with an increased rate of stillbirth, spontaneous abortion, abruptio placentae, prematurity, and low birth weight. There is an increased risk of sudden infant death syndrome (SIDS) in newborns whose mothers have used crack cocaine during pregnancy. Major developmental abnormalities have been described, but these do not occur in the vast majority of exposed babies.

During the neonatal period, there may be transient abnormalities in metabolism and cardiovascular physiology, and evidence of fetal distress, such as low Apgar scores and meconium staining. Neonatal neurotoxicity has been widely described; signs range from subtle to dramatic, and include tremulousness, irritability, decreased interactive behavior, muscular hypertonia, and even seizures. Neonatal neurotoxicity may be transient, but there is increasing evidence that some problems may be long lasting. Recent observations of "crack babies" from the ages of three to five years show attention deficits, poor social interaction, and flat affect of mood. IQ in school age children may be affected only a little if at all by prenatal exposure to cocaine, and it is not surprising that Sandra's first child appears "normal." Behavioral changes may occur, however, that cannot be explained by disruptive aspects of the home environment.[1]

Despite these reports, there is controversy over the precise extent of damage that cocaine produces in the fetus. For example, there is uncertainty over whether moderate or sporadic use of the drug produces any significant harm. The uncertainty is related to confounding variables in subjects of controlled studies, not the least of which is that drug-abusing women often are engaged in polydrug use, so that it is difficult to ferret out precise information about each individual drug. In addition, there are indirect problems associated with drug abuse that can affect the developing fetus and living children. These include poverty, homelessness, and maternal medical problems, such as seizure disorders, sexually transmitted disease, endocarditis, HIV, and other serious infections.[2] A patient who refused to discontinue drug use during a pregnancy is unlikely to discontinue use after the baby is born. Cocaine is transmitted in breast milk, which can cause cocaine toxicity in the infant. Cocaine intoxication has occurred in children from homes where the drug is used, presumably because of accidental ingestion.

2. How will the patient's prenatal care be affected if her drug use is reported to the authorities?

Treating Sandra's drug use as a criminal matter would require a breach of confidentiality. As her obstetrician has stated, this approach might discourage drug-abusing women from seeking prenatal care. Prenatal care in drug abusers has been shown to affect the outcome of the pregnancy positively. A substantial proportion who are shown by urine or meconium testing to have used cocaine deny that they have used it[3]; it is conceivable that the fear of criminal prosecution might discourage these women from continuing their doctor's visits entirely.

In addition to obtaining routine prenatal care and counseling, drug abusing women can gain specific benefits from targeted care, which might include serial screening for drug use, and for infectious disease, such as hepatitis, HIV, syphilis, and other sexually transmitted diseases that are known to occur more frequently in drug-abusing patients, and which might adversely affect the neonate. Such patients might also obtain referral to drug rehabilitation and specialized support services, which have been shown to positively affect the outcome.[4]

3. How would the situation differ if the mother were abusing heroin? Alcohol? Nicotine?

In addition to the expected secondary effects of substance abuse, alcohol, heroin, and other drugs may adversely affect the fetus. Maternal use of heroin and methadone have also been associated with a neonatal abstinence syndrome, characterized by withdrawal symptoms approximately 72 hours or more after birth. The effects of maternal use of marijuana on the fetus are controversial, although there is evidence of a slight but insignificant decrease in birth weight for gestational age. Overall, there appear to be no serious effects on the fetus, but it is difficult to reach definite conclusions about the effect based on studies in humans, which are confounded by variables such as multiple substance abuse and variable methods of marijuana ingestion. Detailed reviews of these subjects are found among the suggested readings.

Because use of alcohol or nicotine is not illegal, these substances tend to be more socially acceptable and are perhaps deemed less harmful by patients, including pregnant women. However, alcohol has potentially severe teratogenic effects (fetal alcohol syndrome). Risk of mental and physical defects is dose dependent; severe damage to the fetus generally is associated with heavy drinking, but some damage is possible when a pregnant woman ingests only two drinks per day (one drink is equivalent to 12 ounces of beer, 4 ounces of wine, or 1.2 ounces of 80-proof liquor).[5] Cigarette smoking has been associated with a higher than expected incidence of low birth weight for gestational age, prematurity, spontaneous abortion, abruptio placentae, placenta previa, ectopic pregnancy, SIDS, and perhaps childhood cancer. In addition to increased infant deaths, the long-term health consequences of smoking may be substantial, if one takes into consideration only the problems associated with low birth weight (see Case 24, "Assisted Reproduction in a Woman with Strong Religious Beliefs"). Moreover, passive smoking is known to have adverse effects on others, which would include the neonate and members of the household. Despite widely publicized information on these adverse consequences, many heavy smokers may be unable to discontinue their habit during pregnancy.

ETHICAL AND LEGAL CONSIDERATIONS

1. To what extent can Sandra's physicians or others intervene in order to protect her developing fetus?

A woman in the United States is given wide-ranging authority over the progress of her pregnancy, at least until the fetus has achieved the maturity to be viable outside of the mother. While physicians may view the pregnancy as encompassing two patients, and the state clearly has an interest in the production of healthy citizens-to-be, this does not automatically give physicians or the state the authority *over* the woman if her actions risk negatively affecting or influencing the developing fetus. Physicians can try to persuade a pregnant patient to avoid activities that may be harmful to the fetus, but it becomes another matter whether inability or unwillingness to heed this medical advice should then merit a coercive or punitive response using the state's police powers, for example.

Before considering whether anyone should have coercive authority over Sandra, the interests of the state need to be more closely examined, for it is the state that would be granting such authority. While there is clear constitutional law that the interests in reproductive freedom of the woman outweigh the state's interests in fetal life and health during the first two trimesters of pregnancy, thus limiting the state's ability to regulate abortions, this does not negate the state's interest in the production of a healthy fetus, an interest that lasts *throughout* the pregnancy. The state may act on this interest in certain ways, such as the positive, nonrestrictive actions of providing free prenatal care or posting warnings concerning the harm caused by alcohol or cigarettes during pregnancy. Whether or not the state can cross the line, however, from positive steps of encouragement to negative steps of restriction or punishment, is an evolving area of the law.

There is some precedent for court intervention during a pregnancy to try to protect a fetus against the wishes of the mother. For example, the courts have addressed this in cases in which doctors, believing the fetus to be at risk, have obtained court authority for forced cesareans. In one Georgia case (*Jefferson v. Spaulding*), the fetus was believed to be at risk but the patient refused to undergo a cesarean section. The physician succeeded in obtaining a court order to deliver the baby by cesarean and the mother was detained in the hospital, but subsequently went into labor and delivered a healthy child vaginally. This case vividly illustrates the reality of diagnostic uncertainty and casts doubt on the argument that the physician should be infused with any authority that might impose severe restrictions on civil liberties.

Some have suggested that a woman such as Sandra should be incarcerated, if, despite education and warning, she continues to engage in illicit drug use that could harm her developing fetus. Although this action would stem from beneficent motives toward the fetus, it would be an extreme use of state authority and difficult to support legally, particularly in light of the obligation to employ the least restrictive and most effective measure to achieve the desired goal (see Case 17, "A House-Bound Woman with Tuberculosis"). While there have been a very few isolated cases of attempts to legally intervene *during* pregnancy, such an attempt and its constitutionality would be very difficult to uphold if other measures had not been tried first. For example, in Sandra's case mere referral to a drug program would have a low chance of success. Few drug treatment programs admit pregnant women because of fears about liability, and entrance into those that do may be long delayed because of extensive waiting lists. It would be difficult to justify incarceration of a pregnant woman when voluntary therapeutic alternatives are not even available to her.

On the other hand, if there were evidence that Sandra resisted serious efforts to assist her in abstaining from drug use, it might be argued that more coercive measures could be employed. Moreover, if the state concern, based on physician warning, is that many activities beyond illicit drug use harm the fetus, then it might be logical to extend coercive measures to those activities. Because more harm can be done to the fetus in the first trimester than in subsequent months, one could argue that coercive measures could be applied even before high risk behavior became egregious, perhaps even before pregnancy. Registration of all women of child-bearing age, and monitoring their behavior for the benefit of producing a healthy fetus, might not be an illogical extension of such reasoning. Obviously, the problem with such elevation of fetal interests is that the interests of the woman carrying the fetus become secondary to those of the person-to-be, whose interests are not yet, in fact, legally akin to those of a born person. Extreme measures to produce unharmed babies could cause substantial harm to the life of an already existing person and would harm fundamental notions of liberty accorded to all persons, whether or not they are pregnant. In view of the uncertain nature of fetal harm, it cannot accurately be predicted whether or not a given mother's drug use would harm the fetus and to what extent. This uncertainty would have to be weighed against potential harm to fundamental principles of civil liberty that extend beyond Sandra to society as a whole.

Even if incarceration were used, it is uncertain that this would achieve the goal of having a healthy baby. There is more uncertainty regarding fetal harm from exogenous substance exposure in the third trimester than earlier in pregnancy, and it might well take that long to prove that the patient's behavior was resistant to all efforts. One woman in South Carolina was convicted of child endangerment charges for crack-cocaine use during pregnancy and she is now serving an eight-year sentence for this conviction. More broadly, since 1985, 240 women in 35 states have been criminally prosecuted for illicit substance use or alcohol use during pregnancy. While most of these prosecutions have not resulted in civil or criminal liability, they do reflect an evolving societal tension between respect for the pregnant woman's autonomy and desire to inflict punitive measures in individual cases, as well as to provide a deterrent to future potential offenders.

Because of the difficulties of elevating fetal interests to legally recognized interests of living citizens, prosecutors have resorted to unusual legal ploys. For example, new mothers have been charged with delivery of drugs to a minor, via the umbilical cord, moments after the child's birth. These charges have been based on laws that were originally intended to apply to drug traffickers. In one case (*Johnson v. State of Florida*), a woman was convicted under such a charge, but the Florida Supreme Court overturned the conviction. Although not denying that the drugs might have been harmful to the fetus, the court held that use of such a law to apply to fetuses or newborns was not contemplated when the law was enacted, and its use in such a case was clearly to deter other pregnant women from drug use, rather than to produce a healthy child in that particular case. As with many of these sorts of converted uses of existing laws, application of the law after the fact and in unintended ways does not achieve the state interest in producing a healthy child. Such use of a law might deter some women from drug use during pregnancy, and it certainly punishes those who have done so, but it is just as likely to deter more women from seeking prenatal care because of concern about the legal consequences for themselves. Thus, coercive actions could be counterproductive rather than promoting the goal of helping women to produce the healthiest fetus possible. In an Ohio case, *Cox v. Court*, a trial court was able to obtain an order to place a drug-using woman in protective custody *during* pregnancy, in order to protect the fetus. This judgment was overturned on appeal.

Similarly, attempts to equate potential harm to the fetus with child abuse have been mostly unsuccessful, since the fetus does not have the legal status of a child. The authority of the state in matters of child abuse is itself limited and generally confined to cases in which the possibility of real harm to the child exists. Given the uncertainty over the effects of drug use on the fetus, coupled with the fetus' lack of personhood on which to base assertions of legal rights, physicians and the state would be unlikely to successfully stop a woman's activities on the grounds of child abuse. There have been cases of attempts to remove the child at birth because of the mother's drug use during pregnancy. In a Connecticut case, *In re Valerie D.*, the court, consistent with other cases in its line of reasoning, refused to accord the fetus-now-baby the same legal status as a child, and thus was unwilling to cut off parental rights for actions taken *during* pregnancy. At this time, several states do have on their books laws which impose civil penalties, including the possibility of termination of parental rights, in situations where prenatal substance abuse is found to be so egregious as to constitute evidence of child neglect after the birth of the child. Thus, it is unlikely Sandra's obstetrician could instigate charges over her actions during the pregnancy based on any theory of child abuse. If the pediatrician or any physician had evidence that Sandra neglected or abused her two-year-old child, that might constitute grounds to take action against her, but on behalf of the child already existing rather than the fetus yet to be born.

In some jurisdictions (New York City, for example), health department regulations require drug testing of newborns, and positive results lead to a further examination of the mother's fitness to care for the child. Such drug use does not itself constitute justification to cut off parental rights, and any coercive action taken against the mother could only follow after a hearing with all due process protections in place to make sure the mother was treated fairly. Again, while coercion could prevent future harm to a now-born child and could in some instances deter women from drug use during pregnancy, it might well cause those most in need of help to avoid prenatal care and counseling. Since the ultimate goal is a healthy child, what must be considered are the most effective measures to achieve that without infringing the woman's fundamental liberty interests.

2. What are the physician's legal obligations in this case?

There is no doubt that illicit drug use is a monumental social, medical, and economic problem in the United States, and an individual practitioner faced with a drug-abusing patient may well feel an obligation to act forcefully. If Sandra's doctors treated her drug use as more than a medical problem and reported to the authorities information learned through the patient-physician encounter, this could constitute a significant breach of the confidentiality that is considered essential to the integrity and success of the relationship. As discussed in Case 16 ("A Married Man Contracts Syphilis"), there are certain legally upheld exceptions to this confidentiality obligation. In most states use of illicit drugs does not fall into these categories. Information concerning drug use is considered highly confidential because of the potential harm caused if this information is released into the wrong hands and because of a strong societal interest in encouraging those with drug problems to seek out help and not to be inhibited by fear of disclosure. Despite these interests, several states have now passed legislation mandating that physicians and other clinicians report positive maternal toxicologies to child protective authorities.

The history of abusive use of medical records by law enforcement officials against drug users led to the 1970 federal Comprehensive Alcohol Abuse and Alcoholism Prevention, Treatment and Rehabilitation Act, followed in 1972 by the Drug Abuse Office and Treatment Act.[6] The purpose of this legislation was to ensure the confidentiality of records dealing with such behaviors and their treatment. These acts, and their accompanying regulations, outline strong prohibitions against the revelation of any information concerning patients *treated* for drug or alcohol use. For example, it is more difficult to obtain records from drug treatment centers than from other medical areas, providers are required to use enhanced measures to ensure security, and these records are not generally susceptible to subpoena. Limited exceptions regarding access to records exist in situations in which a patient has committed a crime or a patient has a medical emergency.

Such protections may not cover patients who are being treated for conditions unrelated to drug use, but who also have drug problems. Thus, Sandra's medical records in the obstetrics clinic are not subject to the same restrictions as they might be in a drug treatment center, even though drug use might be mentioned in her medical record. These protections do underscore the general societal policy that when patients with drug problems are under a physician's care, such problems should be viewed as medical problems rather than illegal activities warranting state intervention. It is in the state's interests that patients troubled by substance abuse seek help for their problems and not be discouraged by the threat of legal intervention, or out of fear that information might be disclosed to a potential employer or others who would discriminate. Thus, Sandra's physician should not "take action" by reporting her to the authorities on the basis of her drug use, unless required to do so under state law, with requisite proof.

3. Under what authority was Sandra tested for cocaine?

Accordingly, the question may then arise as to whether patients may be tested for drug use without their permission. Because physicians in most states have no authority to report pregnant patients with drug problems, a medical justification would be needed to test Sandra.

Testing Sandra would provide *her* with no more information than she already has—namely, that she uses cocaine. The physician should be able to explain the risks to the patient rather than set up an adversarial relationship or take actions without her consent that might be to her detriment. Thus, Sandra's physician should counsel her about drug use as part of her prenatal care and could suggest that she be screened for other harmful substances. If she refused to be tested, the physician would likely have neither the authority nor additional medical justification to proceed with testing in this situation. He might, however, have such authority if there were evidence of harm to a vulnerable third party, for example, if Sandra's two-year-old showed evidence of cocaine exposure, presumably from accidental ingestion of cocaine in the home. Even so, in such a case, the obligation of the physician would be based on mandatory reporting of suspected child abuse. In a true emergency, however, such as a case of drug overdose, diagnostic information available by drug testing might save the patient's life or prevent serious harm, and in such a case testing would be justifiable despite a lack of consent.

REFERENCES

1. I.J. Chasnoff et al., "Prenatal Exposure to Cocaine and Other Drugs. Outcome at Four to Six Years," *Annals of the New York Academy of Sciences* 846 (1998): 314–328.
2. C.E. Cherubin and J.D. Sapira, "The Medical Complications of Drug Addiction and the Medical Assessment of the Intravenous Drug User: 25 Years Later," *Annals of Internal Medicine* 119 (1993): 1017–1028.
3. E.M. Ostrea et al., "Mortality within the First 2 Years in Infants Exposed to Cocaine, Opiate, or Cannabinoid during Gestation," *Pediatrics* 100 (1997): 79–83.
4. G. Burkett et al., "Prenatal Care in Cocaine-Exposed Pregnancies," *Obstetrics and Gynecology* 92 (1998): 193–200.
5. I.J. Chasnoff, ed., "Chemical Dependency in Pregnancy," *Clinics in Perinatology* 18 (1991): 1–191.
6. M. McDonald et al., "Special Issues Involving Highly Confidential Information," in *Health Care Law: A Practical Guide* (New York: Matthew Bender & Co., 1991).

SUGGESTED READINGS

American Academy of Pediatrics. Committee on Substance Abuse and Committee on Children with Disabilities. 1993. Fetal alcohol syndrome and fetal alcohol effects. *Pediatrics* 91: 1004–1006.

American Academy of Pediatrics, Committee on Substance Abuse. 1995. Drug-exposed infants (RE9533). *Pediatrics* 96: 364–367.

Bibb, K.W. et al. 1995. Drug screening in newborns and mothers using meconium samples, paired urine samples, and interviews. *Journal of Perinatology* 15: 199–202.

Campbell, D.E., and Fleischman, A.R. 1992. Ethical challenges in medical care for the pregnant substance abuser. *Clinical Obstetrics and Gynecology* 35: 803–811.

Chavkin, W. 1991. Mandatory treatment for drug use during pregnancy. *Journal of the American Medical Association* 266: 1556–1561.

Chavkin, W. et al. 1998. National survey of the states: Policies and practices regarding drug-using pregnant women. *American Journal of Public Health* 88: 117–119.

Chavkin, W. et al. 1998. Policies towards pregnancy and addiction. Sticks without carrots. *Annals of the New York Academy of Sciences* 846: 335–340.

Chervenak, F.A., and McCullough, L.B. 1996. The fetus as a patient: An essential ethical concept for maternal-fetal medicine. *Journal of Maternal and Fetal Medicine* 5: 115–119.

Condon, J.T., and Hilton, C.A. 1988. A comparison of smoking and drinking behaviours in pregnant women: Who abstains and why. *Medical Journal of Australia* 148: 381–385.

Kandall, S.R., and Chavkin, W. 1992. Illicit drugs in America: History, impact on women and infants, and treatment strategies for women. *Hastings Law Journal* 43: 615–643.

Marwick, C. 1998. Challenging report on pregnancy and drug abuse. *Journal of the American Medical Association* 280: 1040–1041.

Oberman, M. 1992. Sex, drugs, pregnancy and the law: Rethinking the problems of pregnant women who use drugs. *Hastings Law Journal* 43: 505–548.

Schwartz, R.H. 1988. Urine testing in the detection of drugs of abuse. *Archives of Internal Medicine* 148: 2407–2412.

Stjernfeldt, M. et al. 1986. Maternal smoking during pregnancy and risk of childhood cancer. *Lancet* 1: 1350–1352.

Surgeon General. 1983. *The Health Consequences of Smoking for Women: A Report of the Surgeon General.* U.S. Dept. of Health and Human Services. Publication No. 410-889/1284. Washington, DC: U.S. Government Printing Office, 191–249.

Volpe, J.J. 1992. Effect of cocaine use on the fetus. *New England Journal of Medicine* 327: 399–407.

Woods, J.R., ed. 1998. Substance abuse in pregnancy. *Obstetrics and Gynecology Clinics of North America* 25, no. 1: 1–272.

Zimmer, L., and Morgan, J.P. 1997. *Marijuana myths. Marijuana facts. A review of the scientific evidence.* New York and San Francisco: The Lindesmith Center.

LEGAL CITATIONS

Case Examples

Ashley v. Florida, WL 674215 (Fla. 1997).
Manslaughter and murder charges were brought against a 19-year-old woman after she shot herself in the stomach after failing to obtain an abortion. The charges were ultimately dropped. Because state law prohibited Medicaid funds from paying for abortion, the patient was unable to secure money to pay for the abortion until she was beyond the state's 20 week 2nd trimester abortion limit. The court in this case cited common law principles that a woman cannot be prosecuted for hurting her own fetus.

Cox v. Court, 42 Ohio App. 3d 171, 537 N.E.2d 721 (1988).
Court reverses juvenile court order placing a pregnant woman in a "secure drug facility" to protect the fetus from the woman's cocaine use during pregnancy.

Jefferson v. Spaulding, 247 Ga. 86, 274 S.E.2d 457 (1981).
> State case ordering a cesarean section to be performed against the wishes of the woman for the benefit of the fetus.

Johnson v. State of Florida, 602 So. 2d 1288 (1992).
> State prosecution and conviction of woman for delivering drugs to her child through the umbilical cord overturned; statute governing the deliverance of a controlled substance to a minor never intended to apply in such cases.

In re A.C., 533 A.2d 611 (App. D.C. 1987) and *In re A.C.*, 573 A.2d 1235 (App. D.C. 1990).
> Washington, D.C. case of a pregnant woman dying of cancer who was ordered by a court to undergo an emergency cesarean section for the benefit of her unborn child; the patient and baby died, and the case decision was subsequently overturned.

In re Valerie D., 223 Conn. 492, 613 A.2d 748 (1992).
> State Supreme Court rejects the termination of parental rights because of mother's drug use during pregnancy.

Whitner v. South Carolina, 492 S.E.2d 777 (S.C. 1997), *cert. denied*, 118 S. Ct. 1857 (1998).
> Child endangerment charges upheld against a woman who used crack cocaine during her pregnancy, and whose child was born with cocaine metabolites in his system; the woman currently is serving a sentence of eight years for this criminal offense. The United States Supreme Court declined to hear this case and let the decision stand.

Statutory Examples

Examples of state statutes imposing civil penalties on women who use drugs while pregnant:

Minnesota Stat. Ann. Sec. 626.556 (1995).

Oklahoma Stat. Tit. 10, Sec. 7001-1.3 (1995).

Example of state statute requiring physicians to report positive toxicology tests of pregnant women to local welfare agencies:

Minnesota Stat. Ann, Section 626.5561, 626.5562 (West. Supp. 1997)

CASE 27

Tracheoesophageal Fistula in a Newborn with Down Syndrome

Baby Raymond is 7 days old. He was born with trisomy 21 (Down syndrome) and an associated tracheoesophageal (TE) fistula. His mother, Yvonne, is 25 years old, and Raymond is her first child. Her husband owns an architectural firm.

The infant is currently being supported by intravenous hydration in the neonatal intensive care unit at the private hospital where he was born. When the baby's physician approached his mother concerning surgery to repair the TE fistula, she refused to consent. Yvonne stated that her husband was distraught about Raymond's condition and she feared for their marriage. Also, his business has not been doing well and they are concerned about the economic consequences of having a very sick child. Her husband has only said that he would leave the decision to her. Both Yvonne and her husband have stated that they would have been in favor of pregnancy termination if they had known the child would be mentally handicapped.

ISSUES TO CONSIDER

- Life-sustaining treatment in newborns with birth defects
- Parental authority in decisions concerning impaired newborns
- Socioeconomic factors as part of a benefits/burdens analysis
- Late-term abortion

MEDICAL CONSIDERATIONS

1. What serious medical abnormalities may accompany the mental retardation of Down syndrome?

Down syndrome (DS) is associated with a number of severe medical problems that are either incompatible with life or can seriously shorten life span. Between 29 and 44 percent of babies born with DS have associated cardiac defects, 40 percent of which are endocardial cushion defects, such as ventricular or atrial septal defect, and abnormalities in the mitral or tricuspid valves. Less commonly, tetralogy of Fallot, ostium secundum, patent ductus arteriosus, or pulmonic stenosis may be present. Cardiac defects are sometimes multiple. Early diagnosis and corrective surgery have been shown to reduce morbidity and mortality.

Common noncardiac abnormalities include esophageal or duodenal atresia, and tracheoesophageal fistula, as in Raymond's case. Tracheoesophageal fistula generally is seen in conjunction with esophageal atresia, occurring alone in only 4 percent of cases. When no associated atresia is present, less complicated surgery is required, but in these cases it may present only as recurrent aspiration pneumonia, so that the diagnosis of uncomplicated TE fistula may be delayed for weeks or even months after birth.

Patients with Down syndrome have a 10- to 20-fold increased risk of developing acute leukemia in childhood and as adults. The prognosis of acute lymphocytic leukemia is approximately the same as in people without Down syndrome, however, the response to chemotherapy and prognosis of acute myelogenous leukemia is significantly better among DS children than those without DS.

Visual disorders are common and include strabismus, congenital nystagmus, decreased visual acuity, and, in adulthood, cataracts. Other problems include obstructive sleep apnea, seizure disorders, decreased hearing, hypothyroidism, and instability of the upper cervical spine. There is an enhanced susceptibility to infectious diseases, owing in part to T-cell abnormalities, but infections may be a particular problem in patients with heart disease.

2. What is the range of mental and related functional abilities that may accompany Down syndrome?

Older studies suggest that children with DS tend to have moderate to severe mental retardation with IQ ranging from approximately 35 to 55, but IQ and functional abilities sometimes fall outside of this general range. In a few cases intellectual and language function approximate that of normals, and in other cases, patients may be completely mute.

Abilities in abstract reasoning, problem solving, and language (specifically, syntax) generally are worse, but social adaptation is better than among patients of comparable IQ who have other forms of mental retardation. Psychiatric and behavioral problems are common, including anxiety disorders, depression, aggression, and self-injury. Children with DS have the best potential for cognitive growth in the first one to two years of life, after which the rate of intellectual growth declines swiftly.

Many factors contribute to the range of cognitive abilities seen in individuals with DS. Visual and auditory disabilities, cardiac disease, and delayed locomotor development often accompany cognitive deficits and have a significant impact; the extent to which these disabilities are addressed and corrected is likely to modify a patient's capabilities significantly. In addition, DS due to mosaicism is sometimes associated with better cognitive function than in individuals with complete trisomy 21.

The range of abilities among patients with DS is broader than previously believed. With increased recognition that children with DS have the potential to be educated, programs designed to maximize their capabilities have been instituted, and emphasis is often placed on the early period of life when they have the greatest potential for intellectual development. The benefits of early intervention remain controversial; it is uncertain if these interventions benefit the children directly or rather motivate and support the parents to pursue all available treatments and approaches.

Families tend to adjust well to having a child with developmental delay. Today, many children remain at home and many enter group homes as young adults, whereas most were institutionalized in the past. It is believed that children reared at home tend to function better overall than do institutionalized children, but the long-term benefits of educational interventions are not known. By age 40, virtually all individuals born with DS have histopathologic changes in the brain identical to those seen in Alzheimer's disease. Because intellectual deterioration is difficult to quantify in patients with mental retardation, the true incidence of clinical Alzheimer's disease in Down syndrome is unknown. As more individuals with DS survive into midlife, when many will develop Alzheimer's disease, there will likely be a greater appearance of delayed cognitive decline.

3. If surgery is performed, what is Raymond's long-term medical prognosis?

Assuming that he has no other immediate life-threatening birth defects, Raymond has a good chance of living into late middle age if he receives the medical care that would be given to an individual who was not impaired with Down syndrome. Average life expectancy of children born with DS is increasing because of advances in pediatric surgery and increasing use of surgery and medical interventions. Although mortality within the first year is much higher than for the general population, at age 20 a person with DS can expect to live another 36 years, and at age 50 another 11 years. Still, for those over the age of 20, mortality is five times that of the general population. This excess adult mortality, which peaks after the age of 40, is higher than for other individuals with mental retardation and much higher than that of the general population. It is not certain if the excess mortality is due to disease itself, conservative treatment approaches, or other factors, such as the premature development of Alzheimer's disease.

4. How could Down syndrome have been diagnosed prenatally?

The most reliable prenatal diagnosis is made by invasive testing, using chorionic villus sampling (CVS) or amniocentesis, which are associated with some maternal and fetal morbidity, and often delayed diagnosis. These tests are routinely offered to pregnant women over 35 years of age, who are at enhanced risk of carrying a baby with DS. Because she is younger (and if she had received appropriate and timely prenatal care), Yvonne could have been offered blood tests to formulate a risk profile to identify women who would be offered CVS or amniocentesis. This "triple screen" includes measurements of maternal serum alpha fetoprotein, human chorionic gonadotropin, and unconjugated estriol, and is generally performed between 15 and 20 weeks gestation. First trimester screening is not widely used because of lower sensitivity, the fact that many DS fetuses are lost through spontaneous abortion before the mid–second trimester, and limited availability and greater risk of CVS and amniocentesis that early in pregnancy. Amniocentesis is generally performed during 14–18 weeks of gestation, and results are available 2 to 3 weeks later, or at 16–21 weeks gestation, entering the "grey zone" of fetal viability. CVS can be performed as early as 9–12 weeks gestation, and results are available approximately one week later, no later than the early second trimester. Wider use of rapid DNA testing of amniotic fluid could enable these results to be available earlier.[2] CVS is offered less frequently than amniocentesis because it is believed to have a higher miscarriage rate, and possibly a risk of fetal limb disruption.

Ultrasound can detect a proportion of certain fetal malformations associated with DS, including cardiac defects, duodenal atresia, and others. Detection of these malformations might provide useful markers, but confirmatory diagnosis of DS would still require amniocentesis or CVS. Many malformations do not become ultrasonographically apparent until the third or late second trimester of pregnancy, when fetal viability occurs. Parents and physicians are very reluctant to terminate pregnancy at this stage, and there are legal limitations as well (see below).

5. If a late prenatal diagnosis is made for which pregnancy termination is deemed appropriate, what medical options exist?

Pregnancy terminated during the late second trimester or third trimester is called *late-term abortion*. The methods of late-term abortion differ significantly from those used in first-trimester abortion. First-trimester abortion is generally performed on an outpatient basis with suction curettage or menstrual extraction. Pregnancy terminated later requires more complex procedures. Dilatation and evacuation (D&E) involves greater dilatation of the cervix than suction curettage, and use of instruments to evacuate the fetus in parts. After approximately 20 weeks, dilatation and extraction (D&X) may be performed; this procedure, often called by the controversial term "partial birth abortion," consists of cervical dilatation over a few days, instrumental conversion of the fetus to a footling breech, breech extraction of all but the head, and partial evacuation of intracranial contents to enable vaginal delivery. The risk of maternal morbidity and mortality for these methods of late-term abortion are very low, but generally increases with increasing gestational age, and depends on the type of procedure performed. Other methods of late-term abortion include hysterotomy (opening the uterus and removing the fetus), and hysterectomy, which are performed under spinal, epidural, or general anesthesia in the hospital. These procedures are associated with greater maternal risk, but this may reflect the medical indications as well as the method. Late abortions are sometimes performed by inducing labor; if the fetus is deemed potentially viable, fetal demise is produced prior to delivery. This is done by injecting hypertonic saline or urea through the abdomen into the amniotic sac, or by injecting diazepam and potassium chloride intravascularly. Maternal and major morbidity correlates with increasing gestational age and type of procedure used.

6. From a counseling and psychodynamic standpoint, how should the parents' apparent rejection of this child be managed?

Childbirth is a period of adjustment for any family. Raymond's parents' situation is perhaps especially difficult because the father has been undergoing problems with his business. His passive attitude with Raymond's caregivers contrasts with his apparent emotional reaction with his wife. This may indicate a manipulative style that is typical of their relationship.

In any case, social workers will want to carefully assess whether there are ways in which both Yvonne and her husband can be supported so that they might perceive other possibilities in their situation. With their permission, perhaps other family or friends or a clergyman can be enlisted in their support. They should also be apprised of existing community services, such as a support group or a multidisciplinary DS clinic.

Whether or not these possibilities apply to them, every effort should be made not to let Raymond's parents feel that they would lose parental authority after the operation, should it occur without their consent. They must be kept informed and involved every step of the way. If the caregivers and hospital decide to seek a court's permission to proceed with surgery, that decision must be very carefully explained to them; the procedure is something that would be done for Raymond's sake, so that he can thrive and achieve his fullest potential. Counseling interventions must be undertaken to help them retain a sense of control, without which it will be much more difficult for them to develop an emotional attachment to Raymond. In fact, they may be more involved with him than they realize; their very selection of a name for him is evidence of this.

ETHICAL AND LEGAL CONSIDERATIONS

1. Should Yvonne's refusal to consent to surgery be respected by the baby's physicians?

Infants and children, lacking the intellectual skills necessary to consider their choices, are presumed by the law to be incapable of making important decisions for themselves. Historically, they have been placed under the guidance and wisdom of their parents when decisions need to be made about fundamental matters concerning their development and well-being. Because of the natural affection created by biologic ties, and due to the primacy placed on parental authority and family autonomy in the United States, parents have traditionally been given the authority to make these decisions in accord with their own values and determination of what serves the best interests of their children. The state has an interest in ensuring the health and well-being of children and exerts this interest through its *parens patriae* power. The state can only intervene and perhaps supersede parental authority in very limited situations, however, as when the choices made by the parents appear at odds with the societal consensus about what serves a child's interests or a parent's neglect or abuse produces risk or outright harm to the child.

In matters of medical decision making, parents have the authority, and indeed the obligation, to make decisions that promote their child's best interests. In the clinical setting, parents, working with the health care providers, have traditionally been accorded the freedom to make such decisions, even those involving the life and death of their children, without the intervention of outsiders.

Historically, there have been few options for an impaired newborn. In ancient times, and more recently in some societies, the practice of not treating or attending to the needs of impaired newborns was not uncommon, and in some cases permission was given to actively end their lives. Such infants were frequently devalued in terms of their future productivity and the burdens to be borne by those who would have to care for them, or their suffering was regarded as sufficient to justify ending their lives.

With the advent of modern technology, selective decisions have been made to withhold life-sustaining treatment from severely impaired newborns in neonatal intensive care units. Usually made in anguished privacy, without outside intervention, such decisions were arrived at by doctors and parents who together determined that the net benefits to be gained by treatment were outweighed by the burdens that the child would bear either as a result of the intervention or because of the underlying condition. Thus, in some ways the moral arguments entertained in these decisions were similar or analogous to the justifications used in other societies or in earlier times.

The uneasy but private alliance that arrived at such decisions was brought to public light and changed dramatically in the United States by a 1982 Bloomington, Indiana, case involving a newborn whose condition was similar to that of Baby Raymond. Afflicted with Down syndrome and tracheoesophageal fistula, the newborn, known as Baby Doe, was in need of corrective surgery. The parents of Baby Doe declined to consent to the operation, believing that the child would never achieve even a "minimally acceptable quality of life," and concerned about the impact of such a child on the lives of their other two children and their family as a whole. While the parents' obstetrician supported this decision, the pediatrician believed that the infant should be transferred to a facility where corrective surgery could be performed, and the hospital petitioned for court authority to override the parents' choice. The trial court concluded that the parents had the right to make such a choice as one of their medical treatment options. When a district attorney then attempted to pursue the case under parental neglect laws, this effort also failed and the Indiana Supreme Court declined to enter the case. The child ultimately died.

This case garnered massive public attention and led to a regulatory response from the Department of Health and Human Services to prevent parents from carrying out decisions to forgo life-prolonging treatment on the grounds of their child's handicap or future quality of life. A series of regulations and accompanying litigation, coupled with legislative efforts by Congress, led to the system now in place governing decisions to withhold or withdraw life-sustaining care from impaired newborns. Under the current system, these decisions are linked with child abuse; states were directed to institute a regulatory apparatus to investigate such cases, or risk losing federal funds for child abuse programs. These federal mandates, the 1984 Amendments to the Child Abuse Prevention and Treatment Act, are known as the Baby Doe Regulations (Table 7–27.1).

The exception of "virtual futility" gives some room for physicians to exercise their discretion in making reasonable medical judgments, which are defined as those that would be made by a "rationally prudent physician." If nutrition and hydration are not "appropriate," they could be withheld from an infant by a physician using reasonable medical judgment.

Thus, Yvonne's choice to decline treatment on behalf of Raymond would probably not be followed, both because of the prohibitions set out by the Baby Doe Regulations, and because of the current consensus that, despite Raymond's handicap, his best interests would be served by receiv-

---

Table 7–27.1   "Baby Doe Regulations": Instances in Which Treatment May Be Forgone[*]

The infant is chronically ill and irreversibly comatose
The provision of such treatment would merely prolong dying
Treatment would not be effective in ameliorating or correcting all of the infant's life-threatening conditions
Treatment would be virtually futile in terms of the survival of the infant, and the treatment would be inhumane

[*]1984 Amendments to the Child Abuse Prevention and Treatment Act.

ing the surgery and being allowed to mature and develop, albeit as a person with Down syndrome. Clearly, were it not for his handicap, there would be no argument over whether this medically indicated surgery should be done. Moreover, unlike a fetus (see Case 26, "A Pregnant Woman Using Cocaine"), Raymond is a born, living baby with fundamental rights, separate and apart from those of his mother, which must be respected. He is protected by society's and the state's strong interest in the preservation of life and strong commitment to equal treatment of all persons, including those with severe physical or mental impairments and regardless of race or socioeconomic status. Although the extent and severity of his handicap are not yet known, current societal consensus is that handicaps should not stand in the way of a child's opportunity to grow and mature to whatever extent possible. A life with a handicap such as Down syndrome is not one automatically devoid of pleasure or productivity, and it cannot justifiably be asserted that someone with Down syndrome is better off not living. This contrasts with a more severe impairment, such as trisomy 13, which would not warrant overriding a parental refusal to treat that was made in the interests of the child. In this assessment, Raymond's interests would be served by receiving the surgery, and thus his mother's choice, while perhaps on some level understandable, would nonetheless be superseded by state interests in protecting the life of this very vulnerable child.

Despite the establishment of federal regulations, there remains controversy in society over efforts to save the lives of extremely impaired newborns. The Baby Doe Regulations captured a narrow consensus regarding DS, but they have been applied overbroadly, perhaps by being overinterpreted, so that, as some argue, they have led to inappropriate treatment of infants with much more severe impairments than DS.

2. What will happen if Yvonne continues to refuse to consent to surgery?

Yvonne's first response to the issue of surgery is understandable, even though it may not be legally supportable. Like her new son, Yvonne is in a very vulnerable position, in need of emotional support and precise information about her son's current medical condition and current and future needs. Mothers such as Yvonne generally have never been faced with this type of problem and know little about the actual manifestations of DS and what they mean to a child, or about the possible opportunities that may exist for support and assistance. Treatment refusals are often based on misinformation or lack of information, and it is possible that with sufficient support and education, Yvonne and her husband might come to feel that there is value in Raymond's surgery and that they will be able to provide for his needs. Referral of the case to an ethics committee might help facilitate communication with his parents and among Raymond's caregivers and help inform the parents about the availability of resources to provide their son with the best possible future.

The present legal realities, however, might severely limit the parents' options. For example, continued refusal on their part could lead to a temporary suspension of their authority to make medical decisions on Raymond's behalf. Because of federal regulations, the hospital would almost certainly petition and obtain a court order, and a temporary guardian would be appointed for Raymond to make medical decisions for him. This would not constitute a total abrogation of parental rights to make other decisions for Raymond, but would merely be a statement that in this particular situation their choice was so harmful to the child's well-being that their authority to make such a decision has to yield to the state interest in protecting vulnerable children. Despite federal regulations, a hospital might not take such aggressive legal action on behalf of more severely impaired infants, such as those with trisomy 13, trisomy 18, or other lethal disorders.

Whether appointment of a temporary guardian for a baby such as Raymond would then lead to a broader examination of their fitness and willingness to be Raymond's parents is uncertain at this time. If, after the operation, they appeared able and willing to raise Raymond and make decisions for him, despite his impairment, it is likely that when he was discharged, his parents would have the authority to make decisions for him. If they lacked interest in Raymond's condition, however, or demonstrated hostility toward him, this might lead to reconsideration of their role as his parents. This could in turn lead to temporary placement of Raymond in a foster home or perhaps even an adoptive situation; however, a drastic measure such as terminating parental rights would only be used as a last resort.

It is important to note that either of Raymond's parents can consent to surgery for him (see Case 29, "A Religious Objection to a Child's Medical Treatment"). It would be more desirable to seek consensus and agreement from both parents, however, as the selection of one parent over another could exacerbate the apparent difficulties in their relationship and in their subsequent ability to cooperate in Raymond's care.

3. Who will pay for Raymond's long-term care?

Because Raymond's parents are not poor, much of his long-term care will probably be paid for out-of-pocket, though their private insurance may cover some costs of treatment and therapy. The cost of raising a healthy child from birth to 18 years of age in 1993 dollars is conservatively estimated at $192,000. Raising a child with a disability would incur additional expenses for health care, rehabilitation, counseling, and special education. These figures vary greatly from one region of the country to another and among various income brackets. Raymond's parents are obviously worried that the increased costs associated with the care of a child with impairments will be greater than their currently precarious financial situation will allow.

If his parents' worst fears about their financial future are realized, his future medical treatment and subsequent attention from social service agencies would likely be financed or subsidized through publicly funded insurance programs, such as Medicaid. While there is strong sentiment in society in favor of providing acute medical and rehabilitation services to children like Raymond regardless of their economic circumstances, there is also a reluctance to increase funding through public means in order to pay for this care. Thus, while the parents' financial situation is irrelevant in terms of whether Raymond is ensured of receiving supportive services in the community, the widespread inadequacy of those services to disadvantaged children would likely pose practical limitations.

4. If Yvonne had decided to terminate her pregnancy based on a prenatal diagnosis of Down syndrome, would there have been any limits placed on this decision by federal or state laws?

From a legal perspective, the status of a pregnant woman has to date been quite clear, at least in the earlier stages of the pregnancy. A pregnant woman has the right to make choices concerning her health care options, as she determines where her interests lie, even if such decisions cause her to end her pregnancy. In fact, a series of Supreme Court decisions has continuously, and broadly, outlined the freedom of women to make choices concerning their reproductive status. In decisions concerning the availability of contraception and abortion, the Supreme Court has repeatedly underscored the essential right of women to be free of unwarranted intrusions and interventions concerning their decision "to bear or beget a child."

In its seminal 1972 decision *Roe v. Wade*, the Court developed a framework based on the trimesters of pregnancy to examine how the interests of a pregnant woman compare to the interests of a developing fetus during pregnancy. The *Roe v. Wade* decision, though under attack in recent years, is still fundamentally supported by the Supreme Court. Under *Roe*, a woman in her first trimester of pregnancy, in consultation with her physician, has complete discretion as to whether or not to continue the pregnancy. She may have an abortion during this time for whatever reason she wishes, without the intrusion of anyone in the decision-making process. During the second trimester, as maternal risks from abortion increase, the woman's right to obtain an abortion is accompanied by the interests of the state in protecting her health and well-being, and thus ensuring that abortions are performed in accordance with that goal. Beginning in the second trimester of pregnancy, the state is allowed to set restrictions on where, and under what circumstances, an abortion may be performed, although a woman still has a fundamental right to an abortion. This has been the stage of pregnancy on which most of the major Supreme Court decisions have focused, as numerous states have attempted to restrict abortion during this time for reasons other than the health of the woman. Most of these restrictions have been upheld by the Supreme Court, even while it still defines as fundamental the right of a woman to have an abortion. For example, several states have enacted laws limiting abortion by mandating complex informed consent procedures or waiting periods between a request for an abortion and its actual performance. In its 1992 abortion decision of *Planned Parenthood v. Casey*, the Court upheld several restrictions of this sort so long as they do not impose an "undue burden" on a woman seeking an abortion. In *Casey*, the Court upheld Pennsylvania's waiting period and informed consent requirements, but it did strike down the requirement that a women inform her spouse of her decision to obtain an abortion before it is performed.

In the third trimester, the interests of the fetus, which is approaching viability, begin to take hold. Under *Roe* a state can outlaw third-trimester abortions, except to save the life or health of the mother, and most states have done so. This blanket restriction is based on the state's interest in protecting vulnerable parties, and on the consensus that after a fetus achieves viability, its interests in life and health outweigh a woman's procreative freedom, unless her life or health is threatened by continuing the pregnancy. Fetal viability is usually considered to occur at approximately the beginning of the third trimester, even if viability requires advanced technology or life support.

5. How can the interests of the pregnant patient be compared to the interests of the fetus? What happens in cases of conflict between these interests?

While not actually having the same rights and legal interests as a born person, the potential for life of the third-trimester fetus takes on enormous legal importance and has become the source of significant debate concerning what choices a woman may make during the last stages of her pregnancy. For example, there exist court cases involving a woman's refusal to deliver via a cesarean section despite her physician's assertions that vaginal delivery might harm the well-being of the fetus (see Case 26). These cases have engendered great debate. Efforts to compel a woman to have a cesarean section have been criticized as interfering with the right of the woman to control her health care and bodily integrity. Some have argued that forcing a woman to undergo a cesarean puts her in the position of being a "fetal container" rather than an autonomous adult.[3] Yet others strongly argue that the interests of the almost-born fetus are so significant at that point as to trump almost all interests of the pregnant patient.

The interests of the fetus in the potential for life obviously exist throughout the pregnancy; however, such interests do not rise to the level of a legally assertable right to life until after the fetus has reached viability, according to the *Roe* decision, as discussed previously. Before viability, the fetus' potential for life cannot be used as a limit to the patient's reproductive or health care decisions. After viability, this fetal right to life can even be trumped if the life or well-being of the mother is at stake.

Therefore, Yvonne's options concerning the availability of an abortion, and any restriction placed on this access, would be highly dependent on how far along she was in the pregnancy, and what restriction the state in which she lives has placed on abortion at that period in the pregnancy. If Yvonne had been receiving health care through the Medicaid program, her access to abortion might also have been restricted by financial concerns, as Medicaid is not obligated to pay for abortions unless necessary to preserve the woman's life, and thus many states do not pay for abortions of their Medicaid patients.

The later Yvonne had been in her pregnancy, the less access she might have had to abortion, as many states have outlawed access to abortion (except to preserve the health or life of the mother) once the patient reaches the late stage of the second trimester. Recent legislative attempts also have been mounted to further restrict abortion procedures as the pregnancy progresses, by means of outlawing late-term abortion procedures known as "partial-birth" abortions. While these legislative efforts have to date been largely unsuccessful or enjoined by courts of law, they do signal the continuing and profound division that exists in our country, at least among certain political factions, regarding the morality and acceptability of abortion per se, as well as abortion in later stages of pregnancy. Unfortunately, the need for later stage abortions continues to exist, despite early access to abortion and the increasing widespread use of prenatal testing early in the pregnancy. Reasons that women seek late-stage abortions include the following:

- Delay in diagnosis of pregnancy
- Failure to obtain first-trimester prenatal care
- Miscalculation of gestational age
- Delay in deciding whether to have an abortion after diagnosis of fetal abnormality is made
- Difficulty arranging for abortion, usually fiscal limitations
- Concealing pregnancy due to fear of informing parents or partner
- Detection of serious fetal abnormality not apparent until late in pregnancy, including
  - early false-negative testing
  - delay in determining prognosis of previously detected anomaly
  - late onset anomaly
  - late detection in low-risk woman in routine ultrasound late in pregnancy

---

REFERENCES

1. B.J. Lange et al., "Distinctive Demography, Biology, and Outcome of Acute Myeloid Leukemia and Myelodysplastic Syndrome in Children with Down Syndrome: Children's Cancer Group Studies 2861 and 2891," *Blood* 91 (1998): 608–615.
2. L. Verma et al., " Rapid and Simple Prenatal DNA Diagnosis of Down's Syndrome," *Lancet* 352 (1998): 9–12.
3. G.J. Annas, "Pregnant Women as Fetal Containers," *Hastings Center Report* 16 (1986): 13–14.

SUGGESTED READINGS

Annas, G.J. 1984. The Baby Doe regulations: Governmental intervention in neonatal rescue medicine. *American Journal of Public Health* 74: 618–620.

Annas, G.J. 1998. Partial-birth abortion, Congress, and the Constitution. *New England Journal of Medicine* 339: 279–283.

Arras, J.D. 1989. Toward an ethics of ambiguity. In *Ethical issues in modern medicine*, eds., J.D. Arras and N.K. Rhoden, 231–240. Mountain View, CA: Mayfield Publishing Co.

Avery, G.B. 1998. Futility considerations in the neonatal intensive care unit. *Seminars in Perinatology* 22: 216–222.

Cicchetti, D., and Beeghly, M. 1990. *Children with Down syndrome. A developmental perspective.* Cambridge, England: Cambridge University Press.

Committee on Bioethics, American Academy of Pediatrics. 1996. Ethics and the care of critically ill infants and children. *Pediatrics* 15: 283–289.

Dommergues, M. et al. 1999. The reasons for termination of pregnancy in the third trimester. *British Journal of Obstetrics and Gynecology* 106: 297–303.

Duff, R.S., and Campbell, A.G.M. 1973. Moral and ethical dilemmas in the special care nursery. *New England Journal of Medicine* 289: 890–894.

Epner, J.E.G. et al. 1998. Late-term abortion. *Journal of the American Medical Association* 280: 724–729.

Fishler, K. et al. 1975. Comparison of mental development in individuals with mosaic and trisomy 21 Down's syndrome. *Pediatrics* 58: 744–748.

Freeman, S.B. et al. 1998. Population-based study of congenital heart defects in Down syndrome. *American Journal of Medical Genetics* 80: 213–217.

Glover, N.M., and Glover, S.J. 1996. Ethical and legal issues regarding selective abortion of fetuses with Down syndrome. *Mental Retardation* 34: 207–214.

Grimes, DA. 1998. The continuing need for late abortions. *Journal of the American Medical Association* 280: 747–750.

Haddow, J.E. et al. 1998. Screening of maternal serum for fetal Down's syndrome in the first trimester. *New England Journal of Medicine* 338: 955–961.

The Hastings Center Project on Imperiled Newborns. 1987. Imperiled newborns. *Hastings Center Report* 17: 5–32.

Hayes, A., and Batshaw, M.L. 1993. Down syndrome. *Pediatric Clinics of North America* 4: 523–535.

Hijii, T. et al. 1997. Life expectancy and social adaptation in individuals with Down syndrome with and without surgery for congenital heart disease. *Clinical Pediatrics* 36: 327–332.

Janerich, D.T., and Bracken, M.B. 1986. Epidemiology of trisomy 21: A review and theoretical analysis. *Journal of Chronic Diseases* 39: 1079–1093.

Meisel, A. 1989 and 1993 (Supp. 2). Decision making for handicapped infants. In *The Right to Die*. New York: John Wiley & Sons.

Moreno, J. 1987. Ethical and legal issues in the treatment of impaired newborns. *Clinics in Perinatology* 14: 325–329.

National Abortion Rights Action League. 1999. Who decides? A state-by-state review of abortion and reproductive rights (see Appendix A).

Schapiro, MB. et al. 1992. Nature of mental retardation and dementia in Down syndrome: Study with PET, CT, and neuropsychology. *Neurobiology of Aging* 13: 723–734.

Sprang, M.L., and Neerhof, M.G. 1998. Rationale for banning abortions late in pregnancy. *Journal of the American Medical Association* 280: 744–747.

Snyder, E.D. 1996. End of life decisions at the beginning of life. *Medicine and Law* 15: 283–289.

Tubman, T.R.J. et al. 1991. Congenital heart disease in Down's syndrome: Two-year prospective early screening study. *British Medical Journal* 302: 1425–1427.

Van der Heide, A. et al. 1998. The role of parents in end-of-life decisions in neonatology: Physicians' views and practices. *Pediatrics* 101 (3 Pt. 1): 413–418.

Wall, S.N., and Partridge, J.C. 1997. Death in the intensive care nursery: Physician practice of withdrawing and withholding life support. *Pediatrics* 99: 64–70.

Zipursky, A. et al. 1992. Leukemia in Down syndrome: A review. *Pediatric Hematology and Oncology* 9: 139–149.

LEGAL CITATIONS

Case Examples

Grego v. United States, No. 24587, 1995 Nev. LEXIS 33 (Nev. March 30, 1995).
Nevada Supreme Court declared that failure to make a timely diagnosis of gross and disabling fetal impairments, thus not providing a pregnant woman the opportunity to accordingly terminate her pregnancy, constitutes negligence, and justification for a "wrongful birth" lawsuit.

In re Infant Doe, No. GU8204-00 (Cir. Ct., Monroe County, Ind., Apr. 12, 1982).
Newborn with Down syndrome allowed to die rather than have life-saving operation performed to correct TE fistula.

Statutory Example

Public Law 98-457. U.S. Child Abuse Protection and Treatment Amendments of 1984.
Federal mandate, following the death of "Baby Doe," in Indiana, to provide medical treatment to virtually all newborns, despite physical impairments at birth.

CASE 28

Determination of Death in a Newborn

At nine months pregnant, Sharon believed she was in labor and went to her hospital's emergency room. "False labor" was diagnosed, however, and Sharon was sent home. She returned 24 hours later and gave birth to a baby girl, but the infant was cyanotic and unresponsive. The baby was intubated and immediately transferred to the neonatal intensive care unit on life support. After 48 hours, the infant's condition has not improved. The baby is flaccid and unresponsive to painful and auditory stimuli, and brainstem reflexes are not elicited. An electroencephalogram (EEG) showed electrocerebral silence (ECS). The baby has been declared brain dead.

Sharon and her husband are told the news, and advised that the next step is to discontinue life support. When the baby's father realizes what this means, and that life support could possibly be discontinued without his permission, he contacts a lawyer. The attorney, who is known in the community for winning many malpractice cases on behalf of patients, seeks a restraining order to prevent the removal of the baby's life support. A court order will be forthcoming, he says, because he can find an expert who will state that the child is not brain dead. One pediatrician says that this is "an outrageous waste of health care dollars" and an opportunity for "another lawyer to make a buck."

ISSUES TO CONSIDER

- Determination of brain death in infancy
- Prognostication in fetal anoxia
- Withdrawal of life-sustaining treatment in a newborn
- Medical malpractice
- Organ procurement in neonates

MEDICAL CONSIDERATIONS

1. What criteria are used to diagnose brain death in a newborn?

The fundamental issue in this case is whether, in fact, this baby is brain dead. Regardless of age, brain death occurs when there is irreversible cessation of all cerebral and brainstem function, however, accepted criteria used to determine this state in adults may not be as precise when applied to very young children, particularly newborns (see Case 10, "A Religious Objection to the Determination of Brain Death"). In the newborn, especially the preterm newborn, neurologic findings may be inexact. Cortical responses are primitive, and visual, auditory, and tactile stimuli cannot be relied on to determine cortical function. The brainstem examination may also be misleading because many apparently brain dead newborns suffer from undiagnosed developmental abnormalities (although in 90 percent brain death is due to perinatal asphyxia), so that abnormal neurologic findings might be difficult to interpret. This contrasts with the older child or adult, whose previous neurologic status is known, and in whom the proximate cause of coma can generally be ascertained.

Confirmatory tests, such as EEG, apnea testing, and measurement of cerebral blood flow, contribute useful information to the diagnosis, but they cannot be relied on individually. EEG and cerebral blood flow radionuclide angiography determine cortical but not brainstem activity. An EEG may show electrocerebral silence (ECS, an isoelectric or "flat" EEG) in a number of potentially reversible situations, as is possible in adults. In fact, many newborns with neurologic problems are given phenobarbital or other anticonvulsants to prevent seizures, and subtoxic doses are sufficient to reversibly suppress EEG activity. In the newborn, delayed elimination of these agents may prolong ECS even further.

In addition to technical problems associated with performing an EEG in a tiny infant, the developing nervous system may yield different information in the EEG; specifically, electrical activity may be very suppressed, especially in prematurity, and nonlethal insults may produce transient ECS. Finally, laboratory determination of cerebral blood flow in newborns may be misleading. Cerebral blood flow may be very low in non–brain dead newborns and not detectable by the commonly used and otherwise highly reliable cerebral radionuclide angiography. Conversely, cerebral blood flow may be demonstrable in newborns even when brain death has occurred. Four-vessel contrast angiography, which has also not been specifically tested for validation in this age group, is theoretically the only method that can ascertain this.

Because of these dilemmas, a multispecialty national task force developed standards for determining brain death in children that delineate specific historical information, clinical findings, and laboratory guidelines to be followed and specify an observation period linked to the age of the child (see Table 7–28.1). These criteria and those delineated by others have been the subject of critical evaluation.[1,2] It should be noted that these guidelines were established by consensus but with a minimum of hard data. There is insufficient information on which to establish guidelines for infants younger than seven days of age, and even less information for premature newborns. Given these limitations, the reasonable observation period for Sharon's full-term infant would be at least seven and probably nine days after provisional determination of brain death. Since it is not possible, by present standards, to determine in such a short time whether the infant is brain dead, the attorney should be able to find an expert who would state as much.

Table 7–28.1 Brain Death in Children: Observation Period for Physical and Laboratory Criteria

Age[*]	*Recommendation*
<7 days	No criteria established
7 days–2 months	2 examinations and EEGs separated by ≥48 hr
2 months–1 year	2 examinations and EEGs separated by ≥24 hr (or 1 examination and EEG and radionuclide angiogram demonstrating absent cerebral blood flow)
>1 year	2 examinations separated by ≥12 hr (if hypoxic-ischemic encephalopathy, increase observation period to ≥24 hr unless cerebral blood flow is absent)

[*] In newborns, assume full-term infant greater than 38 weeks gestation.

Source: Data from Task Force for the Determination of Brain Death in Children, Guidelines for the Determination of Brain Death in Children, *Annals of Neurology,* vol. 21, pp. 616–617, © 1987, Little, Brown and Company.

It is particularly difficult to determine brain death in newborns with anencephaly, who lack cerebral hemispheres, but who may exhibit primitive behaviors that mimic cerebral functions, such as responses to noxious stimuli or feeding, but that actually reflect brainstem function. Brainstem function may be difficult to determine in the anencephalic because a spectrum of brainstem dysfunctions and facial malformations may accompany the absence of cerebrum, and clinical brainstem responses may be absent, although some brainstem function may still exist. Thus, a clinical diagnosis depends on a period of observation until the disappearance of any preexisting brainstem responses, including spontaneous respiration; this may require up to 48 hours.

An additional problem is that anencephaly encompasses a spectrum of abnormalities, overlapping clinically with other profound neurologic defects at times, and misdiagnosis has occurred. Most experts maintain that the prognosis for survival of the true anencephalic is rarely longer than a few days. There are some cases of diagnosed "anencephalics" who have lived much longer even without continuous life support, perhaps because of the presence of substantial brainstem tissue and function.

Other medical controversies surrounding the concept of brain death are discussed in Case 10 and in the References.[3]

2. If the child is not brain dead, what is her prognosis?

Assuming that this child does not also have a developmental neurologic abnormality as the basis of her condition, the proximate cause of her coma is probably perinatal or fetal anoxia. There is wide speculation that the central nervous system in the newborn is more resistant to anoxic insults than in older children and adults. In infants, anoxic insults are generally due to intermittent rather than severe, acute asphyxia, which may damage the cerebral cortex, but which may spare the brainstem. Coexistent cerebral edema may produce relatively less severe damage in the newborn because the sutures have not yet closed. Other undefined elements of neonatal cerebral metabolism may contribute to the presumed plasticity of the youthful central nervous system. There is evidence, however, that cerebral insults early in life damage learning centers and can result in subtle or overt learning disabilities that would not be noted until several years later (see Case 24, "Assisted Reproduction in a Woman with Strong Religious Beliefs," and Case 26, "A Pregnant Woman Using Cocaine").

Despite these optimistic assertions, in nearly all reported cases children who were clinically brain dead but who "recovered" have had severe neurologic impairments, including the persistent vegetative state (PVS). Cerebral asphyxia is probably the most common cause of PVS in newborns.

3. Can this baby's organs be harvested for transplant?

From a medical perspective, under the consensus surrounding brain death determination in newborns, the organs could be harvested if the baby is determined to be brain dead and vital organs can be perfused. Since it may be possible to maintain the donor newborn for longer than seven days (see Case 11, "A Teenager with Prolonged Unconsciousness"), these criteria could be met.

Organs most often needed in very young children include the heart, lung, small bowel, and multiple organs. Kidneys alone are not transplanted much in infancy because of the availability of peritoneal dialysis, which enables the transplant procedure to be delayed into later childhood when a good outcome would be more likely. Unfortunately, there is a great shortfall of donor organs for newborns awaiting transplant. This may be partly related to the failure of physicians to approach families, or unwillingness of families to donate.[4] However, parents of potential child donors may be much more likely than family of adults to donate.[5]

ETHICAL AND LEGAL CONSIDERATIONS

1. If the diagnosis of brain death is confirmed, can life-sustaining treatment be withdrawn against the wishes of the parents?

In situations in which a clear, undisputed diagnosis of whole brain death has been confirmed, in either an adult or a child, such a determination would constitute a declaration of death for legal purposes, thereby relieving the providers of further obligations toward the now deceased patient, other than to treat the body with appropriate dignity. In such a case, treatment interventions could be withdrawn, despite the objections of grieving relatives. Removal of the life support might be delayed if organ transplantation were being considered or if there were religious objections (see Case 10). Most important, physicians must respect the parents' emotional reaction to the catastrophe that has befallen what should have been a normal child, and act accordingly.

In the current case, additional problems would make it imprudent to rush to remove life support. First, of course, is the dispute concerning the accuracy of the declaration of death. In order to demonstrate reasonable judgment and compliance with the standard of care in such a case, the physicians for this infant would be wise to follow the recommended protocol for declaration of death in an infant so young, including monitoring over several days, rather than the 48-hour period they have used as their standard. Given the controversy surrounding brain death declaration in infants so young, and the specific circumstances that may have led to this child's condition, and may well lead to a malpractice lawsuit, it would be imperative that the providers demonstrate reasonableness and caution. Any actions that stand contrary to accepted practice would only serve to aggravate an already explosive situation.

Finally, given the likelihood of a malpractice charge in this case, it seems highly imprudent to rush to action, which would only inflame the situation. One of the most common reasons that patients or families sue for malpractice is their feeling of anger and misunderstanding. Lawsuits are much less likely to be initiated in cases in which parties believe that they have been fairly dealt with and are knowledgeable about the circumstances.[6,7] In this situation, not only is the malpractice charge potentially legitimate, but the distraught parents have already sought legal assistance.

2. If the baby is not brain dead, could life support still be withdrawn? Who would have the authority to make that decision?

If it became apparent that the baby was not brain dead, but was perhaps comatose or seriously neurologically impaired, her prognosis might be assessed to be so bleak that a decision to withdraw treatment by the parents, in consultation with their physicians, would be legally and ethically supportable. The ultimate decision would rest on a benefits-burdens analysis, as discussed in earlier cases. From a strictly legal and regulatory perspective, the infant's condition is such that it would likely fall within the exceptions of the Baby Doe Regulations (see Case 27, "Tracheoesophageal Fistula in a Newborn with Down Syndrome"). For example, she might be so severely compromised that she would never experience pain and suffering. If the parents wished that life-sustaining treatment be discontinued, there is little doubt that this decision would be supported. At this time, however, the parents have expressed a desire not to withdraw treatment. Given their presumptive roles as the best decision makers for the child, and their challenge to an admittedly uncertain and irrevocable diagnosis, there would not be basis to immediately challenge their decisional authority. If, after a period of time, the diagnosis of brain death is clearly confirmed, or if the infant's prognosis is so poor that continuing life-sustaining treatment would be difficult to justify, then sensitive and reasonable clinicians would work toward helping the parents to accept the reality of the circumstances. At the moment, if the parents insist on continuing what the clinicians regard as futile treatment, and the child is not definitively declared brain dead, then the physicians are obligated to continue treatment, under current standards. An infant bioethics committee might called upon to help facilitate communication with the family and to address the caregivers' distress.

Thus, if there were agreement between family and physicians, life support could be removed, even if the child did not meet strict brain death criteria. It is important to emphasize that brain death criteria have been promulgated not to facilitate termination of life support per se, but largely to facilitate organ retrieval for transplant (see Case 10).

3. What weight should be given to the pediatrician's assertion about this infant's utilization of health care dollars?

Based on published data utilizing 1994 constant dollars low-birth-weight infants in neonatal intensive care units incur higher costs than any other patient group. For infants with a birth weight between 501 and 1,500 grams, median treatment costs across all infants approximate $50,000 for an average length of stay of 49 days, but they can quickly escalate. For example, for infants within this weight range in the 90th percentile of treatment costs, the median cost of care was $130,377 to a maximum of $889,136.[8] These costs would probably even be higher today.

Although these costs are very high, there are several weighty reasons why they are not factored into decisions about life-sustaining treatment. Such overt financial considerations have not been deemed appropriate at the individual bedside, especially given the vulnerability of this patient population. This kind of decision would have policy implications of such enormity that it would demand the broadest possible public discussion. Fiscal policy or treatment rationing cannot be made on a case-by-case basis at the bedside and still be fair and equitable; profound injustices would surely result as infants in similar medical situations might be treated unequally, merely because of the values of the particular attending physician. Moreover, unless they are suspected of abuse or neglect, parents are regarded as the presumptive decision makers for their children. This basic policy standard, too, would have to be changed, with profound implications for all areas of parent-child relations.

If, however, the pediatrician believes that an intervention desired by parents would definitely be a net burden to an infant (such as one that merely created or extended suffering with no conceivable benefit to the child), then the physician has not only a right but a professional obligation to function as an advocate for the child. Resort to administrative procedures, perhaps including an ethics committee, would be appropriate (see Case 4, "Management of Life-Threatening Illness").

4. Why would the attorney in this case counsel the parents to maintain the child on life support, despite the clear indication that her life, if she survives, will be catastrophically impaired?

Given an attorney's obligation to advocate for his or her client as vigorously as possible, there are several important reasons why he or she would counsel that life support not be withdrawn at this time. First, and foremost, if the wishes of the parents are to continue treatment and there is dispute concerning the child's condition (such that reasonable people could disagree concerning the diagnosis of brain death at this time), then the parents, as the decision makers for this child, have valid interests that are worthy of support and protection, through the legal process if necessary. These parents are rightfully asserting their interests in this case and are certainly justified in seeking legal protection of their interests, if it appears that the physicians have chosen not to include those interests in the decision-making process. Their lawyer is doing all he should to put a temporary halt to any actions that might exclude consideration of the legitimate interests of his clients in the treatment decision making or that would lead to irrevocable consequences for their infant girl.

Second, given the potential legitimacy of a charge of malpractice, it would be helpful to clarify, to as great an extent as possible, what happened in this case, what the current problems of the child are, and what her future may hold. Such information is more likely to be developed while the child is still alive, rather than as an after-the-fact assessment as to what happened. This sort of strategy could only be justified if the assumption could be supported that the child was not suffering because of the continued life support.

A third motivation might well be that the potential for a significant malpractice award is greatly enhanced if the child remains alive, rather than if the child's life should end so soon. Compensation for the harm done to such a child and her parents would largely be based on the expenses that would be incurred to pay for the child's resulting impairments, as well as compensation for the lost earning potential of such a child. Given the likely astronomical nature of the expenses if this child were to survive, and the lifetime projections of earning potential for someone so young, had she been born healthier, it is likely that such a malpractice award would be enormous. If the child dies, however, then the award would be more modest, compensating the parents for any pain and suffering the child experienced while still alive, and perhaps exacting some sort of punitive award if the actions of the physicians were considered sufficiently egregious. In addition, in the usual malpractice case, the attorney's fee is contingent, set according to a fixed percentage of whatever award is made (usually one-third of the award goes to the attorney). Thus, it is also in the financial self-interest of the attorney to generate as large an award as possible for this family.

In fact, there has been much criticism of the legal profession for this practice of contingency fees, which is thought to encourage frivolous lawsuits and extraordinary (and perhaps unjustifiable) sums for compensation of harm. Because lawyers earn a fee only if the clients win an award, few attorneys will take on a frivolous case that will not lead to any sizable award. It would not be in the attorney's interest to invest the time and resources needed, although such cases are probably taken up occasionally. Second, the size of awards, while requested by a family and their attorney, are highly dependent on the sympathy a jury feels toward the family. Cases that generate extraordinary sums for compensation are usually highly emotional cases, involving significant impairments, which would logically lead those making the award to sympathize with the family, even if the physicians' actions were not egregious.

Finally, initiating and conducting a lawsuit, no matter what the sort, is a highly expensive proposition, one that would not be available to most people with legitimate claims if contingent-fee attorneys were not available. Few people, on their own, have the resources to conduct an effective investigation and pay for everything necessary to support a jury trial, were it not for the fact that attorneys were willing to gamble with their own resources in order to bring about the lawsuit. Unfortunately, this system sometimes leads to injustice for providers, who are often pressured by malpractice insurers to settle a claim out of court, even if they feel they have done nothing wrong and who may experience enormous anxiety and harmful consequences, even if they are ultimately found to be innocent of the charges.

This dilemma has led to proposed alternative means of settling claims for birth-related injuries. In some states there have been attempts to take cases of impaired newborns out of the traditional malpractice system and into a more objective system of an appointed compensation board, composed of physicians, who would examine the circumstances and determine the probable nature of the child's future and the support that would be needed. Such a compensation board would presumably remove some of the incentives in the current system to inflate numbers and generate sympathy with a jury, yet would legitimately and fairly compensate in cases in which harm has been done. Providers would make annual contributions to the system, rather than pay malpractice premiums that might rise astronomically if a case of malpractice were successfully (or even unsuccessfully) launched against an individual practitioner. One major concern about such a system, however, is that it would not monitor or discipline physicians whose practice is consistently inferior and harmful to patients. In addition to compensating patients and families, the current malpractice system also, in essence, polices the profession in ways that peer review has generally been unable or unwilling to do. The medical profession has historically been lax in weeding out those practitioners who genuinely pose a threat to patient well-being. While the current malpractice system does exact a high cost on many fine physicians, it also contributes to the important goal of removing from practice those who cannot practice at a level consistent with good patient care.

5. Should this newborn be referred for potential organ donor status?

Hospitals are required under federal law to have written policies for identifying potential organ donors, so as to ensure that families of all potential organ donors are made aware of the option of donating their loved one's organs. Further, hospitals are also required to report all deaths to local organ banks, who are in fact responsible for approaching families. These federal mandates were put into place as a way to increase family awareness and willingness to donate organs, an especially important goal given the continuing shortages of available donor organs (see Case 22, "A Man with Alcoholic Cirrhosis Wants a Liver Transplant").

Pediatric organs, in particular, are in scarce supply. It has been reported that 25 percent of all patients waiting for new livers are younger that 10 years old. Furthermore, statistics show that in 1993, more than 400 infants in need of new hearts died while awaiting an available donor organ.[9] As transplant techniques improve, the dire shortage for critical organs becomes more acute. Therefore, it seems imperative to ensure that all potential organ donor candidates are identified for possible consideration.

Family members often find great comfort in the possibility of some positive benefit out of what is otherwise a family tragedy. Ultimately, the parents of this infant may come to feel that way as well. Given their current focus and source of concerns, however—particularly given their challenge to the determination of brain death in their infant—it would seem at a minimum premature and perhaps even highly inflammatory to introduce the concept of organ donation at this time. Until the child's brain function status is clear and no longer in dispute and the goals of future treatment are considered, referral for possible organ donation would not be appropriate. The decision to utilize organs from donors who are not brain dead but whose surrogate decision makers come to the decision to withdraw life-sustaining treatment is very sensitive, given concerns about the integrity of the organ donor process. For more information concerning this practice in the pediatric arena, refer to the Suggested Readings.

REFERENCES

1. S. Ashwal, "Brain Death in the Newborn. Current Perspectives," *Clinical Perinatology* 24 (1997): 859–882.
2. J.M. Freeman and P.C. Ferry, "New Brain Death Guidelines in Children: Further Confusion," *Pediatrics* 81 (1988): 301–303.
3. D.A. Shewmon, "Chronic 'Brain Death.' Meta-Analysis and Conceptual Consequences," *Neurology* 51 (1998): 1538–1545.
4. L.A. Siminoff et al., "Public Policy Governing Organ and Tissue Procurement in the United States. Results from the National Organ and Tissue Procurement Study," *Annals of Internal Medicine* 123 (1995): 10–17.
5. J.A. Morris et al., "Pediatric Organ Donation: The Paradox of Organ Shortage Despite the Remarkable Willingness of Families to Donate," *Pediatrics* 89 (1992): 411–415.
6. H.B. Beckman et al., "The Doctor-Patient Relationship and Malpractice. Lessons from Plaintiff Depositions," *Archives of Internal Medicine* 154 (1994): 1365–1370.
7. G.B. Hickson et al., "Obstetricians' Prior Malpractice Experience and Patients' Satisfaction with Care," *Journal of the American Medical Association* 272 (1994): 1583–1587.
8. T. Rogowski, "Measuring the Cost of Neonatal and Perinatal Care," *Pediatrics* 103 (1 Supp)(1999): 329–335.
9. A. Caplan, "Organ Procurement and Transplantation: Ethical and Practical Issues," *Leonard Davis Institute of Health Economics Issue Brief* 2, no. 5 (September 1995) (see Appendix A).

SUGGESTED READINGS

Ashwal, S. et al. 1992. The persistent vegetative state in children. Report of the Child Neurology Society Ethics Committee. *Annals of Neurology* 32: 570–576.

Brody, B. 1988. Parents who wish to keep their dead baby intubated. In *Life and death decision making*, 200–203. Oxford: Oxford University Press.

Coulter, D.L. 1987. Neurologic uncertainty in newborn intensive care. *New England Journal of Medicine* 316: 840–844.

Koogler, T., and Costarino, A.T. 1998. The potential benefits of the pediatric non heart beating organ donor. *Pediatrics* 101: 1049–1052.

Medical Task Force on Anencephaly. 1990. The infant with anencephaly. *New England Journal of Medicine* 322: 669–674.

Mejia, R.E., and Pollack, M.M. 1995. Variability in brain death determination practices in children. *Journal of the American Medical Association* 274: 550–553.

Sloan, F.A. et al. 1998. No-fault system of compensation for obstetric injury: Winners and losers. *Obstetrics and Gynecology* 91: 437–443.

Task Force for the Determination of Brain Death in Children. 1987. Guidelines for the determination of brain death in children. *Annals of Neurology* 21: 616–617.

Weiler, P.C. et al. 1992. Proposal for medical liability reform. *Journal of the American Medical Association* 267: 2355–2358.

LEGAL CITATIONS

Case Examples

Alvarado v. New York City Health and Hospitals Corporation, 145 Misc. 2d 687, 547 N.Y.S.2d 190 (1989), *vacated and dismissed sub. nom., Alvarado v. City of New York*, 157 A.D.2d 604, 550 N.Y.S.2d 353 (1990).
Order to terminate infant's life support despite parental objections overruled on findings that infant did not meet the brain death criteria.

In re Long Island Jewish Medical Center, 641 N.Y.S.2d 989–992 (Feb. 28, 1996).
Litigation involving the hospital's desire to withdraw life support from an infant determined to be brain dead, over the religious objections of the patient's family. In support for the parents, another hospital offered to accept the infant on transfer, where the infant died several days later.

CASE 29

A Religious Objection to a Child's Medical Treatment

Daniel is a nine-year-old boy being treated for acute lymphocytic leukemia (ALL). It has become apparent that he will require platelet transfusions in order to prevent serious hemorrhage. His hemoglobin is dangerously low and he will also require red cell transfusions. Daniel's parents are practicing Jehovah's Witnesses. While they have consented to his treatment to date and very much want their son to pull through this, they are now hesitant to agree to the needed transfusions because this would violate their strongly held religious convictions. Daniel's doctors insist that the transfusions are critical and that they will obtain a court order if necessary so that this critical intervention will not be withheld from their patient.

ISSUES TO CONSIDER

- Parental religious convictions and the right to refuse treatment
- The involvement of pediatric patients in decisions about their health care

MEDICAL CONSIDERATIONS

1. What are Daniel's chances of survival if he is given a full course of treatment?

Childhood ALL can now be cured by chemotherapy in as many as 70 to 80 percent of cases, but it is rapidly fatal without treatment. In order to obtain a remission, an intensity of chemotherapy is required that will invariably lead to marrow suppression and likely need for transfusions. Without the ability to provide transfusions, the consequences of the chemotherapy could be as life threatening as no treatment at all and could lead to significant additional morbidity.

While the overall prognosis for ALL in children is good, certain poor prognostic subgroups have been identified, for example, age under 1 year or over 10 years, leukocyte count greater than 50,000, and cytogenetic features. Prognostic subgroup might guide decisions about treatment, such as whether to recommend bone marrow transplant during the first remission for a child in a poor prognostic group, but it is unlikely that favorable prognostic group would lead to a decision to recommend less than maximum chemotherapy, which could boost the complete remission rate to 95 percent and reduce the risk of recurrence.

The prognosis for children at age 15 begins to approximate the lower survival rate for adults. Under these circumstances, chemotherapy of greater intensity and greater potential toxicity might be recommended. Thus, decisions about intensity of treatment would have to take into account a variety of medical factors, including possible poor survival rate irrespective of whether the patient receives transfusions. These factors might be of importance to a practicing Jehovah's Witness who is considering treatment options. In general, experts agree that treatment should be initiated for ALL regardless.

2. Are there any alternatives to blood transfusions in this type of case?

In certain medical situations, alternatives to blood product transfusion do exist, and Jehovah's Witnesses are generally well informed about these alternatives and willing to accept them (see Case 1, "A Religious Objection to a Blood Transfusion"). However, blood-conserving techniques are largely applicable to situations involving surgery and other mechanical causes of bleeding, where blood-conservation techniques and minimally invasive surgery might be useful. In Daniel's case, chemotherapy will suppress his bone marrow and blood-producing elements, resulting in anemia, thrombocytopenia, and neutropenia. A nine-year-old child would be more likely to tolerate a low hematocrit than would an adult, but neutropenia and thrombocytopenia would have to be addressed. Erythropoietin reduces but does not eliminate the need for red blood cell transfusion in the long term, and it cannot substitute for an urgently needed transfusion. Erythropoietin may not be acceptable to all Jehovah's Witness patients, and has no effect on non-erythrocyte cell lines. Granulocyte colony stimulating factor (GCSF) is commonly given following anticancer chemotherapy to shorten the duration of neutropenia, but it does not prevent it. Thromboplastin might be useful in the future to alleviate thrombocytopenia, but is not available for use at this time. Because thrombocytopenia can lead to life-threatening hemorrhage, the option to give platelet transfusions would be essential.

Bone marrow transplant in children with ALL is generally reserved for the minority that do not respond to chemotherapy alone. In any case, approximately a month is needed before marrow engrafting occurs, during which time chemotherapy would be needed.

While there are scattered case reports of successful and unsuccessful treatment of leukemia in adult Jehovah's Witnesses who refuse transfusion,[1] it would be essential to have the option of a blood transfusion in order to embark on a successful course of treatment for Daniel. Decisions would have to be made rapidly if counts dropped to a critical level.

ETHICAL AND LEGAL CONSIDERATIONS

1. Should the blood transfusions be withheld from Daniel because of his parents' religious convictions?

Decisions concerning medical treatment for a nine-year-old child would normally be left to the discretion of the child's parents. Presumably making decisions in accord with their view of what serves the best interests of their child, parents have a strong interest in passing on their values to their children and in maintaining the privacy and integrity of their family. It is only in exceptional cases, when the choices of parents put their children at great risk, contrary to what a societal consensus would hold to be in the best interests of the child, that there may exist the opportunity and the obligation to intervene on behalf of the child, even at the expense of deeply held beliefs of the parents. Daniel's case would very likely stand as one of those exceptional circumstances in which resort to legal intervention would be justifiable if an agreement permitting transfusions could not be worked out with Daniel's parents. Young children have not had the opportunity to develop their own religious beliefs and are not the chattel of their parents. For practical purposes, a society must take some position concerning the limits of parental authority. The predominant ethical view in our society is that medically reasonable efforts to preserve a young child's life should be undertaken even in the presence of strong, religiously based objections by the parents.

Although overriding the parents' wishes may be justified in this case, it must be recognized that such a move will have associated costs. The parents will feel that they are being forced to violate their religious beliefs and may feel that they face ostracism from their church community. They may feel anger as they are stripped of their parental authority, and this would seriously damage the therapeutic relationship between doctor and parents. The decision to transfuse this child, against parental wishes, may cause estrangement between parents and child as well and may produce damage within the family structure. Any move to override the parents in such a case would have to be undertaken in a very sensitive manner. The parents must be accorded as much participation as possible, with legal involvement strictly limited to the precise treatment issue in question. This family must also be given emotional support once the threat to the child's immediate health is over. The crucial support and availability of Daniel's parents might be in jeopardy, unless the decision to override their authority is sensitively handled, with respect for the parents' point of view in spite of the disagreement.

In the context of medical care, the greater the risk that parental refusal of treatment would harm the child, and the greater the likelihood that the refused treatment would benefit him, the more justifiable would be an action to override the parents, and in some cases taking such action would be obligatory. In this particular case, treatment of Daniel's leukemia cannot proceed in any effective manner without the option of blood transfusions; avoiding transfusions poses significant risk to Daniel, probably as great as not treating him at all. With appropriate therapy, his chances for remission and successful recovery are quite high. Given the clear benefits of treatment, and the clear harms of not treating, the case to remove parental authority temporarily for this specific treatment decision becomes quite strong.

One might question the authority of the state to override parental choices when such choices are based on deeply held religious convictions, as in this case. Freedom of religion is considered a fundamental right, protected by the United States Constitution. While freedom to believe whatever one wants is fundamental and inviolable in our society, that does not necessarily translate into the freedom to act out one's religious beliefs, particularly if such actions bring about substantial harm to third parties. While the right of parents to instill their values into their children's upbringing is essential to society's strongly held support of family autonomy, from a legal perspective such values must yield if the life or well-being of the child is at stake. As one prominent court decision has ruled on this issue (*Prince v. Massachusetts*), religious convictions may lead a parent to make a martyr of himself, but "he is not free to make a martyr of his child." In fact, numerous court cases have upheld the authority of physicians to override parental refusal of transfusion for the child when the parents were practicing Jehovah's Witnesses and refused on religious grounds. In these cases, however, physicians could not act on their own without some legal authority; this authority would have to be granted by a court of appropriate jurisdiction, and the suspension of parental authority would likely only be temporary and would apply only to the specific medical decision in question. Therefore, if additional treatment decisions needed to be made, there is no reason why the parents would not be the decision makers, unless other choices once again reflected an unwillingness to promote the best interests of the child in cases of substantial risk or harm.

2. In what situations might the parents' religious beliefs supersede physician authority?

If there were several possible treatment options, with varying levels of risk or certainty of success, the parents would, in fact, have latitude to choose from the range of options, even if their choice was not considered the medically optimal one. While different state courts have held differently on such issues, there is a general consensus that parents should be given room to choose among options, so long as there exists some support for their choice among medical practitioners. In the case of Chad Green (*Custody of a Minor*), the parents of a three-year-old child with leukemia wanted him treated with the unconventional drug laetrile instead of conventional chemotherapy. The court in that case prohibited the parents from selecting this option, as it had no support in the medical community. The parents took their child to Mexico for laetrile treatment and the child died. By contrast, in the case *In re Hofbauer*, the parents requested standard treatment plus laetrile for their son who had cancer; because the patient's doctor supported the parents' choice, seeing it as a feasible medical option with some chance of success, the court went along with the parents' wishes. Unfortunately, the child died, although it is not possible to know whether the treatment choice resulted in the death. In short, parents do not have to choose the treatment with the best chance of success, but only one of the offered, feasible treatment options with some chance of success.

If Daniel had a disease with a less certain or poorer prognosis, or with a more ambiguous risk-benefit calculus, the justification to override the parents' choice would become less firm. When the prognosis of a disease is poor and medical treatment is unlikely to cure the patient or improve his quality of life, failure to initiate curative treatment (as opposed to palliative treatment) would be ethically supportable. In such a case it would thus be counterproductive to try to overrule the parents and risk damaging the therapeutic relationship by a divisive court proceeding. The therapeutic relationship would be very important when attempting to design a palliative care plan for a child with fatal illness.

If the circumstances did not involve life-threatening illness, and there were no certain or immediate risks of substantial harm to the child if treatment were refused, a physician would generally be obliged to respect parental refusal of a treatment intervention, even if he or she believed that such a choice was not in the medical best interests of the child. It is only as the threat to the child increases, and the benefits of treatment become more clear, that actions to override parental choices are ethically and legally supportable. For example, members of the Christian Science Church reject standard medical treatment and utilize prayer to restore health. If parents who were Christian Scientists refused to allow their child to obtain standard immunizations, this refusal would generally be allowed. If the parents' chose to forgo treatment of bacterial meningitis, however, for which the risks and benefits are clear, that decision would be overridden. States vary as to the freedom granted to parents based on religious convictions, though as the risks from untreated disease escalate, limits are usually in place. In general, most states permit parents for religious reasons to refuse standard immunizations for their children or to use faith healing as an alternative to traditional medicine. It is only if and when the child's medical condition deteriorates, so that treatment would be essential to ward off an immediate and serious threat of harm, or if faith healing fails to address the child's condition, that physicians or governmental authorities could intervene. Usually courts are hesitant to intervene. An unusual exception was a situation in which a disease caused significant psychological harm. In the case *In re Sampson*, the child's mother, a practicing Jehovah's Witness, refused surgery to correct her child's massive facial deformity; the court ordered the operation to be performed even though the condition was not life threatening because the deformity had deprived the boy of the opportunity for normal social interaction.

3. When parents refuse all medical interventions on the basis of religious beliefs, how should these decisions be handled?

The beliefs and values of such parents are deserving of respect regarding how their children should be raised. It is, once again, only when alternative methods, such as faith healers and nontraditional sources of help, lead to a potential for serious risk to the life or health of the child that there may be authority to intervene. For example, if parents consulted Christian Science practitioners to the exclusion of established medical care, and this resulted in dangerous deterioration in their child's health, parental authority could be overridden to permit traditional medical approaches to be utilized, despite the parents' religious objections. The presumption of parental authority would be rebutted if it were clear that the child, to his detriment, was being medically neglected. Charges of medical neglect on the part of parents could even lead to their criminal prosecution. There have been a few prosecutions in recent years of parents whose children died because the parents avoided established medical treatments in preference of faith healing, and a few couples have even been convicted of manslaughter. In these cases, however, the sentences were suspended and the parents were put on probation, given the suffering they already experienced with the death of their children. In such cases, it must be remembered, parents are acting out of strong and generally beneficent convictions that their choices do promote their child's best interests. In Daniel's case, it is obvious that the parents do not wish their son to die; even so, they believe that his interests lie in accepting the tenets of their religion even at risk of physical harm. Society does not allow vulnerable children to be harmed by their parents, however, no matter how well intentioned the parents are.

While little case law exists concerning circumstances that involve "fringe" religions, for which the beliefs are not well understood or are not popularly subscribed to, there is no reason to believe that any different response would exist in such cases; that is, the decisions of the parents would hold unless and until such choices led to the risk of serious harm to their children. It should be noted that such harm does not actually have to occur in order for intervention to be justified; rather, the serious threat of harm would sufficiently justify actions to override parental authority and to temporarily or more permanently strip parents of their rights to make decisions on behalf of their children.

4. What would happen in this case if Daniel, along with his parents, refused to allow the blood transfusion because of his religious convictions?

While it would be understandable that, given his upbringing, Daniel would support his parents' decision to forgo the transfusion, his authority to make decisions on his own behalf would be quite limited, if it existed at all. The fact that he agreed with his parents would make the situation more compelling and disturbing for all involved, but it would not likely change the outcome of judicially ordered transfusions in this case. Morally, while one should be loath to impose invasive treatment on any vulnerable person, young children have not had the opportunity to develop the judgment and maturity required for grave decisions. They are not qualified to ascertain their own best interests.

Children are presumed by law to be incapable of making health care choices for themselves. Such a presumption, while it can be rebutted in individual cases (see Case 30, "A Teenager Who Wants Cosmetic Surgery," and Case 31, "An Adolescent with Cancer Who Wants To Discontinue Medical Treatment"), is generally consistent with the empirical data demonstrating that children below the age of 14 years rarely possess the cognitive skills, emotional resources, or maturity to comprehend and evaluate their health care choices, and therefore cannot give informed consent as an adult.[2] A child as young as Daniel is most unlikely to have developed strong and firmly held convictions and values that incorporate a view of how his life ought to be lived, not only in the present, but in the future as well. Childhood values tend to be transitory and heavily influenced by parents, peers, or other sources of authority. Thus, it would not serve the interests of the child to respect values that are likely to be revised or may be discarded as the child continues to mature. Further, response to transitory values is not likely to promote a child's as yet immature capacity for self-determination.

Thus, Daniel's interests would best be served, and his self-determination most reliably promoted, if he were provided the opportunity to overcome his current illness so he can become a mature young man. At that time, if he wishes to abide by the tenets of his parents' religion and even refuse vital medical care, he will have every right to do so. At his current age, however, and in his perilous medical condition, his lack of mature decisional capacity and established beliefs justifies overriding his choice as well, though, again, such action should be taken in as sensitive a manner as possible.

REFERENCES

1. I. Kerridge et al., "Clinical and Ethical Issues in the Treatment of a Jehovah's Witness with Acute Myeloblastic Leukemia," *Archives of Internal Medicine* 157 (1997): 1753–1757.

2. Leikin, S.L., "Minors' Assent or Dissent to Medical Treatment," In *President's Commission for the Study of Ethical Problems in Medicine and Biomedical and Behavioral Research, Making Health Care Decisions*: Appendix K. Washington, DC: U.S. Government Printing Office, 1982), 175–191.

SUGGESTED READINGS

Asser, S.M., and Swan, R. 1998. Child fatalities from religion-motivated medical neglect. *Pediatrics* 101: 625–629.

Committee on Bioethics, American Academy of Pediatrics 1997. Religious objections to medical care. *Pediatrics* 99: 279–281.

Davies, S.M. et al. 1997. Unrelated bone marrow transplantation for children with acute leukemia. *Journal of Clinical Oncology* 15: 557–565.

Goodnough, L.T. et al. 1999. Transfusion medicine. I. Blood transfusion; II. Blood conservation. *New England Journal of Medicine* 340: 438–447, 525–533.

Luban, N.L.C., and Leikin, S.L. 1991. Jehovah's Witnesses and transfusion: The pediatric perspective. *Transfusion Medicine Reviews* 5: 253–258.

Pui, C-H. 1997. Acute lymphoblastic leukemia. *Pediatric Clinics of North America* 44: 831–846.

Smith, M. et al. 1996. Uniform approach to risk classification and treatment assignment for childhood acute lymphoblastic leukemia. *Journal of Clinical Oncology* 14: 18–24.

Weinstein, H.J., and Tarbell, N.J. 1997. Leukemias and lymphomas of childhood. In *Cancer: Principles and practice of oncology*, eds. V.T. DeVita et al. 2145–2165. 5th ed. Philadelphia: Lippincott-Raven.

LEGAL CITATIONS

Case Examples

Custody of a Minor, 373 Mass. 733, 379 N.E.2d 1053 (1978).
    Massachusetts case in which the parents of three-year-old Chad Green, a child with leukemia, wished to use laetrile to treat him. The court ordered conventional medical treatment for the child, but the parents fled the jurisdiction and the child ultimately died in Mexico.

In re Hofbauer, 47 N.Y.2d 648, 393 N.E.2d 1009, 419 N.Y.S.2d 936 (1979).
    Administration of laetrile for treatment of cancer under supervision of licensed physician is legitimate exercise of parental decision-making authority.

Lundman v. McKown, No. 91-8197, Dist. Ct. Hennepin Cty. (Minn. 1993).
    Father awarded compensatory and punitive damages for the death of his son from diabetes following treatment for the child with prayer alone. Both the Christian Science Church, as well as the plaintiff's ex-wife and her husband, were held liable.

Nikolas Emerson, No. NEW-98-PC-17, Maine Dist. Ct., Penobscot Cty. (Sept. 19, 1998).
   Mother's refusal of AZT treatment for her HIV-infected four-year-old son was upheld,
   after the mother feared her son's death would result from the treatment. The mother had
   previously witnessed the death of another HIV-infected child who had taken AZT,
   which the mother believed had made the child sicker.

Prince v. Massachusetts, 321 U.S. 158 (1944).
   Seminal U.S. Supreme Court case addressing the right of parents to make decisions for
   their children.

In re Sampson, 328 N.Y.S.2d 686 (1972).
   Court ordered surgery over the objection of boy's mother, who was a Jehovah's Witness, because massive facial deformity of boy prevented him from participating in opportunities of normal life; surgery ordered despite non–life-threatening nature of condition.

CASE 30

A Teenager Who Wants Cosmetic Surgery

Tanya is a 16-year-old girl who has recently left home because of an unstable family situation. Her father is an alcoholic and he has physically abused his wife and children. Tanya now lives on her own in a small efficiency apartment in another city. She works as a typist and file clerk for a small contracting business and she is financially self-supporting. She attends night school and hopes to obtain her high school diploma.

Tanya is interested in having breast reduction surgery. She has been taunted frequently because of her large breasts, which are out of proportion with the rest of her body. She is so determined to have surgery that she visits the surgery clinic of her community hospital for an evaluation. She has even made inquiries about purchasing health insurance, since her employer does not provide health insurance for her.

She tells the surgeons that her body configuration makes her "feel like a freak." She is not obese and is in good health, but asserts that her large breasts cause her low back pain, shoulder pain, and fatigue, which interfere with her long hours of hard work.

The surgeons tell Tanya that she would probably be a good candidate for this surgery, and acknowledge that she may well benefit, but they will require consent from her parents. In particular, they would like at least one parent to be present for the important preoperative counseling that they give patients when they are considering this type of surgery. Tanya explains her situation, and says that she is doing well on her own and that she has not spoken to her parents for almost a year. Despite this, the surgeons refuse to consider acting without parental involvement. Tanya is very distraught over her situation.

ISSUES TO CONSIDER

- Emancipated and mature minors
- Elective surgery without parental consent

MEDICAL CONSIDERATIONS

1. What types of risks would Tanya incur from breast reduction (reduction mammaplasty)?

Reduction mammaplasty is generally well tolerated and is sometimes performed on an outpatient basis. The procedure would likely pose no significant medical risk to a patient such as Tanya, who would otherwise be at low operative risk. There is a small risk of infection; nipple necrosis can occur, and this can lead to nipple loss. Scarring may occur and this may be cosmetically unacceptable to the patient. Women of childbearing age may develop a decreased ability to lactate as the result of the surgery and many complain of altered sensation of the nipple. The risk of significant bleeding is less than 1 percent. Other late complications include delayed healing, fat necrosis, sagging, breast or nipple asymmetry, and nipple inversion.

Additional problems need to be considered. For example, adolescents whose breasts are undergoing rapid change may have regrowth of breast tissue after surgery. An obese woman who undergoes reduction mammaplasty may regain tissue lost if she gains weight. Certain drugs, such as oral contraceptives, can increase breast size and should be discontinued before one contemplates any surgery. Endocrinopathies as a cause of breast enlargement would need to be ruled out. Although mammaplasty does not increase the risk of breast cancer, it does produce parenchymal scarring of breast tissue, which can mimic breast cancer on physical examination and even mammography, and may necessitate diagnostic procedures to ensure that these findings are benign.

It would be important that any candidate for cosmetic surgery such as reduction mammaplasty be fully informed of these perhaps unanticipated problems. In addition to medical problems associated with surgery, there are psychological implications. For example, many patients have unrealistic expectations of what the surgery can provide, particularly from a cosmetic perspective. Even when the cosmetic result is satisfactory to others, the patient may be quite dissatisfied if she had a specific though unrealistic result in mind. It would be important to determine as closely as possible from the outset if a satisfactory result would be psychologically acceptable to the patient, or whether her underlying self-image is such that it would still be bad or worsened if the result were unsatisfactory. Although cosmetic surgery may markedly improve self-esteem in some patients, it may have little or no effect on others; for some, failure to have expectations met could even harm self-esteem further. Postoperative depression or dysphoria is common, as the patient adjusts to a new reality that may not be precisely what she anticipated. It is important to explore psychological reasons for this or other forms of cosmetic surgery; if remediable problems are identified and managed, this may prevent the need for surgery. In other cases, psychological or social motivations alone might be sufficiently strong to justify it.

All these issues require significant preoperative counseling and postoperative follow-up and education. Published series of patients, including teenagers, who have undergone reduction mammaplasty report a high level of patient satisfaction. For a teenager, satisfaction with the cosmetic result might be more important than potential problems that seem far off, such as inability to lactate, or diagnostic difficulties of mammography.

2. Could such a procedure have any medical benefit?

Patients with breast hypertrophy who seek reduction mammaplasty may complain of physical discomfort, bad posture (notably, exaggerated lumbar lordosis), premenstrual breast pain, backache, shoulder pain, and deep grooves in the shoulders related to brassiere straps. Older women, and presumably those with respiratory disorders, sometimes complain of an increased effort of respiration, most likely because of increased strain on inspiratory muscles that raise the chest wall. In extreme cases of juvenile hypertrophy, when rapid, massive enlargement of breasts occurs at the time of menarche, skin necrosis may result from venous engorgement. In these unusual cases, not only are the medical aspects quite well defined, but the psychological impact on the young adolescent is potentially quite dramatic. Other pathology may be misdiagnosed as breast hypertrophy, including a variety of neoplastic conditions and endocrinopathies.

As in most forms of cosmetic surgery, psychodynamic factors are highly individualistic. These cannot be minimized, especially in a young person, whose self-esteem may be tightly linked to physical appearance and social acceptance.

3. Would there be any advantages if Tanya could be persuaded to postpone surgery for two years?

Although this might not make her change her mind in the end, delaying surgery would theoretically reduce the chances of tissue regrowth. Unless Tanya had true juvenile breast hypertrophy, it is unlikely that a delay of this nature would have any long-lasting effects on her physical health. It would be important to explore the nature of any psychological impact her condition has and the likelihood that prompt surgery would be beneficial in this regard.

Delay might give Tanya more time to become financially stable or to establish more reliable social supports; these would be crucial if medical complications were to develop that kept her from her job for an unexpectedly long time. Finally, having reached the age of legal majority, Tanya would be more likely to obtain health insurance—perhaps through a new employer—and to have the latitude to select a policy that would defray some of the cost of this type of surgery.

ETHICAL AND LEGAL CONSIDERATIONS

1. In what circumstances can a minor give consent to medical treatment without parental involvement?

Parents are presumed to be the appropriate decision makers for their minor children. Such a presumption may be rebutted, however, in specific cases in which the circumstances of either the parents or the minor lead to a different analysis of what serves the child's best interests and who should be empowered to determine those interests. There is also a legal presumption of decisional incapacity on the part of persons under the age of 18, but this presumption may be inapplicable in individual circumstances. As children mature and grow closer to adulthood, their own capabilities and cognitive skills develop and come to approximate, if not equal, those of adults when it comes to decision making for medical treatment. Since individual children mature and develop at different rates, it is quite plausible that certain older children, particularly those close to adulthood, might be sufficiently mature to make appropriate decisions for themselves. Thus, there is nothing magical about the age of 18 as the dividing line between minors and adults, although that is the age usually employed from a legal perspective to distinguish which individuals should be empowered to make their own choices and which are still vulnerable and in need of protection. Some states have enacted statutes that specifically permit children under the age of 18 to consent to ordinary medical treatment on their own. For example, in Alabama individuals as young as 14 years of age may be permitted to consent to ordinary treatment, while in other states, minors are so allowed to consent at the age of 16 or 17.

In all jurisdictions, however, either in case law or statute, there are exceptions to the usual decisional authority of parents concerning medical care for their minor children. Such exceptions generally fall into two categories: emancipated minors and mature minors. Minors who fit either of these categories are likely to be able to receive routine medical care without need for any parental involvement. Whether they can receive any treatment, regardless of its reasons or risks, would depend on the specific circumstance.

An emancipated minor is one who has taken on responsibilities usually associated with adults in our society, and has thereby demonstrated the ability to function as an adult. As a consequence this person is presumed legally capable of making all decisions as though an adult, including marriage, signing a contract, making a major purchase, and giving consent to medical treatment. The precise actions that would serve to demonstrate emancipated minor status might vary slightly among jurisdictions, but they generally include actions such as maintaining financial independence from parents, living on one's own, marriage, pregnancy and motherhood, high school graduation, or military service. A minor who participates in these sorts of activities (for whatever reason) would be able to consent to her own medical treatment unless there were specific evidence of decisional incapacity, due, for example, to psychiatric disease or developmental disability (see Case 2, "Determining if a Patient Has Decisional Capacity," and Case 7, "Painful Treatment for a Severely Retarded Man"). On first analysis, Tanya, living on her own and supporting herself, would appear to fit into the category of an emancipated minor.

In contrast, mature minors are not categorically considered decisionally capable, but rather their maturity and skills in a specific circumstance demonstrate that they have sufficient ability to decide on a specific medical treatment decision for themselves. Such children may be quite dependent on their parents for money, shelter, or life's other basics, yet in a given circumstance, they are sufficiently mature to be the appropriate decision makers for themselves. They are in the best position to determine their own best interests, and their abilities are such that they deserve respect as autonomous persons. Decisions about abortion are a frequent example; if a minor understands her options and the implications of her decision, and has the abilities usually associated with an adult who makes this type of decision, she would likely have the decisional capacity to go through an informed consent process. The determination that a minor is sufficiently mature could probably be made with little concern for liability by an individual practitioner, although, depending on the nature of the treatment in question, judicial involvement might be warranted. For example, in cases of abortions for minors, states that require either parental notification or parental consent must also provide the minor a judicial bypass. This option grants the minor patient the opportunity to prove her maturity before a court of law, and thus obtain the right to eliminate parental involvement. In more routine treatment of mature minors, however, where judicial involvement is not generally sought, there are no reported cases of physicians encountering legal problems for giving routine medical care to someone aged 15 or above.

Ideally, parents should be involved in any treatment decision for a minor, even if the child demonstrated maturity. In this way the decision would not only respect the wishes and desires of the maturing child, it would also respect the rightful place of parents in decisions concerning their child's care. Yet, for many reasons, parental involvement in a given case may not be possible or appropriate. In these instances, if a youth were sufficiently mature, treatment could proceed with the minor's consent, even in the absence of parental involvement.

There is no record of any liability on the part of physicians rendering care to minors without parental consent if the following factors have been present: The minor is close to the age of majority (at least 15), the treatment clearly benefits the minor and is medically necessary, there is good justification for not obtaining parental consent, and the procedure is not extraordinary or one involving substantial risk to the child. This practically translates into the ability of practitioners to deliver routine medical care to adolescents without parental involvement if it cannot be obtained. In this way, children living on the street, or those whose parents demonstrate little involvement in their children's lives, would not be deprived of treatment because of lack of parental involvement. In situations judged to be emergencies, every jurisdiction, either by statute or common law, permits clinicians to deliver treatment if the child's life or well-being is at risk, even in the absence of parental consent. In such cases, if the minor is sufficiently mature, a physician may obtain formal consent from the patient, and should attempt to do so.

2. To what extent do these principles apply to other forms of treatment that an adolescent might seek?

Because of the nature of some medical problems and the treatment necessary, certain types of care have been statutorily exempted from the obligation to get parental consent, regardless of patient age or maturity. For example, treatment for sexually transmitted disease or substance abuse, or pregnancy-related treatment, has generally been exempted. In such cases, the policy decision has been that the need for treatment outweighs the need for parental involvement, particularly as these are the sort of medical problems that may be embarrassing or detrimental to the minor, if parental involvement were required. It is believed that minors might not seek out these types of care if they had to get parental permission, and, therefore, minors who need such treatment generally may receive it by their own consent.

3. Is Tanya an emancipated minor? If so, should her surgeons rely on her own consent in order to perform the requested surgery?

At first analysis, it appears that Tanya would categorically be classified as an emancipated minor and therefore would be presumed capable of giving consent to medical care without parental involvement. This presumption would stem from several of her actions: She lives on her own (in fact, not even in the same city as her parents) and supports herself financially. She lives like a self-sufficient adult, working to support and better herself. Her actions seem to demonstrate maturity, so that if her need for medical care were routine and ordinary, there would be little doubt that she could consent on her own, and physicians would invite virtually no risk of liability because of the lack of parental consent.

Even without these features of independence, there is evidence that parental involvement in her health care might not be appropriate. Given the history of abuse from her father, it would be difficult to argue that he can be relied on to act in the best interests of his child. Although there is no information concerning Tanya's mother, given Tanya's move out of the house, there is reason to believe that support at home was insufficient. Therefore, even if Tanya still lived at home, there is legitimate concern over whether it would be appropriate to involve her parents in her health care decisions. Tanya could be classified as a mature minor if she needed treatment while living in her parents' home but felt unable to involve her parents. The reported history of abuse illustrates precisely why statutory exemptions were created for certain types of treatment for minors. Tanya might justifiably fear further abuse from her father were she obligated to get his consent for pregnancy-related treatment or drug rehabilitation, and perhaps for a controversial and potentially emotion-laden treatment such as mammaplasty. If Tanya is in need of protection, it could well be from her father's tendencies rather than from her own immaturity. In any case, evidence of her prior living situation is less important in the evaluation of her maturity than whether she has given evidence of her ability to make decisions as an adult.

Despite the fact that Tanya could be categorized as emancipated, there would still be several reasons why surgeons might decide not to proceed, with or without parental involvement. To begin with, she is a minor who has experienced, at a minimum, physical abuse from a parent. She is also anguished about her physical appearance, which has led to embarrassment, ridicule, and perhaps poor self-esteem. Adolescents, in general, tend to place a premium on physical appearance, perhaps disproportionate to the reality of their circumstances. There would need to be in-depth evaluation as to whether Tanya's judgment and assessment of her situation were accurate, and whether her desire for surgery really reflected other problems that could be addressed without exposure to the risks of surgery. This is important for anyone undergoing cosmetic surgery, especially for a minor who seems to have little support available.

The fact that this intervention is neither urgent, risk free, nor part of routine care for teenaged women would make it prudent for physicians to proceed cautiously in the absence of parental involvement. It is not certain that Tanya's surgery would be categorized as medically necessary. If she were 18 years old, from a strictly legal perspective, there would be no doubt that she would be entitled to consent to this type of surgery, as long as she found surgeons willing to perform it. Furthermore, if she had strong parental involvement and support, physicians might proceed more comfortably. In the ideal, both patient and parents would support and consent to the surgery. In the absence of parental involvement, it would be helpful to see a strong support system, perhaps with other adults functioning as surrogate parents who would at least serve as sources of guidance for Tanya; these could include a sympathetic teacher, school counselor, or even an employer.

Although on the surface Tanya is capable of functioning without parental involvement, she may also be quite alone and in need of other sorts of assistance before, or in place of, this unusual intervention. Reduction mammaplasty is not the sort of standard procedure envisioned to be within the scope of consent for a mature or emancipated minor. Her physical symptoms make the argument stronger that the surgery could be performed on Tanya's consent alone, however, it might be more prudent for the physician to continue to counsel the patient and establish a relationship with her. If, as she continues to mature and reaches majority, she still desires the surgery, then she may be psychologically stronger, and physicians will have more legal certainty that her consent alone would be sufficient. This would also provide the opportunity to address whether medical indications exist above and beyond cosmetic considerations. If so, the patient would be more likely to have support from her health insurance, if she obtained coverage.

4. If Tanya were to have the surgery, who would be responsible for its cost? Could her parents be charged, or their insurance plan?

The costs of this surgery may well be Tanya's biggest practical hurdle. While parents are traditionally liable for the expenses incurred by their minor children, this would normally not be the case if the minor were considered emancipated. The parents could not be held legally responsible if their daughter had, in essence, declared her independence from them financially and in other ways. It is unlikely that the hospital could hold parents accountable if they had no involvement in the decision; thus, were they to pay for the operation, this would stem from their own voluntary decision. Reduction mammaplasty is generally not covered by Medicaid, and private insurance policies either do not cover this procedure or reimburse only on the basis of factors such as weight of tissue removed or other compelling evidence of the need for surgery, such as severe back pain, neurologic symptoms, or perhaps serious psychological consequences of breast size. The insurance company may demand photographs, but a physician might be unwilling to send them without parental consent. Thus, Tanya would have to demonstrate that she was capable of paying for this expensive surgery, either through her own health insurance or her savings; she would need to factor in associated expenses, such as time taken off from work and treatment for possible later complications. It is unlikely that her doctors would proceed without being assured of some sort of reimbursement. For very practical reasons, therefore, the surgical option might be foreclosed for the foreseeable future.

Tanya's lack of health insurance coverage and potential limits on her access to health care services as a result, are common problems for individuals who work for small employers who do not have the financial ability to provide health insurance to their employees. For an analysis of current problems in the provision and availability of health insurance, consult the Suggested Readings.

SUGGESTED READINGS

Buenaventura, S. et al. 1996. Outpatient reduction mammaplasty: A review of 338 consecutive cases. *Annals of Plastic Surgery* 36: 162–166.

Buchanan, A., and Brock, D. 1989. Minors. In *Deciding for others*, 215. Cambridge, England: Cambridge University Press.

Committee on Adolescence, American Academy of Pediatrics. 1996. The adolescent's right to confidential care when considering abortion. *Pediatrics* 97: 746–751.

Corriveau, S., and Jacobs, J.S. 1990. Macromastia in adolescence. *Clinics in Plastic Surgery* 17: 151–160.

Evans, G.R.D., and Ryan, J.J. 1994. Reduction mammaplasty for the teenage patient: A critical analysis. *Aesthetic Plastic Surgery* 18: 291–297.

Ford, C.A. et al. 1997. Influence of physician confidentiality assurances on adolescents' willingness to disclose information and seek future health care: A randomized controlled trial. *Journal of the American Medical Association* 278: 1029–1034.

Holder, A.R. 1985. Minor's consent to treatment. In *Legal issues in pediatrics and adolescent medicine*, 123. New Haven, CT: Yale University Press.

Holder, A.R. 1987. Minor's rights to consent to medical care. *Journal of the American Medical Association* 257: 3400–3402.

Kuttner, R. 1999. The American health care system: Health insurance coverage. *New England Journal of Medicine* 340: 163–168.

Sarwer, D.B. et al. 1998. The psychology of cosmetic surgery: A review and reconceptualization. *Clinical Psychology Review* 18: 1–22.

Schnur, P.L. et al. 1997. Reduction mammaplasty: An outcome study. *Plastic and Reconstructive Surgery* 100: 875–883.

LEGAL CITATIONS

Case Examples

Akron v. Akron Center for Reproductive Health, 462 U.S. 416 (1983).
United States Supreme Court case that held that law requiring parental consent for all unmarried women under 15 in order to obtain an abortion was unconstitutional.

Planned Parenthood of Central Missouri v. Danforth, 428 U.S. 52 (1976).
United States Supreme Court case establishing that the constitutional right to privacy that permits a woman to obtain an abortion is applicable to minors as well; parents

cannot have an absolute veto over their minor child's decision to have an abortion (though not every minor, regardless of age or maturity, has the capacity to decide on abortion on her own).

Statutory Example

Alabama Code Sec. 22-8-4 (1997).

Any minor who is 14 years of age or older, or has graduated from high school, or is married, or having been married is divorced or is pregnant, may give effective consent to any legally authorized medical, dental, health, or mental health services for himself or herself, and the consent of no other person shall be necessary.

CASE 31

An Adolescent with Cancer Who Wants To Discontinue Medical Treatment

Zach is a 13-year-old boy who has osteosarcoma. He presented with leg pain, and after undergoing a course of preoperative chemotherapy, he underwent segmental limb resection followed by placement of an endoprosthesis. This limb-sparing surgery allowed him to remain fully ambulatory, which was important because he was a fairly active child. Three months later, however, he developed pulmonary metastases, for which he underwent preoperative chemotherapy and thoracotomy with wedge resection of three metastatic nodules in the left lung. His postoperative course was complicated by empyema, for which he required chest tube drainage and antibiotics.

Zach recovered from this setback but two months later developed a cough. Diagnostic workup revealed bilateral pulmonary nodules and a mass involving the tricuspid valve and papillary muscle. Despite two courses of doxorubicin (Adriamycin) in the past, Zach has no evidence of clinical heart failure, so his physician believes that further treatment, including surgery, is possible, though its benefit is uncertain at best. At this time, Zach stated that he does not want further treatment. "I'm not going to get better," he asserted, "so why should I go through more treatments?"

The oncologist explained to Zach's parents that the rapid tumor recurrence points to a poor prognosis. Heart function is adequate but excision of the cardiac mass would be essential before further aggressive treatment could be done. The prognosis after bilateral pulmonary lesions is not as favorable as after unilateral lesions. Even with treatment, Zach's chances of surviving another year are "very low."

Zach has remained firm in his wish to stop treatment, even after evaluation and counseling from both a social worker and psychiatrist. His parents comfort him but they are not able to articulate their feelings and anguish to him. Privately, they tell the oncologist that they are strongly in favor of treatment. The oncologist gently reminds them that this is not what their child wants, and that perhaps they should "try to let go." "Are you saying there is no hope?" asks his mother. "There is never no hope," says the doctor, "but we can't dismiss the prognosis."

The parents respond, "We can't let go. We want everything done for our son, even if there is only one shred of hope." Zach's mother tearfully adds that she wishes they had not allowed "that experimental surgery." Zach is their only child.

ISSUES TO CONSIDER

- Participation of a minor in medical treatment decision making
- Determination of a minor's capacity to make medical decisions
- Conflict between parents and minors concerning the course of treatment

MEDICAL CONSIDERATIONS

1. What impact has limb-preserving surgery had on Zach's prognosis?

The traditional surgical approach to malignant bone tumors has been amputation. Limb salvage has increasingly been used, even in young children who have not yet reached skeletal maturity. Although complications occur, such as infection, prosthetic failure, and tumor recurrence, overall outcome and long-term cure and recurrence rates appear to be no worse than results achieved with amputation. The benefits of limb salvage over amputation are substantial for most, though not all, tumor sites. Psychological outcomes for children appear to be approximately the same for those receiving limb salvage as for those undergoing amputation.

Limb-sparing surgery and intensive preoperative and postoperative chemotherapy have improved the outlook for many patients with osteosarcoma. The ability to offer limb-sparing surgery depends on the site of the primary tumor and its extent, and the integrity of the surrounding bone. The use of expandable prostheses may increase the use of this beneficial option for children with incomplete skeletal growth. Surgical resection is also generally recommended for visible pulmonary metastases in osteosarcoma, unless metastases are too numerous.

2. What is Zach's long-term prognosis?

Long-term outcomes depend on the extent of disease at presentation, and whether there is an adequate histologic response to preoperative chemotherapy. Zach had no apparent metastases at presentation, which may confer more than 80 percent eight-year survival, but patients who have an incomplete histologic response following chemotherapy have only approximately 50 percent chance of prolonged survival.[1] The clinical course among survivors may include recurrent metastases, as in Zach's case, local recurrence, or development of second malignancies. Bilateral pulmonary metastases, bone and other extrathoracic metastases also confer a poor prognosis. There are scattered reports of long-term survivors following recurrence, but given the extent of Zach's disease, prolonged survival would be unlikely. Aspects of osteosarcoma and other solid tumors in children are discussed in the Suggested Readings.

3. What are the long-term outcomes in survivors of childhood cancer?

Children who survive childhood cancers generally have a good outcome, although chemotherapy and radiation are not without long-term ill effects. Chemotherapeutic agents increase the risk of damage to many internal organs and may lead to pulmonary, cardiac, or renal dysfunction. Skeletal growth and gonadal function may be impaired. Brain irradiation as well as intrathecal or intravenous chemotherapy may produce neurologic sequelae, including intellectual defects, which appear to be greater the younger the child is at the time of treatment.

In addition, the incidence of second cancers is increased, most commonly nonlymphocytic leukemias, and solid tumors (often radiation-associated osteosarcoma). The incidence of malignant tumors during the fifth through the fifteenth year after diagnosis of the first cancer is approximately 10 times greater among survivors of childhood malignancies than among the general population. It is uncertain if this is a result of anticancer treatment or an underlying cancer predisposition.

ETHICAL AND LEGAL CONSIDERATIONS

1. To what extent can this 13-year-old be involved in decisions concerning his medical treatment?

When the patient is a competent adult, there is a legal mandate and moral obligation to involve him in decisions that affect his care. Patient involvement should also be a guiding principle for physicians who care for children. Of course, the degree of involvement and participation of a minor patient will vary depending on the age and level of capability of the individual child (see Case 29, "A Religious Objection to a Child's Medical Treatment," and Case 30, "A Teenager Who Wants Cosmetic Surgery"). Children may not yet possess sufficient decisional capacity to participate in an informed consent process as an adult would. The involvement of the child may nevertheless serve many other purposes, equally important in the context of the therapeutic relationship.

While parents are usually an integral part of the decision-making process for a minor, it is essential for physicians to remember that it is the child who is their patient and to whom they have the greatest obligation. This obligation includes respect for the person, which for a child may include sensitivity to emerging decisional capacity, as well as protection of those qualities of a child that make him vulnerable and recognition of ways in which he is still immature. All patients, including children, are owed honesty by their physicians. Although the nature, language, and timing of explanations to a child would have to be adapted to the particular situation, dishonesty or lack of candor should be avoided because this may exacerbate the natural tendency of children to fantasize about the causes and consequences of illness and may increase their fears and anxieties.

The older the child, the more likely that he will be able to place his illness in a context and participate in decisions that affect him. For older children, there is no reason that the informed consent process should not approximate the process undertaken with competent adults.

Even for those children who still lack some skills necessary to take complete authority over decisions about their care (and thus not yet able to give legally binding informed consent), there are still strong practical and philosophic arguments that a child's assent should at least be obtained before a treatment is implemented.[2] While some children may send out clear signals that they are unable or unwilling to be a part of the decision-making process, the presumption should exist that they have opinions. These views must be sought out, if possible, and the child's agreement received, even if such agreement may not be as truly informed and voluntary as an adult's consent would be. Soliciting such assent accords the child respect as a person, and it may also lead the child to reveal wishes or thoughts that would be important to consider in the decision-making process. Moreover, treating the child respectfully and providing him with information will likely solicit cooperation and enthusiasm for the course of treatment. In Zach's case, treating him without this assent would be harmful to a treatment goal of palliative care, if that were the option ultimately employed.

2. Can the decision of this 13-year-old patient be honored despite the parents' disagreement?

There are two central issues to explore in this difficult situation involving conflict between parents and their dying child. First, there must be an examination of how much authority Zach's expressed wishes have. Second, the physician must explore the extent to which the wishes of a minor place limits on parental authority.

Whether Zach has the capacity to make the decision to refuse additional treatment would depend on his understanding of his illness and treatment options and how he has processed that information to arrive at his decision. Zach would not be categorically presumed competent, as he is not an adult, and he has not undertaken any of the activities that would categorize him as emancipated (see Case 30). Yet, he may be a mature minor, that is, have the explicit abilities and understanding in the present situation to render a decision that is informed and therefore worthy of respect.

Although Zach may not, to date, have had the ability to give consent (implying his complete authority over the decision-making process), presumably he has been a part of the medical decision-making process up until this point. That is, he has been informed of the nature and progress of his illness, and his willingness to go along with treatment has been solicited and received. For example, it is quite likely that his desire to remain physically active, despite his illness, influenced the decision to perform the segmental limb resection rather than a more radical type of surgery earlier on in his illness.

If Zach has been a part of the previous decision processes, then it is likely that he has also been party to discussions concerning benefits versus burdens. While he may have lacked the maturity necessary to completely comprehend the trade-off of short-term burdens for longer-term gains, he has experienced firsthand the burdens and benefits of those treatments and yet is also well aware that he is deteriorating rather than recovering. While he may not be able to articulate his feelings in sophisticated language, his misgivings about continued treatment seem eminently reasonable, given his experiences to date and the grim outlook. There is no doubt that a competent adult in this situation would have his wishes respected by his physicians. It is only because Zach's parents wish to pursue an aggressive (and perhaps unrealistic) course that the child's expressed choice is being challenged.

While parents have the authority to make decisions concerning their child's care, that exercise of authority should become more of a shared process as the child matures. Moreover, their authority to make such decisions rests on their ability to determine what lies in the best interests of their child. In most cases such a determination is clear and unchallengeable, or at least reasonable, so that third parties would lack the authority to override their evaluation. When the parents' evaluation of their child's interests includes inflicting risks and burdens on him for little likely benefit, then providers may have reason to question or even challenge the parents' choice; a challenge would be even more justified when such a choice could only be implemented against the child's will.

Just as adult patients must have the capacity to make decisions in order for their choices to have authority, so should it be clear that parents have decisional capacity to make decisions before their choice for their child can be respected. In this specific case, there may be several reasons to be concerned about the parents' ability to make decisions for Zach at this point. First, it is not at all clear that these parents have accepted the reality of their son's poor prognosis. Hope provides motivation to continue, but it cannot be allowed to obscure a poor prognosis or the physical and psychological harm that undesired treatment would impose on a child. In a certain sense, Zach may have demonstrated a more mature and rational ability to handle this situation than his parents have. It is understandable that Zach's parents may have difficulty in accepting the reality of the death of their only child. This would be better addressed with support and counseling than with unquestioning adherence to their decision. In fact, it might be argued that, because part of the obligation to Zach is to promote his well-being and do him no harm, the physicians may have no choice but to refuse the parents' request. The oncologist himself is doubtful that further treatment will benefit Zach. Given all these factors, aggressive treatment of Zach might even violate the doctor's professional integrity.

Thus, given the premise that this child comprehends his situation and has reasonably arrived at his decision, a decision that appears to have the support of his physicians, it is unlikely that Zach's parents could impose treatment on him at this time. Of course, respecting Zach's choices at the expense of his parents' wishes is not without consequences. Zach may experience guilt for causing a rift in his family; his parents may feel anguish at being forced to confront a reality that they have tried to put off and anger that their authority is being undermined. Tension may erupt in this family at a point when calm is crucial. These problems underscore the need for increased psychological support for all concerned. A hospice referral, which would provide support and therapy for the family as a unit, beyond the individual patient, might be very valuable at this point. Most hospice programs are able to serve the needs of pediatric as well as adult patients.

3. What would be the place of Zach's wishes if his prognosis were less certain, or perhaps even more favorable?

Part of what makes respect for Zach's wishes so compelling is the likelihood that treatment would not improve his prognosis significantly. In other situations, however, Zach's treatment refusal might need to be more closely scrutinized, for example, if he had a curable malignancy, or if he required dialysis for renal failure. While for the competent adult, requests to forgo medical treatment deserve to be respected regardless of the prognosis or consequences of the choice, there would be serious question concerning a 13-year-old's ability to evaluate whether certain burdens are worth certain benefits. If Zach had chronic renal failure and wanted to stop dialysis, physicians might be more justified in imposing treatment on him temporarily because the outcome was more certain, and it might buy him time to seek kidney transplant, or at least permit him to develop to a more mature state so that his evaluation of the quality of his life would rest on more mature footing. Zach might be able to mount a strong enough defense of his position to persuade his physicians that they should feel obligated to respect that choice, but his youthful benefits-burdens analysis might be more aggressively challenged in light of the outcome of his choice.

Even in this revised scenario, there is still the dilemma of physically forcing treatment against a patient's wishes. While such intervention might feel unseemly or be difficult to implement, it might be more justifiable if long-term benefit were possible. If Zach were educated about these possibilities, his assent might even be obtained. For example, dialysis in anticipation of a possible kidney transplant and better health and vigor might be preferable to Zach than no future at all. Likewise, treatment for an exacerbation of leukemia might provide Zach with good long-term survival.

4. How would the analysis change if Zach's parents were the ones who wished to stop treatment, given the dismal prognosis, while Zach wished to pursue whatever treatment options remained for him?

This reverse scenario does not diminish the virtual certainty that Zach will die in the near future, with or without additional treatment. The discussion should realistically center on what type of death Zach will have, rather than how much longer he may cling to life. As in the original scenario, Zach remains on the cusp of decisional capacity, and in this reverse scenario Zach's understanding of his situation would need to be probed. Does he understand the likely prognosis with or without treatment? Does he have a realistic assessment of his circumstance? Answers to these questions would help Zach's physicians to consider the process that led Zach to his desire to receive burdensome treatment expected to yield little benefit.

Zach's parents, whose decision would now stand in accord with the physician's recommendation, might feel comfortable that their evaluation of the best interest of their child was given respect and authority. Yet, the problem of frustrating Zach's wishes would remain, and the level of despair he might experience, perhaps feeling as though his sources of support were giving up on him, would require significant attention and therapeutic intervention.

Despite Zach's poor prognosis, it is possible that, in this reverse scenario, the child rather than the parent would still garner the most support. Zach's psychological state should be part of the benefits-burdens analysis, and his fervent desire for treatment might in itself serve as a justification to treat, despite the low chance of physical benefit.

REFERENCES

1. A.J. Provisor et al., "Treatment of Nonmetastatic Osteosarcoma of the Extremity with Preoperative and Postoperative Chemotherapy: A report from the Children's Cancer Group," *Journal of Clinical Oncology* 15 (1997): 76–84.
2. S.L. Leikin, "Minors Assent or Dissent to Medical Treatment," in *President's Commission for the Study of Ethical Problems in Medicine and Biomedical and Behavioral Research, Making Health Care Decisions*: Appendix K,175–191 (Washington, DC: U.S. Government Printing Office, 1982).

SUGGESTED READINGS

Committee on Pediatric AIDS, American Academy of Pediatrics. 1999. Disclosure of illness status to children and adolescents with HIV infection. *Pediatrics* 103: 164–166 (see Appendix A).

Committee on Bioethics, American Academy of Pediatrics. 1994. Guidelines on forgoing life-sustaining medical treatment. *Pediatrics* 93: 532–536 (see Appendix A).

Committee on Bioethics, American Academy of Pediatrics. 1995. Informed consent, parental permission, and assent in pediatric practice. *Pediatrics* 95: 314–317 (see Appendix A).

Harrison, C. et al. 1997. Bioethics for clinicians: 9. Involving children in medical decisions. *Canadian Medical Association Journal* 156: 825–828.

The Hastings Center. 1987. Special comments: Children. In *Guidelines on the termination of life-sustaining treatment and the care of the dying*, 33–34. Bloomington: Indiana University Press.

Marcove, R.C. et al. 1994. Limb-sparing surgery for extremity sarcoma. *Cancer Investigations* 12: 497–504.

Marina, N. 1997. Long-term survivors of childhood cancer. The medical consequences of cure. *Pediatric Clinics of North America* 44: 1021–1042.

Meyers, P.A., and Gorlick, R. 1997. Osteosarcoma. *Pediatric Clinics of North America* 44: 973–989.

Moreno, J.D. 1989. Treating the adolescent patient. *Journal of Adolescent Health Care* 10: 454–459.

Pizzo, P.A., and Poplack, D.G., eds. 1997. *Principles and practice of pediatric oncology.* Philadelphia: Lippincott-Raven.

Weir, R.F., and Peters, C. 1997. Affirming the decisions adolescents make about life and death. *Hastings Center Report* 27, no. 6: 29–40.

LEGAL CITATIONS

Case Examples

In re Rosebush, 195 Mich. App. 675, 491 N.W.2d 633 (1992).
In comments in addition to the case holding, the court stated that a mature minor's advance directive that refused life-sustaining treatment should be considered or even enforced when determining whether to terminate such treatment for the minor.

Statutory Example

Illinois Comp. Stat. Ann. 755- 35/5 (West 1993).
State statute permitting an emancipated minor to execute an advance directive.

APPENDIX A

Internet References, Suggested Readings, and Other Sources

CASE CITATIONS

Case 4

www.jcaho.org/index.htm
Joint Commission on Accreditation of Healthcare Organizations.

Case 6

http://altmed.od.nih.gov/nccam/resources/cam-ci/
CAM citation index; international abstracts of research on complementary/alternative medicine.
see also **http://nccam.nih.gov**
National Institutes of Health, National Center for Complementary and Alternative Medicine.

http://www.fda.gov/fdac/features/1998/598_guid.html
Food and Drug Administration Guide to Dietary Supplements: Answers to questions that have arisen in the wake of the 1994 Dietary Supplement Health and Education Act.

Case 13

http://www.facs.org/fellows_info/statements/st-19.html
American College of Surgeons statement on Advance Directives by Patients: "Do Not Resuscitate" in the Operating Room.

see also **http://www.asahq.org/standards/09.html**
American Society of Anesthesiologists.

http://www.nahc.org/consumer/hpcstats.html
Hospice Association of America, Basic Statistics about Hospice.
see also **http:www.nho.org**
National Hospice Organization.

Case 14

http://www.milliman-hmg.com
Milliman and Robertson, Inc. Practice guidelines developed by this actu-
arial consulting firm of the insurance industry, used widely by managed
care organizations.

Case 15

http://www.ahcpr.gov
(click on Clinical Information, Clinical Practice Guidelines, 9. Cancer
Pain)

http://guweb.georgetown.edu/nrcbl/biblios/suicide.htm
National Reference Center for Bioethics Literature, Assisted Suicide- Selected Bibliography.

Case 18

http://www.ama-assn.org/special/hiv/policy/amapol.htm
American Medical Association Ethical Opinions on HIV/AIDS Issues-
HIV Infected Patients and Physicians.

Case 19

http://www.dmv.ca.gov/pubs/matured/dl663toc.htm
State of California, Department of Motor Vehicles, "Tips for Mature Drivers."

http://ostpxweb.dot.gov/policy/aging
U.S. Department of Transportation, Office of the Assistant Secretary for Transportation Policy, "Improving Transportation for a Mature Society."

Case 20

http://www.ama-assn.org/physlegl/legal/termrel.htm
American Medical Association Legal Issues for Physicians: Ending the doctor-patient relationship.

Case 22

http://www.organdonor.gov/facts.asp
United Network for Organ Sharing, Facts about Transplantation in the United States.

Case 24

http://www.asrm.org/current/practice/embryos.html
American Society of Reproductive Medicine, Practice Committee Report, practice guidelines on maximum number of embryos that should be transferred in assisted reproductive technologies (see **www.asrm.org/** for other policy statements).

http://www.asrm.org/current/practice/informedART.html
American Society of Reproductive Medicine, Practice Committee Report, Informed Consent for Assisted Reproductive Technologies.

http://www.cdc.gov/nccdphp/drh/art96/index.htm
Centers for Disease Control. 1996 assisted reproductive Technology Success Rates. National Summary and Fertility Clinic Reports (February, 1999).

Case 25

http://www.ama-assn.org/special/hiv/newsline/reuters/07156232.htm
Interim results of study demonstrating efficacy of nevirapine in preventing vertical transmission of HIV from mother to newborn.

http://www.ama-assn.org/special/hiv/policy/amapol.htm
American Medical Association Ethical Opinions on HIV/AIDS Issues-
HIV Testing.

http://www.aap.org/policy/re9827.html
American Academy of Pediatrics, Policy Statement, Disclosure of Illness
Status to Children and Adolescents with HIV Infection.

Case 27

http://www.naral.org/publications/whod99analysis.html
National Abortion Rights Action League State-by-State Review of Abortion and Reproductive Rights.

For contrasting views on abortion, *see also*
http://www.nrlc.org/
National Right to Life Committee.

Case 28

http://www.upenn.edu/ldi/issuebrief2-5.html
Leonard David Institute of Health Economics of the University of Penn-
sylvania, Issue Brief 2(5): Arthur Caplan, "Organ Procurement and
Transplantation: Ethical and Practical Issues."

CITATIONS THAT APPEAR IN MORE THAN ONE CASE

http://www2.cdc.gov/mmwr/
Centers for Disease Control; Full text of MMWR Morbidity and Mortality
Weekly Reports, MMWR recommendations, and CDC Surveillance and
Summaries.

http://www.ama-assn.org/sitemap.htm (click "policy finder," Ethical
opinions)
Ethical opinions of the American Medical Association Council on Medical
and Judicial Affairs.

http://www.aap.org/policy
Policy statements of the American Academy of Pediatrics.

OTHER USEFUL ONLINE SOURCES

Medical issues

http://www.guideline.gov
National Guideline Clearinghouse; Web site operated by U.S. Department of Health and Human Services, Agency for Health Care Policy and Research (AHCPR; *see also* **www.ahcpr.gov**) for purpose of disseminating evidence-based clinical practice guidelines developed by participating professional organizations.

http://www.healthfinder.gov
Government sponsored site with reliable medical information and numerous links to other government, university, professional, support group, and journal sites.

http://www.managedcareconnection.com
Online managed care resources with extensive links.

http://www.nih/gov
National Institutes of Health home page.

http://www.nlm.nih.gov/databases/freemedl.html
National Library of Medicine (NLM); free Medline using Internet Grateful Med or PubMed. Free access to other online databases, including Bioethicsline.

http://www.ncbi.nlm.nih.gov/PubMed/fulltext.html
NLM collection of Medline journals with full text of many available online.

http://library.nymc.edu/Database/resource.htm
New York Medical College, electronic journal collection with full text of many available online.

www.soros.org/death
Project on Death in America; professional and public education, research, and public policy, and other initiatives on death and dying. Website has links to many organizations involved in death and dying.

http://www.lastacts.org
Website for the Robert Wood Johnson Foundation's Last Acts Campaign, a national coalition to improve care and caring at the end of life. Site content includes discussion groups for both professionals and consumers, electronic newsletter, policy reports and linkages to many other end of life sites.

http://www.update-software.com/ccweb/cochrane/revabstr/ mainindex.htm
Cochrane Database of Systematic Reviews; evidence-based reviews on a wide range of health care issues, by professional contributors (Cochrane Collaboration), updated quarterly. Full text of reviews available by subscription.

http://www.shef.ac.uk/~scharr/ir/netting.html
Netting the Evidence; University of Sheffield (England) School of Health and Related Research (ScHARR); provides many links devoted to evidence-based medicine on a variety of pertinent topics.

http://hivinsite.ucsf.edu/
HIV Insite website of the University of California at San Francisco, with information on medical, prevention, social/policy and statistics related to HIV and AIDS, up-to-the-minute coverage on HIV related news stories, and linkages to an array of additional HIV/AIDS websites.

http://www.ama-assn.org/special/hiv/hivhome.htm
JAMA HIV/AIDS Information Center, providing clinical updates, peer reviewed readings, and other professional and patient oriented information, with extensive links.

http://www.fda.gov/default.htm
Food and Drug Administration home page.

Ethical Issues

http://www.asbh.org

American Society of Bioethics and Humanities (ASBH); multidisciplinary professional society of individuals, organizations, and institutions interested in bioethics and humanities.

http://www.aslme.org

American Society of Law, Medicine, and Ethics (ASLME); Multidisciplinary organization devoted to legal and ethical issues that arise in the delivery of health care. Website contains information regarding the ASMLE, its journals, conferences, news stories, and linkages to an array of additional sites related to ethical and legal issues in health care.

http://www.bioethics.gov

National Bioethics Advisory Commission (NBAC), presidential-appointed body that reports on bioethical issues confronting the American public and submits recommendations to the Executive branch. Site provides access to reports and recommendations of NBAC.

http://www.georgetown.edu/research/nrcbl/

National Reference Center for Bioethics Literature: Website with links to Bioethics Line, Ethics and Genetics, educational and teaching resources, bibliographic resources, and other related websites; Resources referenced include books, journals, legal materials, newspapers, regulations, government publications, and other related materials.

The following websites are a sample of the many sites developed by university-based bioethics centers in the United States. These sites contain information regarding the faculty and ongoing activities of these centers, the availability of online course work, conference and other educational opportunities, policy briefs, news stories, and linkages to other resources related to biomedical ethics:

http://www.med.upenn.edu/bioethics/index.html

University of Pennsylvania Center for Bioethics.

http://www.med.virginia.edu/bioethics
University of Virginia Center for Biomedical Ethics.

http://www.med.umn.edu/bioethics
Center for Bioethics, University of Minnesota.

http://www.pitt.edu/~bioethic/
Center for Bioethics and Health Law, University of Pittsburgh.

http://www.stanford.edu/dept/scbe/
Stanford University Center for Biomedical Ethics.
http://guweb.georgetown.edu/kennedy/
Kennedy Institute of Ethics, Georgetown University.

http://www.mcw.edu/bioethics/
Center for Study of Bioethics, Medical College of Wisconsin.

Legal Issues

http:www.lawcrawler.com/
Search engine with links world wide to an array of legal resources, including court opinions, federal and state legislation, journal articles, etc.

http://supct.law.cornell.edu/supct
Decisions, briefs, and transcripts of proceedings before the United States Supreme Court.

http://lawlib.slu.edu/centers/hlthlaw/
Center for Health Law Studies of the St. Louis University School of Law. Information about the Center's faculty and resources, and research gateway to health law searches on the world wide web, as well as up-to-the-minute health law news, linkages to journals, and other health law-related sites.

http://www.aclu.org/issues/aids/hmaids.html
American Civil Liberties Union site providing the latest information on AIDS-related litigation, legislation, policy statements, news, and linkages with other AIDS-related sites.

http://www.emtala.com
Law firm site with array of information concerning litigation and federal regulations and interpretative guidelines concerning the federal Emergency Medical Treatment and Active Labor Act (EMTALA).

HEALTH LAW TRADE ASSOCIATIONS

http://www.abanet.org/health/home/html
American Bar Association Health Law Section.

http://www.healthlawyers.org
American Health Lawyers Association.

INDEX

E

M

N